Psychological
Factors in
Health Care

Psychological Factors in Health Care

A Practitioner's Manual

Edited by
Michael Jospe
Kaiser-Permanente Medical Center

Joseph Nieberding

Barry D. Cohen
Kaiser-Permanente Medical Center

LexingtonBooks
D.C. Heath and Company
Lexington, Massachusetts
Toronto

Library of Congress Cataloging in Publication Data

Main entry under title:

Psychological factors in health care.

Includes index.
1. Medicine and psychology. I. Jospe, Michael. II. Nieberding,
Joseph. III. Cohen, Barry D.
[DNLM: 1. Delivery of health care. 2. Psychology, Clinical. 3. Dis-
ease—Psychology. W84.1 P974]
R726.5.P79   616'.001'9   77-11395
ISBN 0-669-02076-1

Copyright © 1980 by D.C. Heath and Company

Published simultaneously in Canada

Printed in the United States of America

International Standard Book Number: 0-669-02076-1

Library of Congress Catalog Card Number: 77-11395

To our parents

Gerda and Leo Jospe

Helen and Jack Nieberding

Annette and Monroe Cohen

and to our teachers, colleagues, and patients, who have taught us so much of what we know and understand about the psychology of health and illness

Contents

Foreword *William Schofield*   xi

Preface   xv

**Introduction: A Conceptual Perspective on the
Psychology of Illness** *Michael Jospe*   xix

Part I   *Teaching and Training for Practice: A Trend
                Away from Dualism*   1

Chapter 1   **Training Programs in Health-Care Psychology at
                the University of Minnesota Health Sciences
                Center** *A. Jack Hafner*   5

Chapter 2   **Psychological Internship Experiences in a Family-
                Practice Clinic** *Joseph Nieberding* and
                Michael Jospe   11

Chapter 3   **Psychological Medicine and Family Practice**
                Harley J. Racer   25

Chapter 4   **The Role of Psychology in Baccalaureate Nursing
                Education** *Roberta Ann Smith* and
                Kenneth A. Wallston   39

Part II   *Delivery of Health-Care Services: Psychology's
                Role in Selected Aspects of Medical Practice*   55

Chapter 5   **Clinical Psychology and Health Psychology: The
                Application of Clinical Psychology to Health-
                Care Practice** *Robert D. Wirt*   59

Chapter 6   **Interviewing and Psychological Screening in
                Medical Practice: The Psychological Systems
                Review** *Harold R. Ireton* and
                Donald M. Cassata   67

Chapter 7   **Discussing Emotional Etiology for Illness with
                Medical Patients** *Ronald D. Hilliard*   79

Chapter 8   Psychological Factors in Emergency Medical
               Services *Elaine Wustman*   85

Chapter 9   The Pediatric Health Psychologist, the
               Pediatrician, and Other Caregivers
               Wentworth Quast   103

Chapter 10   Psychological Interventions in Pediatric Oncology
               Jonathan Kellerman   113

Chapter 11   Psychological Aspects of Loss and Grief in
               Spinal-Cord and Other Chronically Disabling
               Injuries *Patrick J. Fazzari*   129

Chapter 12   Behavioral-Medicine Approach to Health Care:
               Hemophilia as an Exemplary Model
               James W. Varni and *Dennis C. Russo*   139

Chapter 13   Pain and Its Management: A Behavioral-
               Medicine Perspective   *Jo Ann Brockway*   169

Chapter 14   Obstetrics and Gynecology: The Well-Being of the
               Total Woman   *Cathie-Ann Lippman*   185

Chapter 15   Health Psychology and Older People: Toward
               Eradicating Agism from Attitudes and Practices
               Richard Steinman   211

Chapter 16   Work Stress: Effects on Physical and Mental
               Health of Patients and Treatment Personnel
               Barbara L. Smith   229

Chapter 17   Interviewing and Identifying Persons with
               Alcohol Problems   *Seth Ersner-Hershfield,
               Mark B. Sobell,* and *Linda C. Sobell*   241

Part III   *Delivery of Health-Care Services: Psychological
               Aspects of Human Sexuality in Health Care*   255

Chapter 18   Responding to Sexual Concerns in Health-Care
               Settings: Brief Sex Counseling and Supportive
               Referrals for Sex Therapy   *Barry S. Reynolds*
               and *Susan Price*   257

Chapter 19   Understanding and Treating Medically Related
             Sexual Problems   *Barry D. Cohen* and
             Michael Jospe   283

Chapter 20   What Health-Care Professionals Need to Know
             about Gay Men and Lesbians
             John C. Gonsiorek   297

Chapter 21   Sexuality and the Health Professional
             Harold Q. Dillehunt   313

Part IV   *Delivery of Health-Care Services: Cross-Cultural
             Factors and the Health Professions*   323

Chapter 22   Psychological Factors in Providing Health Care
             to Blacks   *Robert Mahon*   325

Chapter 23   Overcoming Barriers to the Treatment of the
             Hispanic Patient   *Carmen Carrillo*   339

Chapter 24   Cultural Background of Native American Health
             Behavior   *Luis Kemnitzer*   347

Chapter 25   Health-Care Issues for Asian Americans
             Reiko Homma True   365

Part V   *Delivery of Health-Care Services: Patients and
             Families*   377

Chapter 26   The Doctor-Patient Relationship in the
             Mastectomy Experience   *Win Ann Winkler*   379

Chapter 27   Psychological Aspects of Neurological Diseases:
             A Patient's Efforts to Disprove Being Labeled
             Crazy or Hysterical   *Cynthia Birrer*   391

Chapter 28   Commentary: The Parents' Experience of Health
             Care for the Terminally Ill Child   *Marcia Ross*
             and *Alvin P. Ross*   409

             Annotated Bibliography of Selected Materials
             in Health Psychology   *Linda J. (Tik) Menefee*
             and *Joseph Nieberding*   425

Index 453

About the Contributors 473

About the Editors 481

Foreword

There is an aphorism that asks, "Why is it we grow so soon old and so late smart?" Indeed, why is it? We speak of "the wisdom of the ages." We acknowledge that fundamental truths are slowly arrived at and sometimes lost for a while in the mists of history, but for the most part retained to be part of each generation's heritage as the gift of the experiences and insights of our forebears. Some truths are so immutable, so much an inescapable given of every age of man—the realities of pain and of mortality—that they are always with us. Other truths are so variable in expression and experience—such as the comforting if not curing impact of the human touch—that they are in some social ages all but forgotten and in others exploited irrationally.

Another aphorism is, "There is nothing new under the sun!" When we speak it we are not expressing the principle of conservation, the concept that there are no accretions to the finite total of matter and energy. Rather we are, perhaps wistfully, reviving our humility or preening our arrogance in seeing that many discoveries turn out upon reflective scrutiny to be rediscoveries of what was known in a previous time.

So it is with the underlying premises of this book. There is a new perspective, a new enterprise before us, and it has only very recently received a title: health psychology. In its essential dimensions and proposals, in the path it points, it is as old as the oldest of the healing arts. The famed attorney Louis Nizer has written, "Words of comfort, skillfully administered, are the oldest therapy known to man." But the focus, the content, and the mode of communication of the words to be skillfully administered have come to be founded increasingly on penetrating psychological research. Yet health psychology is new enough as a conscious effort at the investigation of specialized knowledge that we await consensus as to its proper definition.

As a field of specialized study, research, and practice with which many psychologists are objectively identified, health psychology is less than a decade old. Historians may identify its public debut as 1978, when the American Psychological Association established the Division of Health Psychology. This event of public recognition was preceded by several years during which an increasing number of psychologists of varying specialties (notably, clinical psychologists, physiological psychologists, and social psychologists) were finding both opportunity and challenge to apply their instrumentation, their research methodology, and their interpersonal skills to a variety of problems and settings within the arena of medical illness.

The at-first limited and later rapidly expanding opportunities for the discipline of psychology to participate in the health-illness enterprise have been stimulated by several factors. Among these have been (1) growing dissatisfaction by consumers with the quality of physician-delivered health services, especially in light of the progressive increase in scientific medical knowledge; (2) increasing awareness by the medical schools of our country, especially in the post-World War II years and in response to growing consumer protest, that the physicians they trained were proving to be significantly deficient in knowledge of the psychology of physical illness and disability and unprepared to realize the potential of their medical expertise by communicating it in the context of a relationship that was adequately perceptive of and responsive to the attitudes and anxieties of their patients; (3) research that established the impact of certain personality traits as predisposing to specific illnesses and to poor response to medical regimens; (4) research that developed psychophysiological methods by which patients could achieve control over certain symptom-arousing patterns of neuromuscular autonomic activity; and (5) research that pointed to the stress-inducing and illness-disposing quality of combinations of life experiences.

Further impetus to psychology's concern for those behaviors that are part of the patient's total effort to cope with disability has come from a growing recognition of the inadequacies of the traditional medical model for the conceptualization of illness. Psychologists, especially clinicians, have been vociferous in their criticism of this model, and they have not stood alone. Many physicians have perceived the necessity for recognizing that illness is a response by the whole person to the totality of his life situation. George Engel has been a notable proponent of a biopsychosocial model to correct the inadequacies of the too-limited medical model.

As medical schools have increasingly appreciated the inadequacies of their "blood and bone" curricula, they have instituted changes in both content and organization. Courses in behavioral medicine have been introduced; their seriousness of intent is reflected in the addition of a behavioral-science section to the National Board Examination. Of equal if not greater significance has been the establishment of departments of family practice in our medical schools, and residency programs to train primary-care physicians. Such settings and programs provide an excellent medium for cross-fertilization in the training of physicians and health-care psychologists, as attested by one of the chapters in this book.

With respect to graduate education and professional preparation to practice a truly comprehensive approach to health care, the medical establishment is only slightly ahead of psychology, as witnessed by the developments mentioned. It is too soon for the specialty field of health-care psychology to have a generally accepted blueprint for preparing individuals for careers in medical or health settings (other than psychiatric clinics or hospitals) or for many such programs to be in place. Some would argue that all that is required is some revision of the established scientist-practitioner model for clinical psychologists, with special attention to the focus and length of internship training. Others would insist that the health-care psychologist needs a very different curriculum. This field of professional endeavor will necessarily evolve, and we are at a stage when many approaches may be explored.

There is a present need, however, for both prospective students and current practitioners to have a sense of the scope and the particulars of health-care psychology—its practices, its problems, and its promise. This volume is directed to that need. It is a compendium that ranges from philosophy (the problem of our mind-body "apartheid") to practice (for example, screening for the "psychological matrix" of the patient) to specific presenting problems (for example, cancer and hemophilia). It presents the experience with and the concerns for psychological factors in health care—not only by psychologists but by other practitioners—and it includes the perspectives of the consumer.

Those who read this book in its entirety will be rewarded—sometimes by new information, sometimes by validation of their experiences, and sometimes by reorientation and sensitization. This volume will be a useful resource and reference for the health-care practitioner of any discipline who is called for consultation in an unfamiliar area or who may be invited to collaborate in a study of patient care.

William Schofield, Ph.D.
University of Minnesota, Minneapolis

Preface

Psychological factors in health and illness have been acknowledged for a long time. Much more recently, however, the interest and awareness of many disciplines have focused on the significance of these psychological factors in health care. A major purpose of this book is to make information available to health-care practitioners about the contributions of psychological factors in health-care teaching, training, service delivery, and consultation-liaison services.

It seems appropriate at this time to consider the definitions of many terms. First, what is a health-care practitioner? For the purposes of this book, health-care practitioners are workers in a variety of disciplines, including physicians, nurses, psychologists, medical sociologists, medical social workers, and physical therapists. This list is by no means all-inclusive. As interest in an integrated, comprehensive perspective on the prevention, diagnosis, treatment, and rehabilitation of illness increases, so too does the controversy about what to call this emerging field. Terms such as *health psychology, health-care psychology, behavioral medicine, medical psychology,* and *behavioral health* may be recognizable to the reader. What is perhaps less clear are the distinctions among these terms, as well as their similarities. One also must consider the fact that definitions change rapidly. We would like to comment briefly on these terms in current usage. All will appear throughout this book.

Behavioral medicine is defined as "the interdisciplinary field concerned with the development and integration of behavioral and biomedical science knowledge and techniques relevant to health and illness and the application of this knowledge and these techniques to prevention, diagnosis, treatment and rehabilitation" (Schwartz and Weiss, 1978, p. 250). Many see behavioral medicine as a point of convergence for a variety of biomedical and behavioral-science disciplines.

Matarazzo finds that the behavioral-medicine definition presented by Schwartz and Weiss (1978) is too broad when preventive measures are also included with treatment and rehabilitative techniques. Matarazzo (1979) prefers to identify *behavioral health* as "an interdisciplinary field dedicated to promoting a philosophy toward health which stresses *individual responsibility* in the application of behavioral and biomedical science knowledge and techniques to the *maintenance* of health and the *prevention* of illness and dysfunction by a variety of self-initiated individual or shared activities" (p. 1).

The term *medical psychology* has been used for many years. Asken (1979) defined it as "the study of psychological factors related to any and all aspects of physical health, illness and its treatment at individual, group and systems level" (p. 67). There are objections to this definition, primarily because use of the term *medical* may indicate to some a tacit endorsement of the medical model of disease. As Masur (1979) points out, it may be that some of the more significant contributions of psychology to health care have come precisely because of the unique psychological and behavioral-science paradigms, which are in great contrast to a strictly medical approach.

Health-care psychology is a term that avoids the "medical" bias, and it also places more emphasis on health than on disease. It does imply patient care and, in general, a clinical-service orientation.

The most recent of these terms to gain wide acceptance is *health psychology* (Stone, 1979). Matarazzo (1980) also identified *health psychology* as the currently preferred discipline-specific term that encompasses psychology's role as a science and profession in both behavioral medicine and behavioral-health domains. He presented the following working definition: "*Health psychology* is the aggregate of the specific educational, scientific and professional contributions of the discipline of psychology to the promotion and maintenance of health, the prevention and treatment of illness, and the identification of etiologic and diagnostic correlates of health, illness, and related dysfunction" (p. 815).

The editors' intention here has been to share with the reader current thinking about the usage of the various terms that exist relative to the issue of psychology and health care. One can see that some of the terms are more inclusive than others. For example, a health psychologist may be practicing behavioral medicine. However, someone engaged in the practice of behavioral medicine is not necessarily a health psychologist. This highlights the interdisciplinary nature of behavioral medicine, on the one hand, and the grounding in psychological perspectives, research, and practice, on the other. The definitions and discussions reported here are continually evolving. Discussion continues on both the current referents of these terms and their potential implications for the future (Matarazzo, 1979, 1980).

This book is designed as a manual, a practical resource book for health-care practitioners and for those in health-care training. It is designed to inform health-care professionals about the contributions and uses of psychological factors in health care. We hope this book will prove useful in behavioral-science courses in medical schools, in nursing schools, and in other health-related professions programs, as well as in psychology graduate training, as the emerging field of health psychology becomes more carefully studied and explored.

References

Asken, M.J. Medical psychology: Toward definition, clarification, and organization. *Professional Psychology* 10: 66–73, 1979.

Masur, F.T. An update on medical psychology and behavioral medicine. *Professional Psychology* 10: 259–264, 1979.

Matarazzo, J.D. Health psychology: APA's newest division. *The Health Psychologist* 1: 1, 1979.

Matarazzo, J.D. Behavioral Health and Behavioral Medicine: Frontiers for a New Health Psychology. *American Psychologist* 35(9):807–817, 1980.

Schwartz, G.E., and Weiss, S.M. Behavioral medicine revisited: An amended definition. *Journal of Behavioral Medicine* 1: 249–252, 1978.

Stone, G.C., Cohen, F., and Adler, N.E. (Eds.). *Health Psychology—A Handbook*. San Francisco: Jossey-Bass, 1979.

Introduction: A Conceptual Perspective on the Psychology of Illness

Michael Jospe

Illness is the night-side of life, a more onerous citizenship. Everyone who is born holds dual citizenship, in the kingdom of the well and in the kingdom of the sick. Although we all prefer to use only the good passport, sooner or later each of us is obliged, at least for a spell, to identify ourselves as citizens of that other place —Susan Sontag

The drama of being ill—the psychological stresses and adjustments of things going seriously awry—is often hidden under the scientific cloak of modern medical practices. It is easy for us to forget that the practice of medicine entails a great deal more than the practice of the technology of biology. One of the ways in which we can forget that *people* are involved on both sides of the healing enterprise is to view medicine as nothing but an exercise in the application of certain techniques to bodies that are viewed as malfunctioning organisms. Susan Sontag's eloquent words, taken from her essay *Illness as Metaphor,* jolt us into the realization that being ill does indeed have its powerful psychological component in addition to, and interacting with, the physiological one, which we so take for granted. When we look at the ways in which people deal with illness, we cannot help but be impressed with how well many patients do in fact come through, with how well people can survive both acute crises and long-term adjustments to chronic illnesses. This introduction will address itself to some of the psychological mechanisms that people manifest in order to deal with the "nightside of life" about which Sontag writes. I will begin by looking at some considerations, both historical and contemporary, of the healing relationship and then go on to some models within which the psychology of illness can be usefully conceptualized.

We now know that medicine, a recent science, is a young and relatively new branch of the far-older art of healing. When we look at the history of healing, we are able to see how ideas about the causes of illness have changed over millenia from demons, evil spirits, demonic infestation, and all their attendant pseudotherapies to anatomy, chemistry, physiology, and the discovery of microbes. The rise of the methods of modern science meant that ancient medical practices were changed, modified, and, in most cases, abandoned altogether. The science of medicine gradually displaced the art of healing, with specific, recognized causal factors and specific manipulations resulting in specific effects. More and more, the healing process came to be seen as the practical application of scientific knowledge obtained either empirically or through controlled experimentation. Less and less were interpersonal and psychological factors seen as important or even relevant until, finally, they were either dismissed altogether or considered an embarrassment to be tolerated but not acknowledged. The arrogance born of the huge successes of mechanistic science and scientific therapy allows one a dismissing backward glance at the history of healing and therapeutics—a glance both scientifically and psychologically comfortable, since looking askance at things that are difficult to grasp because of their complexity allows us to focus on more easily identifiable variables and more easily measurable outcomes. We now know, however, that any view of medicine that excludes a consideration of interpersonal and psychological variables is bound to be a shortsighted one, one that ultimately will be far less productive and comprehensive than one that takes the trouble to recognize such variables. It is easy to think that when scientific medicine is explicit about its independent variables, it has disposed of other variables that often contribute to any observed therapeutic effect. It is also easy for many health-care professionals to be alienated by the much-bandied-about phrase, "you have to be holistic," often thrown as an accusation that practitioners are not being "holistic," rather than as presenting a desirable philosophy to practice. There are two wide ranges of phenomena that make one realize, on the basis of scientific evidence rather than mere belief, that scientific medicine per se, and particularly allopathic medicine, is simply not a sufficient entity to include alone in the healing equation. The first of these broad classes of phenomena is the placebo effect, in which we recognize the psychological impact of the relationship between healer and patient, and the second is the wide variety of adjustments that people who are ill undergo in the course of their illnesses. We know that we cannot view the psychological processes of illness as being identical with those of health.

Nonspecific and Placebo Effects in Medicine

Scientific aspects of therapy need to be cast in a less-sacred light, one in which the importance of psyche in the healing of soma, as well as the importance of people in the healing of both, is stressed more than is commonly done today. Rather than being an embarrassment to the medical profession, nonspecific and placebo effects can be viewed as an indicator of the power of psychological factors in any therapeutic endeavor. Acknowledging the role of psychology in medicine does not mean acknowledging the ineffectiveness of physical methods of therapy; on the contrary, it indicates how the combination of medical and psychological conceptualizations of healing can lead to extremely powerful results. Each factor alone is powerful, and the interaction of both kinds of factors, being multiplicative rather than merely additive, is bound to be even more powerful.

The term *placebo effect* refers to the changes in the patient produced by placebos or procedures acting as placebos. More precisely, the term refers to that portion of the behavioral therapeutic change in patients that can be attributed to any therapeutic procedure that is without specific activity for the condition to be treated, as contrasted with the behavioral or therapeutic changes owing to mere passage of time, repeated testing, or other influences. Whitehorn (1958) emphasized expectational and relationship considerations in discussing the placebo effect as "all those psychological and psychophysiological benefits or determinants which quite directly involve the patient's expectations that depend directly upon the diminution or augmentation of the patient's apprehension by the symbolic implications of the physician's behavior and attitudes." The placebo effect has been closely scrutinized by Jospe (1978) and Shapiro and Morris (1978), who indicated in their reviews of the research that placebo effects have been found to occur in a wide variety of patients suffering from a wide variety of complaints. Placebo effects manifest themselves in medicine, surgery, and psychotherapy. Despite intuitive feelings about the existence of a type of person whom we might call a "placebo reactor," the experimental literature shows little evidence of the existence of such a personality type. Rather, it now seems likely that even though we cannot dismiss entirely the possibility that some people are more placebo-prone, most people can react to placebos at one time or another. Indeed, in almost any double-blind drug study, a third of the subjects will react favorably to placebo controls. Patient, physician, milieu, and treatment variables can all influence the magnitude of the placebo effect, leading us to a recognition of the importance of psychological factors in any malady. Psychological and emotional factors can never be excluded in any illness or treatment, and the only patient for whom we can safely say the presenting complaint bears no relationship to psychological factors, being due solely to structural disease, is one who is comatose.

During the progress of medicine from early to modern times, there occurred a shift in treatment focus from spirits or demons to some vague inkling of natural causes. The aggregate known as "illness" ceased to exist because physicians spoke of ailments and specific organs and sites—a necessary condition for the ordering and classification that diagnostic categories allowed. The great nineteenth-century pathologist Virchow said that there are no general diseases, only diseases of organs and cells. Every illness, rather than being viewed as involving all aspects of the person's being, was traced to its origin and then assigned to an already outlined and described category. All that then remained was the physician's application of the prescribed therapy to the particular case. Sickness was something that attacked not the whole person but merely an organ or a few cells. Technology allowed huge strides to be made in medicine and surgery. When physicians spoke of "sickness," they were not speaking of a human being with an illness, but of a *case* of disease *x*, of duration *y*, with treatment *z*. We can see how far medicine had moved since Aristophanes considered it to be one of the arts taught to the Greeks by divine poets. However, elements in medicine that constitute the "art of healing" remain, largely in the guise of the placebo effect. The elements that make patients people, not merely collections of malfunctioning cells, will now be discussed in relation to the psychology of illness.

Some Considerations of the Role of Psychological Factors in Illness

The tremendous advances in medicine far outpaced advances in psychiatric thought, and it is no accident that Sigmund Freud was a neurologist first and a psychiatrist later. Essentially, Freud's discoveries and conceptualizations were necessary to fill in the gaps left by a too-mechanistic view of human beings. From Freud sprang the idea that we need to understand psychological mechanisms in every aspect of human existence, and from Felix Deutsch and Franz Alexander came various psychoanalytic speculations about symptoms and their relationships to the problems of the patient. Freud and some of his followers allowed us to take the necessary first steps to reach our current position, in which we try to stop practicing Cartesian dualism and begin acknowledging vulnerability to stress, conflict avoidance and emotions, neuroendocrine and autonomic shifts, and psychosocial and ecological impingements on the total well-being of people. The point that illness is not merely a matter of physiological disturbance was forcefully expressed by Jerome Frank (1973) in *Persuasion and Healing*. Frank wrote about the importance of our acknowledging that psychological and bodily processes can profoundly affect each other. High among the former are the meanings of illness emerging from the interplay of the sick person with his or her family and culture. All illnesses, whatever their bodily components, have implications that may give rise to anxious emotions, raise difficult moral issues, damage the patient's self-esteem, and estrange the patient from his or her compatriots. Chronic illness, especially, causes demoralization. Constant misery, forced relinquishment of the activities and roles that supported the patient's self-esteem and gave his or her life significance, the threat of suffering and death—all these may generate feelings of anxiety and despair. In turn, the anxiety and despair of the patient may be intensified by reactions of anxiety, impatience, and progressive withdrawal in those close to him or her, especially when an illness threatens their security as well as the patient's. Thus illness often creates a vicious cycle by evoking emotions that aggravate it. The nature of some of these emotions and emotional changes will now be discussed.

Kasl and Cobb (1966a, 1966b) distinguished between health behavior, illness behavior, and sick-role behavior. They defined *health behavior* as any activity a person, believing himself or herself to be healthy, undertakes for the purpose of preventing disease or of detecting it while it is still asymptomatic. *Illness behavior* consists of activities that people undertake when they feel ill, attempting to define their state of health and seeking remedy if necessary. Complaining and consulting other people are typical of illness behaviors. People who consider themselves ill and take steps to become well again show *sick-role behavior.* Receiving treatment, perhaps becoming dependent to some extent, and some degree of neglecting everyday activities are typical sick-role behaviors. The continuum from health to disease shows us many changes in behavior, identity, and role performance. I have mentioned some changes in behavior that occur when people are healthy, ill, or sick. In addition, a number of internal emotional changes occur as people move from a state of being healthy to one of illness or sickness. In illness, some degree of psychological distress occurs. Anxiety, depression, resentment, low self-esteem, loss of sense of social support, guilt, and sadness may occur. There is also some discomfort arising from the symptom, which may cause psychological distress, and vice versa. In the sick role, a patient experiences distress, discomfort, motivation to get well, and some sort of performance related to sick-role norms. Both personal needs and environmental and interpersonal incentives and barriers can contribute to and affect motivation to get well. Sick-role norms include commitment to one's social roles apart from being a patient, congruence with self-concept, knowledge and internalization of norms, mutuality of doctor-patient expectations, and willingness to conform.

The perceived threat of the disease and its consequences is the common thread running through health, illness, and sick-role behavior, as well as the way the perception relates to the particular behavior. The perceived value of preventive action is the most important variable mediating the influence of perceived threat. Threat and action both can be influenced by a number of demographic and background variables. Personality and situational characteristics can affect the ways in which people react to the demands of various sick-role norms. Quite clearly, we are dealing with a situation in which people's feelings, thoughts, and actions are simply not the same when they are healthy and when they are experiencing the stresses of illness or sickness.

Such stresses may be both systemic and psychological, the latter constituting the "psychological distress" that is of such importance in illness and sick-role behaviors.

A considerable amount of research has been conducted in the past few years on the psychology of health, illness, and sickness and the ways in which stress relates to these states. Lipowski (1969) says that "to understand how the patient experiences his illness and copes with it one has to know what all aspects of his disease mean to him and what responses to his complaints he obtains from other persons, including health professionals. Psychosocial factors influence the course and outcome of every illness, and it is imperative that their evaluation should be a part of medical diagnosis and management." The book *Advances in Psychosomatic Medicine* (Lipowski, 1972), which deals with psychosocial aspects of physical illness, includes such contributions as recent life changes and illness susceptibility, the personal meaning of illness, somatic perception during illness, coping with severe illness, and the impact of the hospital environment on the patient. Steinhauer, Muchin, and Rae-Grant (1974) address themselves to psychological aspects of chronic illness, including, importantly, the effects of chronic illness not only on patients (particularly children) but also on their families and those treating them. Mechanic's (1972) well-known and outstanding work on psychosocial aspects of illness includes a survey of some of the literature on social psychological factors affecting the presentation of bodily complaints that shows how a host of nonspecific factors can influence the ways in which people perceive and present what ails them. A comprehensive collection of papers on the relationships of stressful life events and physical illness edited by Dohrenwend and Dohrenwend (1974) includes life-change and illness susceptibility, catastrophic illness, and emotional distress. Another recently edited volume (Moos, 1977) deals with coping in the face of severe illnesses such as cancer, cardiovascular disease, burns, chronic conditions, and organ transplants. In Moos's book we see what sorts of factors are involved in such coping, how severe the stresses can be, and what an enormous disruption can occur from a state of illness and its accompanying psychological processes. Once these works have been read and their implications considered, one is forced to recognize some of the absurdities involved in not acknowledging the importance of psychological factors in illness and sickness.

Let us briefly consider some aspects of research on stress that are relevant here. Selye (1956) sees stress as the state of the organism following failure of the normal homeostatic regulatory mechanisms of adaptation. Selye has been the major worker in research on systemic stress. A major key to the understanding of systemic stress has been the distinction between the specific effects induced by one or another stressor agent and its nonspecific effects. The intensity and duration of both specific and nonspecific effects can produce important changes, which, according to Cofer and Appley (1964), "taken together, constitute the stereotypical response pattern of systemic stress . . . [operationally defined by Selye as] a state manifested by a syndrome which consists of all the nonspecifically-induced changes in a biologic system." A large variety of stimulus events (stressor agents), including temperature extremes, infections, hemorrhage, drugs, injury, surgery, and shock, can give rise to such stress. Stressor agents may be both direct (surgical, pharmacological, physical) and indirect (neurogenic or psychogenic). It is interesting to note that illness behavior and sick-role behavior may involve both kinds of stressor agents, and when the local or focal adaptations appropriate to the particular form of the stressor are ineffective, or when the stressor is nonspecific, the general adaptation syndrome (GAS) is invoked. The GAS, which consists of three stages (alarm reaction, stage of resistance, and stage of exhaustion), involves complex interrelations between neurological, hormonal, and metabolic mechanisms.

Psychological stress is somewhat broader than systemic stress. Appley (cited in Cofer and Appley, 1964) proposes that stress is "the state of an organism in any situation where his general well-being is threatened and where no readily available response exists for the reduction of the threat." A condition of insufficiency alone, however, is not enough to produce psychological stress. As Cofer and Appley indicate, the change from innate or habitual behavior to new coping behavior, or the exhaustion of the already existing effective coping responses, permits a change in arousal known as the *instigation threshold.* If something interferes with goal behaviors, or if such an interference is anticipated, and if this interference continues, then the *frustration threshold* is reached. Threat is now perceived, anxiety is aroused, and coping behavior is intensified. Exclusively task-oriented, problem-solving behavior is no longer the only behavior, so ego-oriented, self- or integrity-sustaining behaviors arise. Such behaviors would be involved in the identity and behavior aspects of Kasl's and Cobb's (1966*a,* 1966*b*) conceptualization of illness behavior and sick-role behavior, mentioned earlier. Should task- and ego-oriented behaviors persist for a while without any effective change in the situation, the *stress threshold* is reached. All task-oriented behaviors are eliminated, and only ego-protective behaviors remain. Danger may be perceived and possible desperation or panic might occur before the ego-protective behaviors are in turn eliminated, thereby leading to an *exhaustion threshold* and the perception of helplessness and hopelessness. The latter will not occur in most everyday illnesses, but it is probably what occurs in "giving up the will to live" and in such phenomena as voodoo death.

Psychological stressors may involve either a deficiency or an excess of stimulation as well as ambiguity or conflict of stimuli. When a person is engaged in illness or sick-role behavior, he or she may be removed from the familiar environment, and familiar stimuli may be removed. Cofer and Appley (1964) mention these two types of changes as stress-invoking; in addition, the person may be exposed to a large number of both direct and indirect stressor agents, some of which may well be involved in the therapeutic measures being undertaken. The person's ability to rely on habitual behaviors is disturbed, and he or she moves "up the stress ladder" (Cofer and Appley, 1964) in order to protect his or her orientation, stability, or integrity. Ambiguity is a stressor because the person cannot know what response is required. Conflict is a stressor because the person is required to perform incompatible responses. Both result in uncertainty, restrictions of response repertoire, and, if unabated, stress. In illness behavior, ambiguity may arise, for example, from a lack of information as to the nature, course, and prognosis of the illness. These are only some of the stressors involved in illness; other factors involved in illness, such as vulnerability, also will increase stress. These factors will seldom be present or, if present, will not be of the same magnitude in healthy people as in people who are in a clinical situation for one reason or another or are engaged in illness or sickness behavior.

Moos and Tsu (1977) present a model that neatly ties up many of the things we have been talking about here. A person's response to a physical illness will be a function of background and personal factors, illness-related factors, and physical and social environmental factors. All these in turn, will influence the cognitive appraisal (perceived meaning) of the illness, the adaptive tasks, and the coping skills a person will manifest. Moos and Tsu view serious physical illness or injury as a life crisis necessitating basic adaptive tasks to which various coping skills can be applied. The point is stressed that family members and friends, not just the patient, are affected by the crisis, encounter many of the same or closely related adaptive tasks, and use the same types of coping skills.

There are many background and personal factors, ranging from age, intelligence, and philosophical and religious beliefs to prior experience with various kinds of coping. These will determine the meaning that the illness has for the patient, family, or friends and will affect the psychological and intellectual resources that the person brings to bear to withstand the crisis. Illness-related factors are an obvious set here, and they include the type and location of symptoms. Different symptoms have different meanings; for example, the significance of disfiguring injury to the face will be quite different from an equal amount of physiological and structural damage done to a less-visible part of the body. The considerable body of research on coping shows how it may be affected by physiological processes, and we know from psychosomatic medicine that physiological processes may be affected by psychological ones. The illness-related factors are thus an obvious, but by no means necessarily simple, component of our model. Stress can be worsened or lessened by physical and social environmental factors. Even though hospitals exist to make us better, their environments may be extremely stress-producing. Emergency rooms and intensive-care units may be excitingly dramatic on television dramas, but they are not perceived as such when we are involved on the patient's side of what happens in them—few areas can be as alienating or as stressful. Hospitalization imposes stresses of its own. Volicer (1978) has reported that patients scoring high in hospital stress reported more pain, lower physical status during hospitalization, and less improvement after discharge than patients scoring low in hospital stress. The social environment is essentially the human environment: patients and their significant others, relationships between staff and patients, relationships between patients and community (friends, work colleagues, clergy, social agencies), and the sociocultural norms and expectations we discussed earlier when looking at the work of Kasl and Cobb. Obviously, any stresses in the social environment can lead to greater stress in the patient and can impede the healing process. What we mentioned about Selye's work applies in all these sets of factors influencing coping and adaptation.

Moos and Tsu divide the major adaptive tasks into several general categories. The first set of tasks is illness-related: dealing with pain and incapacitation, dealing with the hospital environment and special treatment procedures, and developing adequate relationships with professional staff. The second set of general adaptive tasks entails preserving a reasonable emotional balance regarding feelings aroused by the illness, preserving a satisfactory self-image and maintaining a sense of competence and mastery, preserving relationships with family and friends, and preparing for an uncertain future in which there is the threat of significant losses. The tasks are encountered in almost any illness but will be variously balanced according to who gets what disease and under what circumstances. Pain, discomfort, self-image, and the future will vary according to the predicaments in which people find themselves. It is important for all of us (not only patients and their significant others, but helping professionals as well) to recognize how important the adaptive tasks are and to understand that all patients and their families will have to face them to one degree or another.

Many types of coping skills are necessary to allow people to deal with the preceding adaptive tasks. Coping is a positive psychological process that can be learned and can be flexible in relation to situational demands. One such set of coping skills involves denying or minimizing the seriousness of a crisis, which enables people to handle significant psychological trauma while still performing other tasks necessary for daily living. Many people engaged in medical psychology are concerned that such denial is too often seen as a maladaptive rather than a temporarily adaptive mechanism. It is often important to deny, minimize, or dissociate oneself from situations that could otherwise be quite overwhelming, while allowing oneself to gather other personal coping resources or to dispose of matters that need to be taken care of immediately.

The effective use of intellectual resources and the search for relevant information constitute another important set of coping skills. We tend to be anxious when we are uncertain or ill-informed, and getting information about illnesses can serve both to correct misconceptions and to give patients something constructive with which to fill time that might otherwise be spent pondering those misconceptions. We should not underestimate the role that hospital, clinic, or library medical informational and educational services can have here.

People who can request emotional support and reassurance from concerned family, friends, and medical staff are displaying another set of coping skills. People who can do this are generally less tense and stressed than those who cannot. Encouraging patients and families to express their feelings allows them to cope better than when they hold everything inside. Significant emotional support can often be obtained from other people in similar situations, hence the success of self-help groups and organizations, ranging from cancer-patient support groups to large national organizations for epileptics. Physicians sometimes insensitively scoff that "every little disease now has a national group," without appreciating the informational and supportive coping with which such groups help patients and those concerned about them.

Many illnesses require learning specific illness-related procedures, such as injecting one's own insulin, monitoring one's own blood pressure, or managing one's own diet or complex medication regimen. Such a set of tasks is another coping skill, effective mastery of which allows the return of a sense of control in situations that otherwise often represent the exact opposite.

The setting of concrete limited goals, such as walking again or attending one's grandson's graduation, often allows patients to achieve realistic, attainable, and reasonable goals without causing further stress by setting themselves up for inevitable failure. Doing such things can change some problems from overwhelming ones to difficult but still-manageable ones, particularly when they are broken down into specific behaviors and the small, achievable goals that are part of larger, more ambitious goals.

Many diseases require the rehearsing of alternative outcomes, such as preparing oneself for procedures by using anticipation and mental rehearsal—and even the anticipatory mourning process, in which an expected death or other loss is acknowledged before it occurs.

People under stress often try to find a general purpose or pattern of meaning in the course of events, and patients will often benefit by talking to someone with whom they can have existential discussions of this nature.

The usefulness of the preceding models lies in their ready translatability into behavior; rather than being merely philosophical conceptions of an ideal or belief about how people react to the crisis of illness and sickness, they tell us what specific things to look for in a patient and how we can help redress the balance when things go awry. They also set the psychological tone for the rest of this book. We are concerned with what happens to *people* in health care, not just to bodies. In the final analysis, we are concerned that health-care professionals once more become healers, recognizing the many dimensions in which human beings operate and the many dimensions in which we can intervene in order to allow a recapturing of "bedside manner" and the true concern with suffering that made so many of us enter the helping professions in the first place. The placebo effect and the complexities of the psychology of illness surely attest to the enormity of the beneficial powers that we can exert in our manifold capacities as people to whom others turn for help.

References

Cofer, C.N., and Appley, M.H. *Motivation: Theory and Research.* New York: Wiley, 1964.

Dohrenwend, B., and Dohrenwend, B., eds. *Stressful life events: Their nature and effects.* New York: Wiley, 1974.

Frank, J. *Persuasion and Healing.* Baltimore: Johns Hopkins Press, 1973.

Jospe, M. *The Placebo Effect in Healing.* Lexington, Mass.: Lexington Books, D.C. Heath and Company, 1978.

Kasl, S., and Cobb, S. Health behavior, illness behavior and sick-role behavior: I. Health and illness behavior. *Archives of Environmental Health* 12: 246–266, 1966*a*.

Kasl, S., and Cobb, S. Health behavior, illness behavior and sick-role behavior: II. Sick-role behavior. *Archives of Environmental Health* 12: 531–541, 1966*b*.

Lipowski, Z.J. Psychological aspects of disease. *Annals of Internal Medicine* 71: 1197–1206, 1969.

Lipowski, Z.J. (ed.). *Advances in Psychosomatic Medicine,* Vol. 8: *Psychosocial Aspects of Physical Illness.* Basel: S. Karger, 1972.

Mechanic, D. Social psychologic factors affecting the presentation of bodily complaints. *New England Journal of Medicine* 286: 1132–1139, 1972.

Moos, R. ed. *Coping with Physical Illness.* New York: Plenum, 1977.

Moos, R., and Tsu, V.D. The crisis of physical illness: An overview. In *Coping and Physical Illness.* R. Moos ed. New York: Plenum, 1977, pp. 3–22.

Selye, H. *The Stress of Life.* New York: McGraw-Hill, 1956.

Shapiro, A.K., and Morris, L.A. The placebo effect in medical and psychological therapies. In *Handbook of Psychotherapy and Behavior Change: an empirical analysis,* eds. S. Garfield and A. Bergin, New York: Basic Books, 1978, pp. 369–410.

Sontag, S. *Illness as Metaphor.* New York: Farrar, Strauss and Giroux, 1978.

Steinhauer, P., Muchin, D., and Rae-Grant, Q. Psychological aspects of chronic illness. *Pediatric Clinics of North America* 21: 825–840, 1974.

Volicer, B. Hospital stress and patient reports of pain and physical status. *Journal of Human Stress* 4: 28–37, 1978.

Whitehorn, J.C. Psychiatric implications of the placebo effect. *American Journal of Psychiatry* 114: 662–664, 1958.

Part I
Teaching and Training
for Practice: A Trend
Away from Dualism

Until recently, there has been a dearth of readily available collections of readings in the field of health psychology. One cannot help being fascinated by the things one sees in health psychology, the observations one makes, and the questions one asks, as well as by some of the answers one is able to find. One of the things that emerges from a consideration of the field is the clear realization that there are as many opinions regarding the psychological nature of illness as there are patients. And always in this area one encounters the extraordinary relationship between healers, such as physicians or nurses, and patients. One is sometimes frustrated by problems observed in the patient-healer relationship, sometimes amazed in the most positive ways, sometimes appalled, and sometimes moved.

On the side of patients, one frequently observes a phenomenon no different now from what it has been for centuries. The great Hippocrates, in his *Precepts,* said that some patients, although conscious that their condition is perilous, recover their health simply through their contentment with the goodness of the physician. Jehudah Halevy, medieval philosopher, mystic, and physician, remarked that every ill person fears death and hopes for a cure, and when told the physician is coming, the person feels happy and longs to wait for what the physician will say. Halevy said any fool and inexperienced person finds it possible to be a physician. In truth, we know that this is not so, but we know too that what Halevy said means that there is a great deal more to dealing with illness than merely combating an infection or surgically excising an offending organ. We are talking here about bedside manner, and it is bedside manner, or the lack thereof, that so impresses or offends.

In this section, some of the front-line providers of health care are addressed: physicians, nurses, and psychologists. An attempt is made to show how training programs can allow professionals to develop a heightened awareness of psychological issues, with a clear emergence of a gradually more holistic view of people that diverts focus from the dualism that persists in most training in both the applied biological sciences and the applied social ones. Medicine, once a great social art, continued to be one until the advent of the bacteriologists of the previous century (King, 1962). Medical practice then became more and more entrenched in the biological sciences, and it is only now that we are beginning to be able to observe the first glimmerings of a new era, with "a fusion . . . taking place between

1

these two phases in the history of medicine, so that it may be spoken of more properly as a practice that is biosocial in foundation" (King, 1962). We think it is extremely important for people to understand that mere frustration or scoffing at a physician's or nurse's lack of bedside manner or psychological sophistication is an inappropriate response when, because of the biological emphasis, one considers how many medical and nursing professionals were never trained to be sensitive, caring, or concerned. Too often we notice stereotyping or categorization of such health practitioners. In the following four chapters, we look at ways in which a full complement of people in the health-care professions can be taught to work with one another and develop a fruitful, pragmatic interdisciplinary understanding that allows the old barriers and stereotypes to either disappear or, failing that, to assume proportions that are so much less than they have been in the past that they no longer interfere with a consideration of whole persons being treated. A few different perspectives on innovative approaches to training health-care professionals are offered.

Racer (chapter 3) views the family physician as having equal responsibility for both discerning the emotional situation of patient and family and diagnosing and healing organic disorders. Family practice is an area of medicine in which there is a heavy interdisciplinary melange of individual psychology, family structure and dynamics, developmental psychology, community medicine, and medical sociology. Included as an essential ingredient in the training of family practitioners can be regular contact, in a number of ways, with behavioral/social-science practitioners. Such contact increases the learning of psychological medicine by the family-practice resident through increasing the effectiveness of the training and immediacy of the behavioral-science clinician. There is a heavy reliance on modeling, and Racer puts this well when he writes that in both practice and teaching, modeling must show the natural confluence of behavioral and organic approaches in the comprehension of the need of patients for care. By introducing psychology interns into the family-practice residency, we see the development of a collegial rather than merely delegatory or referral relationship between two professionals working collectively.

Nieberding and Jospe (chapter 2) show what it was like to be the innovators on the psychology-intern side of the preceding collective working relationship. They show how a multifaceted relationship emerged, being collaborative, supervisory, and consultative. The relationship fulfilled both the consultation and liaison functions that Lipowski (1974) characterizes as the necessary and mutually complementary activities of mental-health professionals in the wide range of the nonpsychiatric areas of medicine: clinical, teaching, and research activities.

That nursing is now and has for some time been in the forefront of the health-care professions in adopting a holistic approach is shown clearly by

Smith and Wallston (chapter 4). Their chapter discusses how psychology can provide an integration of theory and research to provide clinically applicable knowledge. Smith and Wallston go on to provide some specific illustrations of the clinically applicable knowledge offered by psychology. We begin to see a conceptualization of patients as people and people as part of the larger, interacting social systems. A biopsychosocial orientation is the direction in which we are progressing. Nurses have closer and more frequent contact with patients than any other member of the health-care professions. They can clearly teach us a great deal by showing us how they treat "the total person," how they are trained to do so, and how physicians and psychologists can work with them to reinforce the trend away from dualism that this book seeks to promote.

References

King, S.H. *Perceptions of Illness and Medical Practice.* New York: Russell Sage, 1962.

Lipowski, L.J. Consultation-liaison psychiatry: An overview. *American Journal of Psychiatry* 131: 623–630, 1974.

1

Training Programs in Health-Care Psychology at the University of Minnesota Health Sciences Center

A. Jack Hafner

Over the past ten years, the internship training program in clinical psychology at the University of Minnesota Health Sciences Center has shown a gradual transition from a more traditional emphasis on experiences related to patients with primarily mental-health problems, particularly psychiatric populations, to a broader group of patients reflecting a variety of different sorts of psychological dysfunction, particularly problems related to their physical illness. This broadening of training experiences also has meant that interns get experience with different professionals in the health area, including physicians in a variety of medical specialties, as well as working with professionals in various areas of allied health.

The emphasis in the training program has shifted to what has now come to be called *health-care psychology.* It might be helpful to define what we consider health-care psychology to mean in this broader training context. Schofield (1969) defines health-care psychology as "the application of psychological principles and techniques to understanding and management of psychological problems arising in the context of physical illness. It is the introduction and utilization of psychological dimensions in the treatment of medical illness. It provides attention to the cognitive, affective and behavioral problems of medical patients so that a treatment regimen may be truly comprehensive. It is the application of psychology to health care behavior including both prophylactics and therapeutics. It is the broad practice of psychology in general medical settings and is concerned with patients who have problems of physical illness and handicap."

The internship training program in health-care psychology at the University of Minnesota Health Sciences Center is a 1-year full-time program designed for doctoral students in clinical psychology to gain competence in psychological assessment, intervention, and consultation, as well as experience in supervising psychology clerks and teaching clinical material to medical and allied health personnel. The training experiences emphasize the practice of psychology in a comprehensive medical center and in community health-care delivery. This training program has been approved by the Committee on Accreditation of the Education and Training Board of the Ameri-

5

can Psychological Association. Students in this training program come from graduate schools throughout the United States. While enrolled in the program, interns are registered as full-time students in the medical school as psychology fellow specialists. Eight stipends provide financial support for the interns. Funding for these stipends comes from the university hospitals and from a National Institute of Mental Health (NIMH) training grant. In the past several years, there have been over 100 qualified applicants for these eight stipends.

The internship program in health-care psychology is a rotational program, whereby the intern spends blocks of time, usually 12 weeks, on a particular service and then rotates onto another service, so that during the internship period individuals are given exposure to a number of different settings as a part of their training. The shift to a health-care psychology emphasis has resulted in an increase in the number of available experiences provided to interns. The training program allows for specialization in the child, adolescent, or adult areas. An intern selecting one or the other area for emphasis, however, is given some experience with the populations of all these age groups. The program provides more placement opportunities than time available for any particular intern. What this means is that there is a certain amount of individualization for each intern in the program. An effort is made to try to accommodate, whenever possible, particular training interests of an intern.

Some of the traditional training experiences that are available during the internship include adult psychiatry, both inpatient and in an outpatient psychiatry clinic. Also provided are experiences in child and adolescent psychiatry, both inpatient and outpatient. Other training opportunities pertaining particularly to the mental-health area include the student mental health service at the University of Minnesota, where the intern has a chance to do therapy with university students. A similar experience is available at the student counseling bureau at the university, which emphasizes additional concerns regarding student interests and vocational planning. We have a health-care psychology clinic, and this provides opportunities for working as an independent and autonomous health-care professional in the child, adolescent, and adult areas. The emphasis in training in this clinic is on psychological evaluation and brief psychological intervention procedures. Our interns get some training in the area of chemical dependency, in terms of both doing screening evaluations and experience with rehabilitation programs for chemically dependent persons. Another training opportunity for the interns is in rural community mental health.

Training experiences that reflect a broader health-care psychology emphasis include neuropsychology, where the intern works with patients from neurology and neurosurgery. Here the intern learns to deal with test instruments and procedures for assessing patients in regard to clinical neuropsychology. The intern also has a chance for direct consultation with neurologists and neurosurgeons on this rotation. A pediatric neurology placement is also available, and this provides experience in assessment and intervention with children with developmental, behavioral, and learning problems. The intern participates as a member of a multidisciplinary team that includes pediatric neurologists and speech pathologists.

Another health-care psychology area is that of the children's service in the Department of Physical Medicine and Rehabilitation. Here the intern becomes familiar with a patient population and patient problems encountered in a medical-rehabilitation setting for physically handicapped children. The intern is also exposed to interdisciplinary team functioning and deals with both assessment and intervention procedures. The adult physical medicine and rehabilitation rotation for an intern provides training with psychological problems related to adult disability and rehabilitation. The intern becomes familiar with assessment, treatment, and rehabilitation of patients, particularly with chronic-pain problems. Again, as on the child service, the intern is exposed to an interdisciplinary health-care team and learns to identify the role of the psychologist on this team.

The medical consultation service provides another experience for interns in the broader health-care psychology domain. Here the intern acts as consultant to the various medical services at the University of Minnesota Hospitals. The intern is involved in consultation with staff and in evaluating medical patients. The intern makes recommendations regarding how the psychological functioning of the patient may relate to the patient's physical problems and the course of treatment.

The rotation available to interns in the Department of Pediatrics is one that emphasizes the health-care psychology area. The intern is provided training experiences on the inpatient wards of pediatrics and on the outpatient services. The kinds of experiences provided on the pediatrics rotation include working closely with medical staff in the treatment and care of children with medical problems, such as cystic fibrosis, leukemia, bone cancer, and other oncological disorders. The intern learns to provide therapeutic assistance to children experiencing adjustment problems related to their primary medical illness. The intern also assists parents who are experiencing difficulties in coping with their child's illness. On the pediatrics rotation, the intern has opportunities for working with dying patients. This involves dealing with parents who are trying to cope with the issue of death and dying as well as working with dying patients themselves.

A training placement that would seem to particularly characterize training in health-care psychology is the family-practice medicine rotation (see chapter 3). This placement offers interns the opportunity to work in a more general medical setting rather than in particular medical-specialty areas that some of the other health-care psychology placements offer. The intern on the family-practice medicine rotation is given an opportunity to become familiar with general medical settings, both outpatient and inpatient, within the community. With this rotation the intern learns to identify the psychologist's role in working in a general medical setting. The training on the family-practice medicine rotation involves both assessment and intervention procedures with medical patients. The intern also learns to work as a consultant with family practitioners in their daily practice.

In reviewing with the interns their training experiences of the past several years, the interns have been particularly positive about the training experiences in the areas of health-care psychology. The intern evaluations indicate that training in health-care psychology affords unique occasions for innovation. The health-care psychology placements seem to provide the opportunity for interns to demonstrate their resourcefulness in applying their training in human behavior on health problems.

With the change in emphasis in the internship training program to provide broader health-care psychology experiences, we also have emphasized this aspect of the training program in the internship brochure and in the selection process for new interns. We are now selecting interns on the basis of their interests in the area of health-care psychology in particular. We have noticed in the past several years appreciably more interest in health-care psychology training experiences on the part of applicants.

In 1972, a committee was appointed in the Division of Health Care Psychology at the University of Minnesota to review the possibilities of developing a new doctor of psychology degree in health-care psychology. Interest in developing such a new degree program was an outgrowth in part of the internship training experiences in health-care psychology. The result of this committee's work was a formal proposal for a professional degree program leading to the doctor of psychology in health-care psychology that was presented to the Graduate School of the University of Minnesota and is currently under review.

Some particularly influential factors in the development of the proposal for such a degree in health-care psychology came from the American Psychological Association's conference on levels and patterns of training in professional psychology, held at Vail, Colorado in 1976 (Korman, 1976). Another important development influencing the proposal was the American Psychological Association's Task Force on Health Behavior Research (1976), which was chaired by Dr. William Schofield. The reports of both these groups were given careful consideration in the development of the proposal.

It might be helpful to present some of the underlying thinking for the proposal of the new degree in health-care psychology. Psychology's role as both health science and health profession has, up to the present time, been reflected in its close relationships with psychiatry and the field of mental health. This limited identity with mental health can be seen particularly in training programs of clinical psychology. However, with a current emphasis on an improved system for delivery of comprehensive health care, increased attention is likely to be directed toward prophylactic education and psychological factors that impinge on general health-related behaviors. The comprehensive health care afforded through such mechanisms as health maintenance organizations will require a considerable broadening of service and research activities in the area of psychological factors that relate to the predispositions to illness, attitudes affecting health practices, resistance to medication, cooperation in treatment, response to therapy, atypical course, delayed convalescence, and abuse of insurance coverage. The psychology of physical illness has received relatively little systematic study; yet rarely is a physically ill person without some psychological concomitants, even though not of psychiatric proportion. The program in health-care psychology was designed to prepare students to be professional psychologists whose primary employment would relate to health care. Graduates of such a program would be expected to become practitioners in health-care psychology and render a variety of psychological services to individuals and to social institutions providing health and psychological care.

The curriculum for the new program proposed in health-care psychology would include required basic knowledge areas of psychology, such as psychological measurement, differential psychology, learning, and statistics, as well as developmental psychology, psychological problems of the aged, vocational psychology, descriptive psychopathology, physiological psychology, and personality. Additional required courses would be in the areas of pathophysiology of disease, interdisciplinary studies in drug problems, principles of organization and management of health-service organizations, and fundamentals of epidemiology. An important new course to be developed for the program would be that of the psychology of disease and disability, and this would cover such areas as the process of adjustment to disease and disability, family adjustment problems related to disease and disability, the social psychology of disability, problems of living with chronic illness, and the vocational psychology of disease and disability.

The professional-skills training in this new program would come through specifically designed laboratory courses that would provide the students with the technical skills for appraisal and management of patients with psychological problems accompanying illness. Additional professional-skills training would be provided that relates to consultation and to program development and evaluation in health-care settings. Theory and method of psychological techniques would be presented in conjunction with laboratory and field-placement experiences. These particular laboratory courses would follow a competency-based curriculum, whereby identified competencies and the training requirements to obtain these competencies are specified, followed by an evaluation of whether or not a particular level of competency has been obtained by the student.

The early involvement of students in practicum work emphasized in this new program follows the Vail conference recommendations. The students would begin working in field settings early in their graduate training. Initially they would observe professionals, who would provide role models for them. Then the students would be involved in field applications of the professional-skill areas taught in the laboratory course. Field-placement experiences would include, in particular, general medical settings. The fourth and final year for the students in the program in health-care psychology would be devoted to a full-time internship in a comprehensive health-care delivery setting. During the internship, the student would have an opportunity to function at a junior staff level and apply and develop skills in the areas of assessment and intervention, consultation, program development and evaluation, and training.

In summary, psychologists are now being employed in growing numbers in health-care settings. The specific competencies of these psychologists have been developed through working experiences or through some of the internship training programs in health-care psychology, such as the one at the University of Minnesota Health Sciences Center. The proposal for a professional degree program in health-care psychology just described is an effort to provide a more comprehensive and systemic training of professional psychologists with competencies to function in general medical or health-care settings, where the concern is directed primarily to dealing with a broader spectrum of health-care behavior. With additional opportunities for training in health-care psychology offered by internship programs, and possibly through new doctoral programs, it can be expected that psychologists will significantly broaden their contributions to health-care delivery.

References

American Psychological Association Task Force on Health Research. Contributions of psychology to health research. *American Psychologist* 31: 263–274, 1976.

Korman, M., ed. *Levels and Patterns of Professional Training in Psychology.* Washington: American Psychological Association, 1976.

Schofield, W. The role of psychology in the delivery of health services. *American Psychologist* 24: 565–584, 1969.

2

Psychological Internship Experiences in a Family-Practice Clinic

Joseph Nieberding
and *Michael Jospe*

Historically, the clinical and research activities of psychologists in the fields of health and medicine generally have been limited to problems associated with mental illness. Until recently, the training and subsequent research and employment of psychologists have perpetuated this restriction of the profession. Schofield (1969) remarked that the potential contribution of the professional psychologist outside the realm of mental health is limited unless the current pattern of training the scientist-clinician broadens in scope beyond that of psychiatric illness and psychiatric services.

Recently, there have been significant developments in training programs and professional degree programs that attempt to prepare psychologists for work in the health-care field. The Division of Health Care Psychology of the University of Minnesota has proposed the establishment of a professional degree program leading to the Master of Science and Doctor of Psychology degree in health psychology (Wirt, 1974). The University of Minnesota also offers a predoctoral internship training program in health psychology (see chapter 1). The internship provides traditional training experiences in adult and child inpatient psychiatric units, psychological assessment, and outpatient psychotherapy, along with other possible rotations frequently found in predoctoral internship programs. However, the interns also can choose from an array of innovative placements that stress psychology's role in a comprehensive health-care service system. Several of these rotations include consultation throughout most of the university hospital's medical and surgical services, pediatrics, an inpatient pain-treatment program utilizing behavior-modification techniques, a crisis-intervention unit connected with the emergency room of the general hospital, and placement in a family-practice setting (Ireton, Racer, and Hafner, 1978; Jospe, 1976).

The following is an account of the experiences of the first two psychology interns to be placed in a local family-practice clinic and community hospital. Before actually describing the types of experience each had, a brief description of the family-practice clinic and nearby hospital will be presented (see chapter 3 for additional details).

The family-practice clinic was located in a medical office building in a middle-class suburb of Minneapolis. A nearby 470-bed, private hospital provided the inpatient medical and emergency room services. Ten family-practice residents, who were each at various stages of their 3-year residency program, provided the medical treatment. The clinic also was staffed with a full-time medical director, whose primary responsibility was consultation with the family-practice residents and administration of the family-medicine clinic. Approximately three physicians of various specialties were available to the residents for consultation when the clinic director was not available. Also, a clinical psychologist who was an associate professor in the Department of Family Practice and Community Health would consult with the family-practice residents regarding psychological aspects of patient care in addition to psychological methods, such as psychological testing, short-term intervention techniques, and interviewing skills. The psychologist would be available for individual consultations with the residents, to review video tapes of doctor-patient interactions, and to interview clients and families with the residents upon request. Additionally, weekly patient-care conferences were collaboratively taught by the family-physician director and the psychologist, who served as models of an interdisciplinary approach to patient care for the residents. Both the psychologist and the medical director strongly supported the request presented to the director of the internship training program that the family-practice clinic serve as the location for a psychology internship rotation.

The following objectives were drawn up for the internship placement. The most central, underlying goal was to train psychologists to effectively consult to family physicians and other primary-care physicians regarding the psychological aspects of health and illness. In the process of this training, interns would become familiar with the operation of a community medical clinic, as well as develop cooperative working relationships with family-practice residents and other medical personnel. Some of the more specific goals were to observe physicians at work, study the medical model and system of diagnosis, learn about the problem-oriented medical record, conduct psychological assessments of patients, provide short-term therapy and counseling for patients, work as a member of a comprehensive health-care team, and become familiar with the psychological resource network available within the clinic, hospital, and community (Ireton, Racer, and Hafner, 1978). Dr. Jospe was the first psychology intern at the clinic, spending approximately 24 hours per week over a 3-month period. A 4-month period elapsed before Dr. Nieberding began a 2-month full-time rotation. (Although this internship is customarily a predoctoral one, both Dr. Jospe and Dr. Nieberding had already taken their Ph.D. degrees when they began working at the family-practice clinic.) Dr. Jospe's experiences will be presented first, followed by those of Dr. Nieberding.

Clinical Experience as a Health-Care Psychologist

Dr. Jospe began the rotation at the family-practice clinic by spending 2 weeks accompanying the family-practice residents in all their patient contacts, either at the clinic or at the nearby hospital. He was introduced to the patients either as Dr. Jospe, function unspecified, or as a psychologist who was learning about medical practice, depending on the wishes of the physicians he was accompanying. In all cases, patients were asked whether they would mind his presence, and no one ever did. Over the first 2 weeks, he had the chance to observe about fifty or sixty physician-patient interactions at the clinic and in rounds at the hospital. This allowed him to begin forming impressions as to which physicians related most warmly to patients, which ones dealt with difficult psychological questions with ease, and which were able to answer their patients' psychological questions with only minimal assistance from him. Following the initial 2-week period, he began to see more patients for evaluation, therapy, and supportive care, while still seeing patients with the residents when his schedule permitted. Since the following experiences with medical patients differ from those which most interns and psychologists encounter in more traditional psychiatric settings, the experiences will be described in some detail.

The age range of the patients and their present complaints, diagnoses, and treatment modalities utilized were comparable to standard general practices in similar urban settings across the country. Their problems ranged from a sudden, traumatic heart attack to those of an obsessive-compulsive schoolteacher who had been coming to the clinic for many years during the summer. The teacher, unable to fill his time constructively when his pupils were on vacation, developed a host of psychosomatic complaints and usually gained 30 to 50 pounds. Another patient had just had spinal surgery and was referred to Dr. Jospe for treatment of a sexual dysfunction that had troubled him for many years before he finally confided in his family physician. (Perhaps it was this man's vulnerability during the post-surgical stress that made him able to confide in someone. Both he and his wife were treated successfully.) One of the most striking experiences for all the staff was the sudden and unexpected death of a young man hospitalized for the treatment of pulmonary emboli. Dr. Jospe had had several brief contacts with this man earlier and found that such a sudden death produced a shock in him that made him able to more fully understand how traumatic this incident was for the resident who had been treating the man. Dr. Jospe was part of the supportive team that rallied around the resident, enabling him to share his feelings of grief, guilt, and confusion following his patient's death. This experience demonstrated the effect of loss or grief on those in the helping professions who care about their patients. Not only the patients' families, but also the helping professionals have to cope with practically the same issues of loss, grief, anger, and other difficult emotions.

One patient remembered with great fondness was a woman in her late seventies who had recently had both her legs amputated following the gangrenous deterioration of those limbs owing to diabetes. Her physician thought it might be a good idea for her to discuss her feelings of loss of autonomy following her surgery and the question of residence in a special facility for handicapped older people. She had seen Dr. Jospe several times before, when he had accompanied her physician on rounds. When he went to see her to "discuss her feelings," she gave him a long lecture on how terrific her physician was and how she did not need any "youngster" coming to talk to her about what was necessary and unalterable. He suddenly saw himself in a much clearer perspective in relationship with this particular client. He realized that indeed he was a youngster in her perspective as a seventy-year-old woman. The exposure to human suffering from the perspective of a medical practice provided him with a richer appreciation for this facet of human nature than one might otherwise have obtained, particularly if the training had been restricted to a psychiatric facility. This exposure to such a broad range of human problems and coping styles gave him an idea of how some people are very vulnerable and others much less so in the face of great crisis and loss. This enabled him to develop an appreciation for the real ability some people have to cope with situations they might not be expected to be able to handle.

Some of the outpatients also provided valuable first-hand experiences in dealing with a number of relatively "heavy" situations. Once, a middle-aged man was gently and skillfully informed by his physician that he had diabetes. The man took it in stride, while Dr. Jospe felt anxious because he was still learning how difficult it can be to transmit such news. Another time, when a woman was told she had cancer, her stunned reaction was something he learned to cope with only later in his internship when working with leukemic children, a situation that became a matter of fast coping, with much support from his supervisor.

For the most part, the contact with outpatients was brief and supportive when they were there for physical complaints. It was with those who had psychological complaints that he had the most contact with and with whom, in fact, he ultimately spent the majority of his time at the family-practice clinic. Some of these patients continued to be seen for further psychotherapy during the remainder of Dr. Jospe's internship.

In view of Dr. Jospe's expectations that the time at the family-practice clinic would be devoted largely to the psychological aspects of physical illness, he was at first disappointed with doing so much non-medical-related clinical psychology. However, an important point must be made here, and that is that if psychology is viewed as a health science, then Dr. Jospe was really in the right place to be doing what he was doing. The way in which each intern was operating was not merely as an adjunct to people who might, by some standards, be viewed as the real professionals, that is, those administering to the physical needs of the patient. This was not the case in this setting because at all times the interns felt that they were accepted as colleagues involved in as comprehensive and integrated a health-care delivery system as possible. This is in marked contrast to many interns who are trained in other settings. In this respect, each intern was quite fortunate, for each later found himself or herself in positions where psychology, whether clinical or health care, was seen as a service to be provided for medical personnel primarily and patients secondarily.

Dr. Nieberding was the second psychology intern to rotate at the family-practice clinic. The major portion of his first month there was spent accompanying the residents in their contacts with outpatients and hospitalized patients. As was described earlier, this team approach to patient contact enabled each intern to utilize his or her skills as trained observers while also participating in the unfolding process of patients interacting with and communicating their needs to their physicians. Each intern was continually impressed by the ease with which patients could talk about significant issues in their lives other than the medical problems that "brought them in." It seemed so simple, natural, and appropriate for the resident to ask "And how are things going with you?" after first listening to the presenting medical complaints. Patients usually seemed quick to respond to the openness and responsiveness of the physician. Since many of the clinic experiences were similar for both interns, Dr. Nieberding will describe in greater detail four hospital experiences: two very different emergency room experiences, an anxious woman during the delivery of her child, and a surgery patient.

A number of weekends and evenings were spent in the emergency room with the family-practice residents. As was the case in other settings, the introduction of the intern to the patient was by name, without any accompanying label or explanation of background or profession. This enabled both the physician and the psychology intern to operate very smoothly as a team, permitting a shifting of responsibilities and role modeling depending on the medical and psychological needs of the patient. Early one Saturday afternoon, a 28-year-old woman presented to the emergency room with complaints of lower back and stomach pain. Since the medical examination and laboratory tests revealed no organic component, the possibility of an emotional basis for the pain was presented to the woman by her physician. In a very accepting tone of voice, the physician asked her how things were going with the rest of her life. She immediately responded with tears and quivering statements describing her difficulty as a recently separated woman who had full responsibility for a 5-year-old diabetic child. As an integral part of the treatment team attending to the needs of this woman, the transition from assessment and treatment of her medical needs to treatment of her emotional needs was easily facilitated. Owing to a backlog of patients waiting to see a physician, case responsibility was transferred to Dr. Nieberding. The physician had participated in the identification of the real source of the disturbance: the reality of her pain and the precipitating causes. The smooth transition in this case eliminated the frequent awkwardness encountered in making a referral to a mental-health professional; it also eliminated the problem frequently encountered in such referrals when so much time elapses between referral and consultation that the patient's defenses are again erected around the painful feelings and psychological intervention becomes more difficult, despite its necessity. In addition, the immediacy of the medical and psychological intervention reduced the likelihood that the patient would feel labeled as having the problem "all in her head." On other occasions when the family-practice residents did not have a backlog of patients waiting to be seen by a physician, they would proceed by addressing the underlying emotional determinants of the patient's physical complaints.

When Dr. Nieberding saw aforementioned patient alone, he assisted her in arriving at a deeper understanding of the ways in which she had dealt with stresses and feelings of inadequacy related to her life situation. Her defenses were sufficiently lowered to allow her to gain insight into her long-standing pattern of displacing her anxiety and pain onto her body. This openness coincided with both the accepting approach by the health-care team handling the case and the "opportunity" to integrate the information presented to her. She could see how she literally pushed back her own needs and would not "listen" to her body's attempt to make her more aware of the inadequacies and deficiencies in her life. When asked to make suggestions about what a woman in her present situation could do to help herself feel better while attempting to integrate her new realizations, she responded immediately with a sparkle in her eye that such a woman should treat herself to a special favor. She immediately asked if she could phone a close friend she "had been too busy to see" to arrange a luncheon date. The nursing and medical staff remarked about the discrepancy between the sad, pitiful woman who had entered the emergency room and the smiling, spirited woman who left. The importance of this emergency contact was that the patient was able to leave with an increased awareness of the way in which she somatized feelings of loss and isolation. She was able to make her visit a positive, insightful experience rather than one that was potentially demoralizing.

The preceding example described the role of a health-care psychologist working with a patient to integrate medical findings with the patient's own subjective experience of pain and anguish. The following is a situation involving an anxious, suicidal person, and it illustrates the role of the health psychologist in facilitating medical procedure. One Friday evening, an agitated, mildly disoriented, 22-year-old woman was brought into the emergency room by her sister and father. She stated that she had ingested 100 aspirin approximately 7 hours before coming to the emergency room, during which time she had vomited twice. Immediately, the emergency room staff mobilized to treat the life-threatening emergency at hand. The patient was quickly helped into a gown, while the other staff literally ran to call additional staff from other areas of the hospital and to bring the necessary equipment. Dr. Nieberding was a part of the health-care team because the physician he was accompanying had primary medical responsibility for the case. The staff, under the director of this physician, began converging on this woman to begin an IV, to pump her stomach, and to draw blood. She started to panic when she realized that a needle would be "poked into her," and she actively fought the staff's attempt to approach her. In view of the fact that her life was threatened, requiring prompt efficient action, her cooperation with the physicians and nurses was crucial. In a loud voice, Dr. Nieberding caught her attention and told her that he would be with her to explain all that was to happen before any medical procedure took place. He also told medical personnel that he would first have to understand what was to happen so he could communicate it to her in an attempt to reduce her anxiety. While the staff waited, he grasped her hand and firmly explained that her cooperation was most important. Although very frightened and skeptical, she stated she was ready to begin. Step by step, each medical procedure was explained from the cleansing of her arm with the cotton swab to the removal of the needle, all the while directing her to breathe slowly and evenly. As the medical procedures were efficiently being carried out, she was able to begin laughing at her fear of needles and doctors. After the medical personnel had left the immediate area following the completion of their life-saving procedures, she began to discuss how upset she had been earlier in the day, prompting the ingestion of the aspirin. She was able to ventilate the hurt and anger she felt when her recently separated lover called to say he was having an affair with another woman. She also began to reconstruct her pattern of similar impulsive, self-destructive behaviors following feelings of rejection. Since the laboratory tests indicated that the aspirin level in her bloodstream was of critical proportion, she was hospitalized overnight. Referral for therapy was made, and a home visit by a county social worker was arranged for the following Monday.

Reports of psychology interns who shared similar responsibilities as psychiatric residents in handling psychiatric consultation requests in an emergency room setting demonstrate the value of emergency room placements for psychologists (Barlow, 1974). Barlow (1974) reported that psychology interns broadened their clinical experience, sharpened their assessment skills, and were better able to formulate treatment plans under stress as a result of emergency room duty. Another advantage was the opportunity to apply intervention procedures while in an urgent situation which necessitated the close cooperation of nursing staff, psychiatric physicians, families, and community workers. The skillful functioning of psychology interns in the emergency room positively affected the perception of psychology's potential contribution to comprehensive health services by nonpsychiatric physicians (Barlow, 1974).

Another experience requiring the utilization of rapid assessment skills and intervention techniques to facilitate medical procedure involved a hysterical, frightened woman in the labor room. Upon Dr. Nieberding's request to observe the delivery of a child, an obstetrician invited him to meet a woman who was in labor. He was introduced as a psychologist who was learning about medical practice. The expected child was to be the second born of a 27-year-old married factory worker and his 26-year-old wife. While in labor for her first delivery, which lasted approximately 28 hours, she reportedly became hysterical and "lost her head." She reported that she had to be "slapped" by her obstetrician so she would not "flip out." Even though her husband was with her in the labor room, he was not able to provide her with much support. In fact, he contributed to her general sense of panic by making statements such as "Well, you could be having twins," or "I hope the doctor doesn't go home for dinner," just as she would begin her contractions. Even though the nursing staff had very carefully instructed the woman in the appropriate breathing techniques so she would not "bear down" during contractions, she became too anxiety ridden to follow their instructions. Upon reviewing her repeated inability to follow the breathing instructions given by the nursing staff, Dr. Nieberding intervened by attempting to direct her breathing. Throughout the contraction, he told her when to inhale and exhale, while continually reinforcing her attempts to restrain from exerting pressure on her abdominal muscles during contractions. Upon screaming that she could feel the baby coming, the nurse examined her to find that the baby's head had crowned. The staff then immediately rushed her into the delivery room. While in the delivery room, she was again instructed in rapid, panting-like breathing so that she would exert as little pressure as possible until the physician came. Even though she was panic-stricken and reacting in her characteristic hysteroid fashion, she did respond to very directive, reinforcing statements regarding her breathing.

Stemming from a desire to both observe a patient's coping mechanisms when faced with major surgery and watch a surgical team in action, Dr. Nieberding was invited to meet Bill, a 34-year-old married father of three children who was in the hospital for exploratory abdominal surgery to remove his spleen and several lymph glands. He had previously been diagnosed as having lymphosarcoma and had been unsuccessfully treated with chemotherapy for several months. The treating physician introduced Dr. Nieberding to Bill as a psychology intern who was interested in observing major surgery while striving to understand how individual's cope with the meaning and implications of such a surgery. The warmth and openness in Bill's approach to others became readily apparent as he expressed his eagerness to share his experience of the surgery. As a result of Bill's extensive reading on lymphosarcoma, combined with the lengthy question and answer sessions he had previously had with his physicians, he was able to give a very clear explanation of the cancerous process. Essentially, enlarged lymph glands in his neck and throat region had been discovered at a very early stage, which meant that there was an excellent prognosis for eliminating the disease process from his body. Following the "introductory overview" of his medical history, Bill reiterated his hope that meetings would serve as an opportunity for him to gain greater insight into himself and into the way he copes with stress. Bill invited open, honest feedback throughout each stage preceding and following surgery. About that time, his wife, Diane, entered the room. Following instructions, Diane pulled out a thermos of coffee and said, while offering a cup of coffee, "I hope you're not afraid of catching any germs." Each of us laughed aloud; her remark was important in setting the mood of the following several days.

Bill began to describe the surprising calm he had experienced during the week prior to entering the hospital and reported that he had only been unable to fall asleep for about 1 hour several nights previously. As we discussed Bill's style of interacting with others, and particularly his reluctance to "burden" his friends with his concerns and fears about his cancer, it became clear that Bill not only was seen as a leader in his large circle of friends, but also was protecting them from feelings that were of concern to him. Diane explained how over the past several years, she had tried very hard to help him both recognize and then verbalize the feelings that would churn inside him. She told of how it had been difficult for her to understand that the reason Bill could not express how he felt was that he was not even aware of the feelings he was having. Both had worked very hard over the preceding years to help each other not only to identify the feelings they were having, but also to begin to comfortably express those feelings to each other. A difficult feeling for each of them to express, but particularly for Bill, was anger. Bill explained the importance of feeling that he was in control of his emotions. This was also true of his way of relating to his feelings about the cancerous process inside him, in that he could easily talk about the feelings he had had previously concerning his cancer. However, he found it very difficult to share the feelings he was having at any given moment concerning his cancer. He viewed the meetings as one way of helping him begin to feel more in touch with the feelings he knew to be difficult to express.

Throughout the several days preceding the surgery, a considerable amount of time was spent with both Bill and Diane. Although Bill was quite open from the start, he became increasingly more able to verbalize his feelings. Moreover, during his presurgical period, he had received feedback from his physicians that the cancerous process had not entered the bone marrow, thereby improving the prognosis. He appeared more relaxed as the feedback from his physicians became more optimistic.

On the morning of his surgery he appeared relaxed and excited about my opportunity to observe his surgery. As a result of the opportunity to observe his surgery, coupled with conversations with the surgeon and anesthesiologist during the surgery, I made several important observations that helped me understand how Bill had internalized his stress. At several points during the course of the operation, the surgeon requested that the anesthesiologist administer more anesthesia because Bill's stomach muscles would occasionally spasm. The surgeon remarked that this could only occur for two possible reasons: (1) that the person was an extensive alcohol user, which was not the case with Bill, or (2) that the person had considerable anxieties that could only be expressed somatically.

When Bill had sufficiently recovered from surgery to feel capable of talking about the surgery, we discussed my experience of the surgery. I shared my amazement and sense of awe at the beauty and complexity of the internal organs of his body. Also, we discussed the surgeon's remarks that there was a strong probability that he was suppressing many of his feelings about the surgery. A sense of amazement came over him as he began to explore the feelings he had during the several days prior to the surgery that had been impossible for him to identify or verbalize. He remarked about a vague, inner, unsettled feeling he had noticed the week preceding the surgery that he had experienced as different from previous feelings of anxiety or tension. This unsettled feeling was in the pit of his stomach, which was ironically where his feelings were manifested behaviorally during the surgery.

The surgeons were able to reassure him that all the pathology reports were negative. Following a course of radiation over the succeeding months, the cancerous process was eradicated.

The opportunity to share the process of major surgery with a relatively well-adjusted individual provided a model of how a potentially life-threatening disease process can be integrated. It also pointed out the importance of using the information obtained from the anesthesiologist and surgeon to assist an individual in his or her attempt to integrate previously unexplainable and unreachable feelings that were manifested somatically.

Reflections on the Benefits of Physician-Psychologist Collaborative Work

As previously stated, the primary purpose of the family-medicine rotation was to train psychologists to skillfully consult with family-practice residents and other primary-care physicians regarding the psychological aspects of their patients' health and illness behaviors. To achieve this end, psychology interns were enmeshed into the daily routines of the family-practice residents. First in the role of an observer, the psychology intern accompanied the family-practice staff, preceptors, and residents throughout the hospital and during visits with patients in the outpatient clinic. As the intern became more familiar with the primary-care providers, in addition to the medical and psychological needs of the patients, the role of the intern gradually shifted from that of an observer to that of a consultant and collaborative team member.

The immediate presence of psychologists operating from a health-care perspective allowed a number of things to happen. First, the work with family-practice residents offered the opportunity for psychologists to provide input into the treatment-team discussions and strategies, in an atmosphere where the particular expertise of each team member was recognized for what it was rather than as a competitive threat to the autonomy of another member or professional group. The successful functioning of two different professional groups, physicians and psychologists, resulted in the gradual breakdown of professional stereotypes and rigid role expectations. Of greater benefit was the sensitive and comprehensive health care the patients received when the complementary expertise of family physicians and psychologists was mutually acknowledged and integrated into daily clinical practice.

Second, patients in distress were able to be seen immediately, or at least on the same day, in a clinic or hospital setting in which they were familiar. Particularly in the emergency room and outpatient medical clinics, where the resident and psychology intern often saw patients as a team, the patients seemed to respond with an increased willingness or ability to understand the psychological aspects of their physical complaints.

Third, the psychology interns gained experience in assessing a much more diverse patient population while in a family-medicine setting than is typically the case in more traditional mental health treatment settings. As the psychology intern developed increased medical knowledge through direct experience, consultation with senior medical staff, and attendance at internal medicine, pediatrics, surgery, and family-medicine conferences, as well as others, the intern developed a deeper appreciation of the biological factors involved in adaptation skills and coping mechanisms used in response to the threat of physical illness or disease. The interns gained direct experience as to the range and scope of special competencies that clinical psychologists can bring to hospitals, outpatient medical clinics, and other health-care facilities. Schofield (1979) elaborates in much greater detail regarding the assessment techniques, therapeutic intervention procedures, consultative services, and research contributions that health psychologists are making to improve the treatment and recovery of medical patients.

Fourth, the family-medicine residents increased their understanding of human behavior, particularly the emotional aspects of illness and health-seeking behavior. Residents developed a more realistic assessment of the potential benefits of consultation from a health-care perspective, combined with greater skills in referral. The physicians also saw how a psychologist could have an important therapeutic impact on a patient, thereby reducing the burden on the treating physician (Barlow, 1974; Ireton, Racer, and Hafner, 1978; Jospe, 1976; Lothstein, 1977; and chapter 3 of this text).

Occasionally, psychologists, social workers, and other allied health professionals are overheard complaining about difficulties experienced in establishing open channels of communication with primary-care physicians. What factors contributed in making the family-medicine rotation a viable, working model of mutual respect and collaboration? The single most important determinant was the fact that the senior staff of the family-medicine clinic conceptualized patient care from a multifaceted, multidisciplinary perspective. The usefulness of psychological consultation in treatment planning and health-care provision was preestablished by the presence of a senior psychological consultant functioning as a team member. Staff physicians and psychologists had been able to previously establish a working relationship built on cooperation across traditional professional role boundaries, thereby serving as a role model for residents and psychology interns.

However, the presence of working role models does not ensure the success of subordinates, trainees, or peers in adopting or successfully utilizing that model of collaboration. Previous literature underscores this point by stressing that successful collaboration depends on psychological or psychiatric consultants proving their usefulness to the medical team (Kaufman, 1953; Lipowski, 1967, 1974). The consultant must be available when needed, possessing a familiarity with medical procedures and able to communicate clear, pragmatic suggestions to the medical personnel. Kaufman (1953) underscores this point by stating that the role of the psychological consultant must be "of practical assistance in the total evaluation and furtherance of treatment of any given patient." The examples given in this chapter serve to illustrate a number of ways in which health psychologists can be "of practical assistance" in the provision of health care.

References

Barlow, D.H. Psychologists in the emergency room. *Professional Psychologist* 5: 251–256, 1974.

Ireton, H. Racer, H., and Hafner, A.J. A health care psychology internship rotation in family medicine. *Journal of Clinical Child Psychology* 61–62, 1978.

Jospe, M. Psychological internship experiences in a family practice setting. Paper presented at a symposium on Health Care Psychology and Family Practice Medicine: New Disciplines, New Relationships, Graduate Education of Psychologists and Medical Residents, 84th Annual Convention, American Psychological Association, Washington, 1976.

Kaufman, R.M. The role of the psychiatrist in a general hospital. *Psychiatric Quarterly* 27: 367–381, 1953.

Lipowski, Z.J. Review of consultation psychiatry and psychosomatic medicine. *Psychosomatic Medicine* 29: 201–224, 1967.

Lipowski, Z.J. Consultation-liaison psychiatry: An overview. *American Journal of Psychiatry* 131: 623–630, 1974.

Lothstein, L.M. Role of the clinical psychiatrist and psychologist in primary care medicine. *Primary Care* 4: 343–354, 1977.

Schofield, W. The role of psychology in the delivery of health services. *American Psychologist* 24: 565–584, 1969.

Schofield, W. Clinical psychologists as health professionals. In *Health Psychology – A Handbook,* ed. G.C. Stone, F. Cohen, and N.E. Adler. San Francisco: Jossey-Bass, 1979.

Wirt, R. Proposals for professional degree programs leading to the master of science and doctor of psychology in health care psychology. Unpublished proposal submitted by the faculty of the Division of Health Services Center, University of Minnesota, January 1974.

3

Psychological Medicine and Family Practice

Harley J. Racer

The Family-Practice Movement

The family physician, among all the practitioners of medicine, uniquely personifies and personalizes the confluence of biological, physiological, pathological, psychological, and behavioral approaches in the care of the patient.

With the explosion of medical specialization in the United States after World War II, the ranks of general practitioners were steadily diminished both by reduced entry and by steady attrition of established general practitioners until less than 20 percent of active physicians were in general practice by the opening of the 1960s. What had always been the hallmark of the healer in tribal societies—the accessibility to all comers, with all kinds of illnesses, injuries, or health-seeking concerns—had begun to show signs of becoming a rarity. Most of all, people who saw themselves as needing help from a person with the attributes and skills of a healer began to find their medical care increasingly fragmented as they sorted themselves into several special categories in order to be sure that the medical specialists who diagnosed and treated their illnesses would be soundly trained scientifically and especially skillful in each area of their need.

It became commonplace in the late 1950s for a young family with parents nearing 30 and two children below the teens to be employing the services of an obstetrician, a pediatrician, and perhaps an internist (who did annual "executive physicals" for the father). From time to time, such a family would need the services of an orthopedist, a surgeon, a psychiatrist, or another medical specialist. Sometimes they were able to obtain such care from other members of medical group practices that were beginning to proliferate. However, there was often a yearning for some one physician who would be like their old family doctor and would care for them for most of their medical needs, but who would, most of all, *know* them and be *known* by them (Stephens, 1975) and, because of that broad, lasting, and growing relationship, would care about them as he or she would give them care or would guide them to other doctors for those special medical needs.

General practitioners felt their own dissatisfactions with their role among many medical specialists in that era of fragmented care. They themselves did not yet fully understand that they were the *people specialists* among their certified specialist colleagues. They often settled for a kind of medical drudgery of gnawing away like an earthworm at an insurmountable mountain of episodes of illness and injury, only by accident accumulating a sequential story of an individual and of that person's family. Such general practitioners frequently lived a short and burdened life, dying out in their forties and fifties with the feeling that they had been overworked and underpaid—or leaving general practice for a specialty with more defined limits and greater rewards for what seemed to be a higher echelon: more respect, prestige, and dollars. However, some of the old workhorse general practitioners in the sentimental pictures of the country doctor on calendars (and his city counterparts) began to lift their heads up from the endless episodes of service and develop a new perspective. So it was that family practice was reborn.

Leo Levin (1970), in an address to those who became members of the newly recognized specialty of family practice, paraphrased Albert Einstein in trying to understand what was happening in the development of this new discipline:

> The development of new theory is not like tearing down the old buildings on a farm and putting up new buildings, so much as it is like climbing up a hill on the farm and suddenly seeing the lay of the land and its surroundings in an entirely new way. . . .

So it was that without abandoning their commitment to be, first of all, good *physicians,* with sound and ample medical knowledge and skills with which to meet all kinds of patients with all kinds of needs competently and safely, these general practitioners developed a new awareness of the relationships that give their medical work for people the rewards of meaning and the dignity of comprehension—of understanding between the patient and the physician.

The new emphasis for the family physician began to reveal that the episodes of care were really events in the continuing saga of biochemical, psychological, and social life of the patient in his or her family and in the community, and that only when those events are understood together is the patient revealed as a person and his or her needs met sensibly and sensitively by the family doctor (Lipowski, 1969; Curry, 1975).

Where general practice had depended on the accidental accumulation of one episode after another, significance could often only be found in retrospect. Family practice, however, intends to offer, from the beginning, a relationship embedded in the whole context of the patient's life: physiological, intrapersonal, and interpersonal.

General practice typically perceived the patient as a victim of illness or injury that had already become a crisis brought to the family doctor for reversal of disaster, with the implication that the patient would be healed by the superior power of the physician. An underlying notion of family practice is that both the patient and the physician assume responsibility for active participation in discovering the earliest antecedents of disorder, whether in tissue cells, the style of the individual's life, the dynamics of his or her family, or the larger environment of the community.

A New Approach to Patient Care: The Family Physician

Family practice as a specialty was at first considered a compilation of the basic information necessary to all the other specialties, with the family physician dipping into each or many of the other specialties as a jack of all trades, master of none—a specialist in ambiguity. It was felt that family physicians would need training in all the other 19 earlier-certified specialties, and that in some cumulative way, or because of the centering of access to the other specialties, family physicians would be special largely by virtue of the *breadth* of their abilities (Core Content, 1966).

Certainly, the family doctor must continue the tradition of accessibility that was part of the problem in that era of fragmented care. Dr. John Millis, reporting for the Citizens' Commission on Graduate Education of the American Medical Association (Millis, 1966), identified the need for development of a "new kind of physician, namely, the primary physician." This would be a physician who would correct the fault of medical care that had become most obvious: its lack of "continuity and comprehensiveness." These ideas have been the cornerstone and the words have become the banner of family-practice physicians.

The primary physician is not only the physician of first contact, but the doctor who will assume primary responsibility for the patient "in sickness and in health, in simple disease and in complex disease." The idea of primary physician, therefore, obviously includes the element of accessibility as a first-contact physician, but also must convey the commitment of the doctor to *continue* in the care of the patient and to *comprehend* with the patient what his or her needs are. Recent introduction of the term *primary-care physician* has much more to do with the nature of the care given, the limits of the care given, or the place the care is given than it has to do with the description of the relationship between the family doctor and the patient.

If the family doctor's relationship with the patient is to have continuity and comprehensiveness, then the training and function of a family doctor as a physician must provide for those elements. In addition to the breadth of family practice, and in order to provide for continuity and comprehensiveness in approaching patient care, the family doctor has taken on responsibility for learning and doing in areas that are indeed special to family physicians among all the other specialties.

The inclusion of knowledge and skills in basic communication techniques is changing the catch-as-catch-can style of the old general practitioner into a more accessible, more accurate, more open, more self-aware approach by the new family physician.

Responsibility for understanding the logical bases of the scientific method is now required in many family-practice graduate curricula. Fundamentals of the management of one's practice, with emphasis on the balance between personal and professional goals and commitments, are now taught as basic to family practice (rather than being left to chance).

Strong programs of learning in psychology of the individual and of the family have been developed, and new family physicians are as responsible to discern the emotional situations of their patients and their families as they are to diagnose and treat organic disorders (Conroe, 1978; Ireton, 1976). Family practice now draws both for learning and for practice on research in individual psychology, family structure and dynamics, family development, family function, community medicine, and medical sociology.

The impact of the community, not only its physical environment, but also its institutions (political, educational, religious, and social) and the impingement of social mores and sanctions on the lives of the patient and the physician—all these have become grist for the mill of the family doctor.

New Approaches to Education for Family Practice

If family practice is indeed a specialty, it must be able to identify the body of special knowledge that can be taught, learned, and used by its practitioners. Education for family practice developed rapidly since 1970, with more than 300 graduate residency programs approved and 5,500 family-practice residents in graduate training in 1978. Old and young general practitioners who are themselves in the process of becoming family physicians of the new breed have formed the nuclei of faculties for teaching the new discipline. Nearly 20,000 physicians, from both the ranks of general practice and the new graduates of family-practice residencies, were examined and certified as specialists in family practice by the American Board of Family Practice by the end of 1978. Large numbers of undergraduate students now elect tracking in family practice, and nearly all of them now seek graduate training in family-practice residencies.

Psychological medicine has been one of the foundation stones for the development of family-practice education for these large numbers. At first there was a period of awkward struggle to balance and "integrate" traditional medical curriculum, which is largely organic and disease-oriented, with the new elements, which are largely behavioral.

Behavioral scientists were added to young faculties to teach both the new physician teachers (general practitioners in metamorphosis) and the new family-practice residents about psychology, the family, and sociology. Seminars in the behavioral areas were developed and were often received reluctantly by young family-practice residents who perceived them as add-on appendages designed to distract from the eager pursuit of applying their already-learned organic medicine to clinical problem solving.

The behavioral scientists (psychologists, psychiatrists, social workers, counselors, and sociologists) were then brought into the clinic centers as preceptors offering supervision to family-practice residents in the process of clinical problem solving in patient care. Now, on site in the very center of the family-practice resident's clinical learning, they could alert and awaken the resident to psychological and behavioral issues that had been overlooked in the eagerness to solve the fascinating "medical" aspects of the patient's problem array. This was a salutary move, increasing the learning of psychological medicine by the family-practice resident by increasing the effectiveness of the timing and immediacy of the behavioral-science clinician at the point of need (Ireton, 1976).

Gradually the expectations of behavioral-science teachers, family-practice teachers who were learning along with their residents, and the family-practice residents themselves began to become aligned. Where there had at first been great confusion—were family doctors now to be trained as minipsychiatrists, junior psychologists or quasi-social workers?—now there began to grow an understanding of how family doctors would express their new awareness of psychological medicine in practice. It became clearer that family doctors need not be trained to "do" psychotherapy in depth any more than they would need the consummate skills of the referral surgeon or any other consultant, but they must be competent to recognize the psychological causes and effects at work in their patients and be able to offer in their own capacity some of the intervention needed by the patients.

If the patient's needs are relatively acute, and if the family doctor's sensitivity and skill make early intervention possible, then brief psychotherapy soundly offered by the family physician may suffice (Conroe, 1978). Moreover, the family physician must be able to recognize more serious, deeper-rooted disorders that will require more expertise and will need to be knowledgeable about those resources and how they can be mobilized to serve the patient's needs. Such a collaboration with other specialists in behavioral areas is exactly like the teaming-up family doctors do with specialist consultants giving service in organic disease for which skills are needed that exceed the personal abilities of the family doctors. This ad hoc formation of a team uniquely assembled to assist the individual patient will always be one of the really special skills of family doctors and, rather than returning the patient to fragmented care, serves as the integrative process that weaves continuity throughout the care of the patient by each person. The role and the function of each member of such a team is continually monitored and interpreted to the patient by the family physician (Stephens, 1975).

New Designs for Family-Practice Education

Most educational designs for the teaching of family practice have been built around the family physician as the primary teacher, just as many of the events in patient care in family practice are correlated and integrated by the function of the family doctor. Heavy reliance on modeling by the family physician, commitment to the development of rapport between family-practice residents and their primary family-practice teachers, and adoption by the family-physician teacher of those principles of psychological and behavioral medicine that are fundamental to the specialness of the new specialty—these characteristics are common in the developing of educational programs across the nation.

The family doctor as a teacher must present first and always as a competent, well-informed medical scientist who will not overlook any of the important biological and organic elements in patient care and teaching. Just as important for the development of the new kind of family physician, however, is that the family doctor doing the modeling demonstrates awareness and competence in dealing with the psychological and behavioral issues in the patient's situation. As in practice, so also in teaching, the modeling must show the natural confluence of behavioral and organic approaches in comprehending the patient's need for care.

The family doctor as a teacher must demonstrate the need for continual self-directed learning, both in updating his or her clinical skills in biological medicine and in acquiring new insights and horizons in approaching patients and their families (Stephens, 1978). Increasing experience in family-practice faculties has underlined the need for continuing concomitant practice by the family-practice teacher as well as patient contact while serving as a preceptor to residents.

This kind of experiential address to the needs of the teacher as well as the student has served to enhance the rapport state between them; the joint venture of learning together (at different levels and perhaps emphasizing different content) has nevertheless increased the bond of a common need. It becomes ever more apparent that the kind of learning needed for the family doctor's best eventual function surpasses specific content to achieve a resilient flexibility that McWhinney (1975) characterizes as a "method of thinking and feeling" quite necessary to the adaptation of a physician who seeks unselected patients with unselected conditions and attempts to develop management that in itself determines the therapeutic relationship over long periods of time (Stephens, 1975).

The next important change in family-practice education has been the reformation of the selection process for family-practice residents. Where academic durability, research genius, or sheer intellectual superiority had been the desirable hallmarks of those residents selected for many of the choice programs in the older specialties, family-practice residencies have more and more sought and attracted medical school graduates who have preserved their humanism, who continue to care most about other persons and about caring for them, and who can find their rewards in relationships more than in performance. As family-practice residencies have developed some maturity and have become more attractive, large numbers of applicants make this kind of selection possible from among highly competent, academically strong medical students.

With the most important activity of the family-practice residency taking place in the family-practice clinic, the development of clinic staffs responsive to highly flexible, innovative, and yet managerially sound policies for patient care supports the holistic learning of the resident. More and more of the model careers identify significant contributions by the clinic staff, from the receptionist, through nursing and bookkeeper, to the clinic manager and laboratory technicians, as critical in the learning of practical knowledge and skills needed by the family doctor.

Some residency programs added a social worker to their clinic staffs, more at first because of the socioeconomic factors important in certain patient groups commonly served. Some clinic staffs included clinical psychologists or other trained counselors to provide service and direct teaching in psychological medicine for the family-practice residents.

Many family-practice residency model clinics have served as learning stations for other members of the health-care team (for example, medical and nursing students; nurse practitioners; clinical psychology interns; physicians' assistants; pharmacy, laboratory, and x-ray technicians; and patient educators) to the end that the model clinic has become hospitable to different kinds of learners with different needs.

One of the most successful experiences with shared learning in the context of conjoint care of patients in the family-practice clinic has been the opportunity for psychology graduate students in a health psychology internship training program to have some of their experience within the family-practice clinic that serves family-practice residents as their model center for learning patient care (Ireton, 1976; and chapter 2 of this book).

A New Collaboration: Psychology Interns and Family-Practice Residents

One of the practical methods to emphasize unity of psychological and biological issues in patient care has been to design collaborative learning, with the health-psychology intern and the family-practice resident brought together in the care of the patient under the supervision of the family-physician preceptor. Both psychology interns and family-practice residents are offered an opportunity to give and take, to become associates, to learn each other's strengths and limitations, and to learn how to work together in the patient's interest (Schofield, 1975).

The health-care psychology intern works daily in the family-practice clinic alongside the family-practice resident. The psychology intern attends hospital rounds, emergency room visits, labor and delivery, and even surgical operations undergone by patients from the clinic practice. From these experiences and from patients, residents, and staff, the psychology intern gets a frame of reference for the goals and possibilities as well as the limitations of medical care. He or she gets medical information, clarification of the "secrets" of scientific medicine, and a picture of the constraints that define the role of the family doctor.

The family-practice resident, however, gets from the psychology intern an alerting about psychological factors that are causes or effects of medical or surgical illnesses. The family-practice resident gets an opportunity to understand the use of psychometrics, psychological diagnostic techniques, the development of therapeutic plans for psychological intervention, and an appreciation of other resources, what they can offer the patient, and how they can be used. Most of all, the family physician, during his or her formative training time, gets an opportunity to experience the benefit for the patient of having a psychological resource person immediately available within the clinic.

The health-psychology intern and the family-practice resident learn to work together, sometimes as cotherapists, or with the psychology intern serving as consultant to the family-practice resident, or with the psychology intern undertaking brief psychotherapy or assisting with the bridging of a referral to another resource for ongoing therapy as indicated.

In the delivery of service to patients and in their interchange with each other, both psychology intern and family-practice resident are supervised by the family-practice preceptor and by the clinical-psychology preceptor, both of whom remain available to both the psychology intern and family-practice resident and to their patients as well. Each preceptor maintains a regular schedule of review with both family-practice residents and psychology interns.

This collaboration raises the learning activity for supervising preceptors as well, with the family-physician teacher especially capitalizing on the repeated demonstration of skills in psychological diagnosis and treatment by the clinical psychologist. In addition, the clinical-psychology supervisor has developed more insight into the medical perspectives of the family physicians and has been able to focus his or her teaching more directly on the needs of the family physician. It has become more clear that the answers to some of the earlier questions can be perceived from examining this combined learning of psychological medicine and family practice:

Family doctors need to be aware of psychological issues both as causes and as effects of patients' problems.

Family doctors need to be skillful in collecting psychological and behavioral data from their patients in order to make comprehensive approaches to problem identification and solution.

Family doctors need to be able to organize and to interpret data of psychological nature (individual, family, and community) in assessing the patient's need for psychological interventions.

Family doctors need to be able to recognize and deal effectively with acute psychological crises in their patients, to assist the patient in recognizing significant psychological needs, and to help the patient establish appropriate psychological interventions.

The presence of the health-psychology intern within the daily life of the family-practice clinic has repeatedly demonstrated ways in which the family physician's increased awareness and responsibility for an integrated approach to holistic patient care can be enhanced by the direct involvement of the clinical psychologist in the family-practice clinic.

Case Studies: Family-Practice Resident and Psychology Intern Collaborating in Patient Care

Patient Disrupts Nursing Home

A.B., age 80, had been an extremely powerful and domineering husband and father until his wife's death 10 years ago. He had been a successful farmer and heavy-equipment dealer until retirement 5 years ago. He became a resident in the nursing home after his second stroke 4 years ago left him with some residual paresis and some organic brain dysfunction.

Although he had been a model patient, even a pet of the nursing staff at first, he had for the past 6 months evidenced increasingly disruptive behavior, for example, salt dispensers in toilets, tableware secreted in storage cupboards, doors taken off their hinges. When confronted by nurses, he became irritable, combative, and his behavior seemed increasingly inappropriate.

The family-practice resident examined him carefully and ascertained that there had been no demonstrable change in his medical condition. Attempts to improve his adjustment by the use of minor and major tranquilizers or sedatives resulted in unacceptable side effects (for example, respiratory depression, extrapyramidal dysfunction, and falls owing to postural hypotension).

The psychology intern established rapport with the patient in the process of a thorough psychometric evaluation. The patient demonstrated increased performance and memory deficit in comparison with earlier measurements. He was able over several hours of interview to admit that much of his behavior was an intentional revolt against administrative rules that he felt were silly or unnecessary.

The family-practice resident and psychology intern were able to help the patient negotiate with the nursing home administrator, nursing staff, and family to establish ways to clarify rules and to remind him of their purpose when his memory did not serve him well.

Nursing staff and administration adjusted their expectations, requests for chemical management of his misbehavior directed to the family-practice resident ceased, and the patient's remaining months of life in the nursing home were significantly improved in quality.

Obese Woman Needs Gallbladder Surgery

C.D., a 59-year-old grade school teacher, had ballooned to 200 pounds when she began to have painful gallbladder colic at several-week intervals. She was mildy hypertensive and moderately depressed.

The family-practice resident, in consultation with the surgeon and the patient, agreed that weight reduction would be highly desirable in reducing surgical risk and morbidity.

Many programs and plans for weight reduction had been tried over the years with negative results (increased weight). The family-practice resident saw the patient regularly over the next 4 months in an attempt to assist her with a successful approach to weight reduction since colic attacks were increasing in frequency and intensity. She became more depressed and her weight reached 286 pounds.

The psychology intern befriended her during one of her hospitalizations. He established contract with her for assessment of her depression and a strongly structured program of behavior modification that included exercises in self-esteem and socialization as well as physical conditioning and calorie restriction. He and the family-practice resident agreed on an alternate-visit plan that enabled psychological approaches to ventilation and development of insight with respect to her depression and the use of stringent calorie restriction monitored by demonstrated ketosis and close tracking for azotemia, hyperuricemia, hypovolemia, and hypokalemia.

Over the next 4 months she gave up 91 pounds and her gallbladder with no significant complications.

Mentally Retarded Couple Complains of Sexual Dysfunction

E.F., age 38, and G.F., age 28, had begun to show more security in their function as first-time parents as their baby daughter H. passed her first birthday and evidences of "failure to thrive" began to decrease, although some developmental landmarks for the girl were still 2 to 4 months delayed. It was at this time that the couple appeared with a shy but urgent request for help with E.F.'s loss of libido. When the couple resumed sexual activity 2 months after the birth of the baby, he developed a pattern of premature ejaculation that persisted for 2 to 3 months, after which he was unable to maintain a sufficient erection for vaginal penetration.

The family-practice resident conducted brief medical evaluations of both husband and wife. They were both in excellent health except for the 40 pounds of excess weight G.F. had retained over the year since her pregnancy. History revealed that E.F. was indeed having spontaneous nocturnal erections, but that he had been unable to maintain erection for intercourse for about 6 months.

The psychology intern undertook sexual counseling with this challenging couple, whose total I.Q. is estimated to approach 170. After 3 hours, with little more accomplished than the nearest approach possible to an adequate data base for sexual counseling, rudimentary suggestions for verbal and noncoital pleasuring were made, with the result that the couple canceled subsequent sessions because sexual satisfaction had begun to flourish.

During the sexual history-taking sessions with the psychology intern, however, some elements of sadistic violent behavior in their relationship were noticed, and when the family-practice resident was given a tangential cue by the mother during a subsequent well-baby visit (denial, unsolicited: she and her husband were not beating the baby with a belt as a neighbor had alleged), he was able to respond and mobilize social work intervention in the home promptly. The psychology intern's contribution had a secondary payoff 6 months after he had completed his rotation.

Dependency Needs Presented as Renal Colic

I.G., age 40, was first seen in the emergency room by the family-practice resident with a classical picture compatible with real colic. He gave a history of having passed at least 10 kidney stones, some from each kidney, over the past 4 years. He was seeking a new physician in his pain crisis because he felt his previous physician had missed the last stone, which he was convinced was still lodged in his right ureter, even though a stone had been retrieved by cystoscopic manipulation from the left ureter. He expressed an almost intolerable anger toward doctors, against his employer, and against members of his family, with whom he was locked in a 2-year-long legal battle over his mother's estate. He was hypertensive. He volunteered concern that he had been abusing alcohol and depending on analgesics to control his pain in order to be able to fight off just about everyone in his world, lately including his long-suffering wife.

Thorough evaluation of his urinary tract and metabolic status by the family-practice resident indicated no renal disease and confirmed essential hypertension. When the intensity, range, and chronicity of his anger was reflected to him, along with the idea that his pain might be a somatic expression of distress, his reaction was explosive, and his scorn for "shrinks" and the implication of humiliating need by patients who use them was clearly and forcefully expressed. When he understood that the psychology intern was present in the clinic as an integral member of the team, however, he very grudgingly consented to accept some inital evaluation—even though he had another level of difficulty when he discovered that the intern was a woman as well as a psychologist.

After initial interviews that included some psychometrics (MMPI and the Holmes Stress Scale) and the interpretation of the test results, the patient almost eagerly contracted for and participated in 6 hours of therapy with the psychology intern. Concomitantly, he had one or two visits with the family-practice resident for supervision of antihypertensive therapy and strictly structured, tapering use of analgesic medication (codeine, 30 mg, and acetaminophen). The visits were directed chiefly at helping him to identify his anger, to accept it, and to choose more constructive ways of dealing with defeat and frustration than with alcohol, analgesics, or by crying "pain." His wife attended the interviews with the psychology intern and the appointments with the family-practice resident when requested by any of the parties.

He is currently using no analgesic medication, complaining of no pain, using alcohol only socially (confirmed by his wife), and looking back on his disrupted relationship with his relatives and his employer as having been in great part his own responsibility.

The Health Psychologist and the Family Physician Working Together

The experience of collaborative teaching and learning in the midst of a family-practice clinic has demonstrated a model for practical use in future practice. More than the kind of internal organization referral *from* medical clinicians *to* psychologists in large medical group practices or within the provider panels of prepaid health plans, this experience depends on close personal involvement of the psychologist and the physician, constant interweaving of actions, clear and close alignment of therapeutic goals and plans, and a truly collegial rather than delegatory or referral relationship between two professionals working collaboratively. Friendship, trust, respect, and rapport between persons working together on behalf of another is a better description of the kind of transaction that can produce this sort of benefit for people seeking help either in distress or in the search of an even higher level of well-being.

It remains for both family physicians and psychologists who are interested in such collaboration to move ahead and to explore the pratical working-out of the problems, such as cost, communication, integration of efforts, and more equable compensation than the wide disparity that currently holds.

References

Conroe, R.M., Cassata, D.M., and Racer, H.J., A systematic approach to brief psychological intervention in the primary care setting. *Journal of Family Practice* 7: 1137–1142, 1978.

Core content of family medicine: A report on requirements for certification. *General Practitioner* 34: 225–246, 1966.

Curry, H. Family practice, its nature and scope. Unpublished paper presented at the Methodist Hospital Symposium: The Physician Teacher and Family Practice, St. Louis Park, Minnesota, June 1975.

Ireton, H.R. Health care psychology and family practice. Unpublished paper presented in the Advanced Workshop Series at the American Psychological Association Convention, Washington, September 4, 1976.

Ireton, H.R., and Cassata, D.M. A psychological systems review. *Journal of Family Practice* 3: 155–159, 1976.

Levin, L. American Academy of Family Practice Annual Address. Unpublished paper presented at the American Medical Association Scientific Assembly, Chicago, Illinois, June 1970.

Lipowski, Z.J. Psychosocial aspects of disease. *Annals of Internal Medicine* 71: 1197–1206, 1969.

McWhinney, I.R. Family medicine in perspective. *New England Journal of Medicine* 293: 176–181, 1975.

Millis, J. *Report of the Citizens' Commission on Graduate Medical Education.* Chicago, Ill.: American Medical Association, 1966.

Schofield, W. The psychologist as a health care professional. *Intellect* 103: 255–258, 1975.

Stephens, G.G. The intellectual basis of family practice. *Journal of Family Practice* 2: 423–428, 1975.

Stephens, G.G. The integration of family practice into today's medical education. *Rural Health Communications* 3: 2–9, 1978.

4 The Role of Psychology in Baccalaureate Nursing Education

Roberta Ann Smith
and *Kenneth A. Wallston*

Introduction

The purpose of this chapter is twofold: (1) to assert that psychology has, perhaps uniquely, integrated theory and the research process to provide clinically applicable knowledge, a goal nursing has held for many years; and (2) to illustrate more specifically some of the clinically applicable knowledge that psychology offers.

Most people who have had minimal contact with nurses (or who only know about nurses through brief encounters in doctor's offices, hospital corridors, or as portrayed by the popular media) cannot begin to fathom the amount of knowledge nurses need in order to carry out their complex roles in today's health-care delivery system. Whether one conceives of nursing as a science unique unto itself or as an applied science drawing the knowledge base of practically every scientific discipline known, one is impressed by the breadth of information needed by the nurse to care for his or her patients and assist them in achieving their optimum state of healthfulness. In carrying out the steps of the nursing process—assessing the state and needs of the patient, planning for and implementing nursing care, and evaluating the effectiveness of the care plan—the nurse gathers a wide variety of data and makes use of a vast array of theoretical principles from the biological, behavioral, and social sciences. Psychology, of course, is only one of the many disciplines with which the nurse must be conversant; yet it is our contention that psychology plays, or ought to play, a unique role in the education of student nurses.

Specifically, our thesis is that in addition to the specific applicable data from psychology, the field of psychology is one of the more advanced branches of the social sciences in both developing and synthesizing theory and research, which is aimed at both testing theory and generating new theories.

What are some of the nursing tasks for which a knowledge of psychological theories and research is especially helpful? The following list is meant to be suggestive rather than all-inclusive:

1. To assess patients' perceptions, feelings, motivations, capabilities, deficits, and interpersonal relationships.
2. To help patients cope with the stress brought on by acute, chronic, and terminal illnesses.
3. To help patients adjust to new situational demands and enforced alterations in lifestyles.
4. To motivate patients to engage in health-promoting activities and to encourage patients to assume responsibility for their own health.
5. To lead groups of other health-care providers.
6. To recognize how nurse's attitudes, values, and feelings influence their reactions to patients and to overcome any possible negative influences their behavior may have on the patient's well-being.
7. To plan appropriate nursing interventions based on a consistent, logical conceptual framework that takes into account individual differences among patients and situations.
8. To gather data systematically to evaluate the effectiveness of a nurse's interventions and to communicate the results of these evaluations in order to contribute to the knowledge base of the nursing profession.

Nursing is in the forefront of the health-care professions in adopting a holistic approach toward understanding and dealing with individuals as part of larger, interacting social systems. Often called a biopsychosocial orientation, this holistic approach involves a conceptualization and treatment of "the total person." In order to actualize this approach, nurses cannot (and do not) attend only to the individual's "body," but also must attend to the individual's "mind" and, most especially, to the interaction of the mind and body in the context of the individual's ecological environment.

The field of psychology, however, is also by and large antidualistic, although there are some specialty areas within psychology that are more narrowly focused. The goal of psychology as a scientific discipline is to understand the determinants and consequences of human behavior. Being a relatively new scientific discipline, psychology is far from having reached that goal. Each new "discovery" appears to raise more questions than it answers; yet, if psychologists have learned one thing from all their efforts, it is that the ultimate answers are far more complex than originally conceived. Human behavior is variously determined, that is, influenced by genetic, biological, cognitive, social, cultural, and environmental factors singly and in combination.

These factors can be understood as interrelating in a transactional model. Such a model

1. Rejects the usual designations of stimulus and response, since they are often not distinguishable from each other and are instead mutual parts of a circular process.

2. Views causality as multidirectional and multidetermined.
3. Focuses on interrelationships of factors, rather than on static characteristics of variables.
4. Recognizes that factors mutually affect each other over time so that a system is in a continual state of change.
5. Acknowledges that any interventions or persons intervening are part of a transactional process.

Thus both nursing and psychology, in trying to understand human behavior, must take into account a wide variety of data existing within a very complex system.

The similarities between nursing and psychology do not end merely with trying to understand human behavior. Many psychologists are health-care practitioners (as are practically all nurses) and, in this role, share identical goals with nurses and other health-care providers. Admittedly, psychologists as practitioners are primarily concerned with individuals' mental health; yet, as every psychologist is fully aware, a person's mental and physical health are closely interrelated. Since psychologists are unique among behavioral and social scientists in terms of being health-care providers, this also serves to underscore the importance of psychology to nursing education.

Historically, psychiatric nursing and clinical psychology were the two specialty areas in their respective professions that were viewed as having the most in common. In traditional nursing education, content from the field of psychology was reserved for presentation to nursing students during a course labeled "psychiatric nursing" (as opposed to "medical," "surgical," "maternal," "pediatric," or "public health" nursing). During such a course, students had experiences taking care of patients who had psychiatric diagnoses (for example, schizophrenia) and who were located in psychiatric institutions (such as state hospitals) or on psychiatric wards of general hospitals.

When students referred to such a course as "psych" nursing, they meant "psychiatric" not "psychological." Thankfully, the influence of this old medical model is now greatly diminished, and most nurse educators no longer design curricula based on the patient's medical diagnosis or location. "Psychiatric nursing" has now become "psychiatric/mental-health nursing," and in many schools of nursing, content from psychology is now integrated throughout the curriculum. There is still, however, a tendency to emphasize content from clinical psychology and psychiatry as being most central to the informational needs of nursing students.

Nursing, although a service profession, can benefit from wider knowledge of both the basic science and applied components of psychology, especially if one accepts a transactional model within which to view behavior. Examples from areas of psychology will be used here that (1) illustrate the synthesis of theory and research, (2) are applicable to nursing practice, and (3) are essential components in analyzing data within a transactional model. The four example areas are developmental psychology, psychology of personality, social psychology, and theories of maladaptation or psychopathology. In less detail, we will discuss some areas in which psychologists have contributed to specific modes of intervention with people in situations common to nursing practice.

The remainder of this chapter focuses on these selected areas from psychology. Since space is limited, we offer them as illustrative examples rather than as an exhaustive compendium of relevant areas in psychology. In the final section of the chapter, we will offer our thoughts as to the placement of psychological content in the total nursing curriculum, how and by whom psychological content should be taught, and the interrelatedness of psychological content with content from other disciplines.

Developmental Psychology

In order to understand complex behavior transactionally, one needs to know the issues important in the processes of development. Knowledge of growth and development is no longer only a yardstick to determine a child's physical, motor, and verbal development. Developmental psychology has provided an understanding of the development of cognition (for example, Piaget's work), morality (for example, Kohlberg and Piaget), and object relations (for example, Freud and the neo-Freudians), especially from birth through adolescence. Eriksen's concept of epigenesis has sensitized us to the fact that all persons deal with various developmental tasks that have preeminence at certain times, but which are of lasting and repeated importance at various stages of life.

Because of Schaie's (1965) developmental model, we now recognize that differences between persons of different ages may result not only from differences in developmental stages, but also from the differences in being 65 in 1979 as opposed to being 35 in 1975 (a time of assessment variable) or from the difference resulting from being in different cohorts (that is, being a toddler during the Vietnam war as opposed to being a young adult during that era).

In the last several years, along with continued research on the developmental processes of children, the field has provided a new and timely focus on adults in the middle and later years of life. It has become life-span developmental psychology. Growing research in gerontology has revealed that as age increases, the degree of variability within a given age group increases (Seigler, 1977). Thus our stereotypes of middle-aged or elderly person must be questioned. For instance, it is no longer valid to equate old age and chronic brain syndrome. Although this serious disease most often strikes the elderly (just as chicken pox is found mainly among the young), most older persons do not suffer from chronic brain syndrome. When they do, it is not just because they are old.

There are, however, changes in functioning that accompany aging. Changes in the elasticity of the lens of the eye affect vision, often by age 40. Perception of high-frequency pitches decreases with age. Although changes in intellectual functioning occur, the changes are complex. Previous work showing that I.Q. declined as aging progressed (Weschler, 1944, 1958) is now being questioned. Seigler (1977) suggests that changes in intellectual functioning among the aged may be related to years of formal education (a cohort variable), terminal drop, (a phenomenon of I.Q. dropping within a few years of death), and health status rather than to "normal aging."

In relation to intelligence and many other performance variables, research can be designed to maximize or minimize differences between the young and old. From the perspective of life-span development psychology, one can begin to conceptualize functioning as related to *competence* (that is, are the needed structures or components available for functioning?) or *performance* (that is, are the capacities that exist being utilized?). Nurses who daily are assisting persons to optimize their well-being need to understand these concepts and need also to ask how much capacity is truly needed to maintain function. Developmental psychology provides an excellent body of methodology and content to deal with issues of competence, performance, and essential capacity.

Psychology of Personality

Personality theories, some of which emerge from developmental theories (for example, psychoanalytic theory) provide a body of knowledge from which nurses can understand the patterns of behavior that make each person an individual. *Personality* may be defined as those traits of a person that can be observed in a variety of situations and which define the uniqueness of the person. A classic text by Hall and Lindzey (1970) states that "a theory of personality should consist of a set of assumptions and definitions to permit their interaction with empirical or observable events." As a transactional model indicates, no one approach provides sufficient data for a complete understanding of the complexity of human behavior. Therefore, while developmental psychology provides us with understanding of how we all develop to be more or less similar human creatures, personality theories help us to comprehend the factors that make us unique beings and can provide a more general conceptualization of human behavior.

An example of one personality theory is learning theory. This is also a larger and more highly refined specialty within psychology. The basic tenet of the theory is that behavior is learned. Behavior can be elicited, maintained, increased, shaped, or extinguished by means of giving or withholding reinforcement or rewards. Personality is consequently understood as the aggregate of all learned behaviors. The theory and related research indicate that some learning is more resistant to change than others, but behavior is changed by a learning, relearning, or unlearning process.

Classicial conditioning and operant conditioning are two important processes by which learning occurs. Knowing these processes as well as other principles by which individuals learn enduring behavior patterns can be very useful in nursing practice. Often nurses, both knowingly and unknowingly, utilize these principles. For example, the nurse in the labor and delivery area, working with a Lamaze-trained woman, employs the effects of classical conditioning when he or she coaches the woman. The nurse trying to enable a mother to instill healthful eating habits in her children may utilize knowledge of operant conditioning to establish a behavior-modification program. The more sophisticated the nurse's knowledge of this and other personality theories, the more likely that he or she will plan an effective strategy with lasting results.

Understanding personality as enduring traits of an individual leads to questions relating to the ways in which those traits, also called *individual differences,* interact with the environment to alter behavior. In other words, the psychology of personality postulates that behavior is a function of both the situation in which a person finds himself or herself and the individual traits of the person. The situation includes the natural environment or a set of circumstances created to achieve a given goal, for example, a nursing intervention. Growing evidence indicates that individual differences interact with behavioral interventions in such a way as to alter the effects of the intervention (Endler and Magnusson, 1976).

Two examples of such individual difference traits are the type A coronary-prone behavior pattern and coping style. The type A coronary-prone behavior is characterized by competitiveness, achievement-striving, and time-urgency. Persons assessed to be type A respond differently to stressful situations than type B persons (that is, persons not characterized by the preceding behaviors). One difference is their desire to be with other persons. While awaiting a stressful experience, type A persons tend to desire the company of others. However, during the stressful experience itself, they prefer to work alone (Dembroski and MacDougall, 1978). Nurses often plan nursing care in terms of interpersonal support before and during stressful experiences. This and other research would lead one to believe that planning such intervention requires knowing about both the person and the situation.

A second kind of individual difference is coping style, that is, an individual's characteristic means of actively dealing with stress. Ways of characterizing a person by his or her coping style are as avoiders, sensitizers, or nonspecific defenders (Goldstein, 1973). *Avoiders* are persons who deny the existence of a threat or maintain emotional distance from the threat. *Sensitizers* respond to threat, in general, with vigilance and more intense emotion. *Nonspecific defenders* demonstrate neither of the other patterns consistently.

This individual trait has been found to affect the usefulness of information of patients. Andrew (1970) found that among male surgical patients, avoiders, nonspecific defenders, and sensitizers used preoperative information differently. Studying outcome variables, she found that the nonspecific defender group responded to information with less usage of pain medication and shorter hospitalizations. Avoiders in the information group did not differ in length of hospitalization, but required more pain medication. Information did not affect either length of stay or analgesic usage for sensitizers. Smith (1976), studying reactivity during endoscopy, also found that coping style interacted with a patient's ability to comprehend preparatory information. In general, sensitizers receiving information were more reactive than sensitizers without information, whereas nonspecific defenders who received information were less reactive than those who did not. The nurse who understands the frequent importance of individual differences in planning interventions is a professional who is knowledgeably individualizing patient care, an important nursing goal.

Social Psychology

Brown and Fowler (1971) define *nursing* as "a process of verbal and nonverbal interaction directed toward the healthful status of the recipient within an institution, an agency of the community." They go on to state that "verbal and nonverbal interaction not only occurs between the nurse and the patient, but includes other members of the health team and others such as the patient's family and friends; however, all of the interaction is goal-directed in the area of the subject's health" (Brown and Fowler, 1971). By its very nature, then, the nursing process involves interpersonal behavior. Since "social psychology is the field of study concerned with interpersonal behavior" (Wrightsman, 1977) and "the social psychologist's primary activities are the acquisition of knowledge and the application of it to the problems of our world," it is not too difficult to see the relevance of social psychology to nursing students, especially if they wish to understand behavior within a transactional model.

Social psychologists, having recognized the vast importance of learning while also seeing the limitations of the traditional learning approaches, have attempted to broaden the learning theories. Rotter's social learning theory (Rotter, 1954) proposes that a behavior in a given situation is a function of the expectancy of reinforcement for the behavior and the value attached to tue reinforcement. One can further propose that the expectancies and values of both the cost and reward of a given behavior should be taken into account. What might this mean to a nurse?

For example, a clinic nurse who wanted to utilize social learning theory to increase the likelihood that a hypertensive man would adhere to his medication regimen might

1. Point out to the patient that medicine taking is the most effective means of lowering his blood pressure (increased expectance of reward).
2. Help the patient recognize the importance he places on being healthy (increased value of reward).
3. Show the patient how he can build medicine taking into his daily routine, thus minimizing disruption of his lifestyle (decreased expectancy of cost).
4. Work with the patient so that he no longer attaches such importance to certain countertherapeutic elements of his lifestyle (decreased value of cost).

In addition to assessing and modifying an individual's specific expectancies about a particular health-related behavior, social learning theory also adresses the locus of control of reinforcements, which nurses may find helpful in understanding patients' behavior. Persons who believe that their own health status is directly a function of their own behavior (termed *internals*) may need to be treated differently than persons who believe that their health is controlled by external factors (see *Health Education Monographs,* 1978).

Person perception, a subarea of social psychology, contains additional implications for nursing, especially in understanding how nurses form impressions of patients and the possible way these impressions might influence nurse-patient interactions. A series of recent studies has shown that nurses are prone to stereotype patients on the basis of diagnostic labels (for example, cancer, alcoholism, psychosomatic conditions) or other characteristics (such as patient's sex or personality style) (DeVellis, Wallston, and Wallston, 1980). While these studies have not yet demonstrated that the stereotypes that nurses hold affect either their willingness to attend to patients or their ability to respond to patients in a person-centered manner, nurses must be aware of how their impressions of patients get formed if, indeed, they wish to treat each patient as a unique individual. On the other side of the coin, nurses must be aware of how they, as nurses, are perceived by patients, other health professionals, and the community at large. Nurses, too, are often stereotyped. While this sometimes works to their benefit, it often limits their effectiveness.

Maladaptive Behavior

Many areas of psychology, including personality and learning theories as well as knowledge of neuropsychology and human adaptive processes, converge in the study of maladaptive human behavior or psychopathology. Let us take as an example one of the most common problems of mental health today—incapacitating depression. This common human problem has been understood in many ways. The psychoanalytic theorists describe it as a disease state resulting from developmental difficulties in the oral and anal stages that have produced lasting defects in self-esteem (Fenichel, 1945).

Various schools of thought within psychology have contributed models which differ from a disease model to explain depression. One of these, the learned-helplessness model, emerged from laboratory research in which dogs that were exposed to inescapable shock were later significantly impaired in their ability to learn adaptive behaviors (Seligman, 1975). From this work it was hypothesized that the behavior of depressed individuals might also be a result of learning that their behavior did not produce reduced tension or increased gratification. Since there is evidence to support this, the implications for treatment are clear. The depressed person needs to experience that positive reinforcement or gratification is contingent upon his or her own behavior. Therefore, the goals of intervention are to teach skills that will achieve the person's goals and motivate him or her to use those skills.

Another related model of depression that has its roots in psychology is that depression results from chronic, infrequent occurrences of positive reinforcement (Lewinsohn and Libet, 1972; MacPhillamy and Lewinsohn, 1974). Depressive behavior is partly accounted for by limited social reinforcement resulting from limited social skills of the depressed person. Although there are many issues, such as the role of cognitive mediation and the individual's expected rate of reinforcement, the model again points to clinically applicable interventions.

This behavioral approach does not conflict with a biochemical view. in which drugs are used to alter the biochemistry in the brain. In fact, a transactional model in psychology can easily accommodate the notion of multiple causation and multiple interventions.

The nurse who views human beings in a holistic way and is knowledgeable of these models of depression will endeavor to incorporate many techniques in her or his interaction with a depressed person. Similarly, various understandings of other patterns of maladaptive behavior may be found in psychology, and these nonmedical approaches can broaden the number of alternative actions open to the nurse.

Modes of Intervention

Psychopathology is an area of psychology that clearly bridges the gap between the basic and applied components of psychology. Let us now focus on several areas of applied psychology that have direct relevance to nurses. The list could be endless, but three areas seem to be of special importance: therapeutic relationships, group dynamics, and adaptation to stress.

Rogers (1967) defined empathy, congruence, and unconditional positive regard as the critical components of a helping relationship. Carkhuff (1969a, and 1969b) and his associates have further refined and described the key elements of helping and have developed ways of training helpers and assessing the effectiveness of these helpers. The nurse who develops the skills of communicating core conditions, such as empathy, concreteness, positive regard, genuineness, self-disclosure, confrontation, and immediacy, will be able to define fully the problem areas facing his or her patient and will then be able to assist the patient to solve the problems at hand. These researchers/trainers have demonstrated that the "helpees" cannot achieve levels of functioning higher than the helpers and, in fact, may decline in functioning if the helper is less skillful in communicating than the patient.

The problem becomes even more complex when dealing with behaviors of persons in groups. Nurses find themselves as part of not only patient groups, but also collaborative work groups such as the health team. Psychologists have, over many years, defined the types of leadership most effective for specific kinds of goals and have identified predictable patterns of process that occur as a group forms and develops cohesiveness (Cartwright and Zander, 1968). They have described means of conflict resolution in groups as well as ways in which groups handle tension maladaptively. The nurse who understands and has had first-hand experience with these various issues of group process can be an effective facilitator, whether the group is a task-oriented peer group or a process-oriented therapy group.

The nurse who has been able to comprehend and integrate psychological principles can effectively reduce the stress resulting from interactions with both patients and coworkers. Stress involves attending to experiences that are appraised as threatening and responding to the threat in any of a variety of ways. Psychologists (some of whom are nurse psychologists) have identified several ways of effectively reducing the negative effects of stress experiences. Information giving, especially about the subjective experiences likely to occur, has reduced distress in endoscopy (Johnson, Morrissey, and Leventhal, 1973) and cast removal (Johnson, 1975) and has decreased the time needed to pass an endoscopic tube into the esophagus (Smith, 1977). Johnson (1975) suggests that decreased distress occurs because there is congruence between expectations and actual experience. Lazarus (1966) proposes that cognitive reappraisal of an event as nonthreatening could enable persons to respond with behaviors different from stress responses and has demonstrated this in laboratory studies (Speisman, Lazarus, Mordoff, and Davison, 1964; Lazarus and Alfert, 1964).

Psychologists have been active in the development of specific techniques such as progressive relaxation (Bernstein and Borkovec, 1973) and biofeedback (Fuller, 1977) to enable individuals to control physiological responses to stress, such as pulse rate or muscle tension.

The nurses who have been able to incorporate knowledge such as that just mentioned into their armamentarium are effective resources for their patients. They can communicate effectively, work well with a team, and provide a variety of alternatives for dealing with stress. They are truly an ally to their patients.

These are by no means all the psychologically relevant concepts needed by the nurse. Anxiety, pain, and crisis theory and intervention are major examples of areas not included here. Their omission occurs not because they lack importance—we believe they are extremely important—but because they are frequently and thoroughly reviewed elsewhere in relation to nursing.

Research Process

The evaluation of the effectiveness of nursing-care intervention strategies is one area where psychology plays an important, but often indirect, role. Psychologists, as behavioral scientists, are committed to carrying out systematic research investigations. Those psychologists who are also health-care practitioners usually, because of their training, recognize the need to gather outcome data to determine if their interventions have made a difference. While it often comes as a surprise to those relatively unfamiliar with the profession of nursing, nurses are (or ought to be) researchers too. The field of nursing research has blossomed over the past 25 years, and much of the research conducted by nurses is psychological in orientation. Training nurses in psychology gives them an appreciation of the research process, which, in turn, reinforces and strengthens the evaluation component of the nursing process.

In this chapter, we are not proposing formalized research projects involving large samples of subjects, rigorous controls, and tight methodology, rather we are suggesting that the case-study approach (or single-subject design) is the appropriate analogy for how a baccalaureate-prepared nurse goes about the business of examining the care she or he gives to patients one at a time. Obviously, most nurses are too busy to carry out full-blown case-study investigations on each and every patient (only student nurses have the time and the external pressure to do so), but periodic assessment of the patient is an integral part of the nurse's role and, as such, lends itself rather nicely to a systematic evaluation framework. What is necessary is that the nurse view herself or himself as an investigator and recognize the great similarities between the nursing process and the research process.

Most nurses do not hesitate to use reliable and valid tools (such as a clinical thermometer or a sphygmomanometer) to gather data about a patient's vital signs or to rely on the results of a host of laboratory tests for other information relevant to the patient's physical health status. Yet, when it comes to assessing and evaluating the patient's psychological health status, nurses tend to use far less sophisticated methods. While the tools that psychologists have developed are maybe not as reliable and valid as those of the physical sciences, such tools do exist (or could be constructed) and are available for use in a systematic manner. Instead of using standardized psychological instruments, however, most nurses gather psychological information about the patient in a more haphazard manner, making inferences about the patient's psychological status on the basis of unstructured observations of the patient's behavior or verbal responses by the patient made during interactions with the nurse. In many instances when the patient's ability to accurately report information verbally is hindered (for example, comatose patients, patients in shock, patients without the requisite verbal facilities to respond reliably and validly to more standardized approaches), observation becomes the primary means available to the nurse to gather psychological data. If the nurse is trained properly in the techniques of making psychological inferences from clinical observations (which, in turn, entails knowing which patient behaviors are critical indicators of various psychological states), then this procedure can yield results that are suitable for evaluation purposes. The more nursing students are trained in psychology, the greater is the likelihood that they will be attentive to critical patient behaviors and the more reliable and valid will be their inferences.

Curriculum Models

There are a number of different curriculum models employed by schools of nursing that introduce psychological concepts to nursing students. One approach is based on the belief that nursing students should learn about psychology from courses offered and taught in departments of psychology.

Schools utilizing this approach usually set aside the first 2 years of college for students to enroll predominantly in nonnursing courses in the physical and social sciences and humanities. Such students are generally required to take an introductory psychology course and may be encouraged to elect one or more additional psychology courses (for example, developmental, social, personality, and so forth). In the students' last 2 years of college, they enroll predominantly in clinical nursing courses, where they are hopefully able to apply what they have learned from their earlier course (or courses) in psychology. One of these clinical nursing courses is usually labeled "psychiatric nursing," during which additional content relevant to persons with maladjusted behavior patterns is presented by nursing faculty who have specialized in psychiatric nursing at either the masters or doctoral level.

The preceding approach, which was previously the norm among nursing schools is now being displaced by what is typically referred to as the "integrated curriculum." Each school of nursing utilizing the integrated approach operationalizes it in a somewhat different manner. However, the basic idea involves incorporating content from psychology along with content from other disciplines in most, if not all, of the nursing courses in order to impress upon students the holistic philosophy mentioned in the introduction to this chapter. This philosophy is quite consistent with a transactional understanding of behaviors. Nursing students in an integrated curriculum are usually encouraged, but not required, to take courses offered by psychology departments as electives. Additionally, the nursing faculty assumes the responsibility for presenting the relevant psychological content that is usually begun in the freshman year and builds sequentially in subsequent years. Schools of nursing that adhere to an integrated curric- ulum usually, but not always, have done away with the traditional "block" nursing courses based on patients' location within an institution, agency, or community. Instead of teaching courses labeled "pediatric nursing," "medical nursing," "psychiatric nursing," "surgical nursing," and so forth, integrated curricula often include courses bearing titles such as "health problems of children," "nursing in primary-care settings," or "management of patients with chronic diseases."

Both the preceding approaches have their respective pros and cons, and as already stated, the differences among schools in their employment and actualization of curricular models are great. Depending on a given school's philosophy, more or less psychological content is presented and labeled for the student as "pure" psychology or nursing content. In the long run, the important thing is not that the students are trained as academic psycho- logists, but that they can utilize their knowledge of psychology to assist them in caring for their patients.

One of the best methods of aiding student nurses in applying their knowledge of psychology to patient care is to directly link their learning of concepts to actual field experiences in clinical situations. Here is where the integrated curriculum model, if it is carried out successfully, has a definite advantage over the less integrated approaches. Not only are students more motivated to learn when they can see the relevance of that learning to direct care of patients, but knowledge from many disciplines can be presented concurrently to help students understand and explore the interrelatedness of scientific knowledge. A biopsychosocial orientation means that no single body of knowledge has greater value than the others, but that each type is necessary, although not sufficient, for the total picture to be complete.

Conclusion

It is, of course, unrealistically utopian to expect nurses to be as well-grounded in all facets of psychological knowledge and theory as even the average undergraduate psychology major, much less a psychological practitioner at the masters or doctoral level. Clearly, therefore, nurse educators must be selective in the content from psychology they choose to present to their students. It is not unreasonable, however, to aim nursing education toward helping student nurses begin to incorporate psychological theories and constructs into their thinking and to integrate this view of the world into their nursing approach in every situation they encounter. Nursing students must be able to deal with abstract concepts as well as concrete realities, examine their own behavior as well as the behavior of their patients, and adopt systematic, empirically based, investigative approaches toward patient care rather than moving from one problem-solving situation to the next without regard to commonalities.

References

Andrew, J.M. Recovery from surgery, with or without preparatory instruction, for three coping styles. *Journal of Personality and Social Psychology* 15:223–226, 1970.

Bernstein, D.A., and Borkovec, T.D. *Progressive Relaxation Training: A Manual for the Helping Professions.* Champaign, Ill.: Research Press, 1973.

Brown, M.M., and Fowler, G.R. *Psychodynamic Nursing: A Biosocial Orientation.* Philadelphia: Saunders, 1971.

Carkhuff, R.R. *Helping and Human Relations: A Primer for Lay and Professional Helpers,* Vol. I: *Practice and Research.* New York: Holt, Rinehart, and Winston, 1969a.

Carkhuff, R.R. *Helping and Human Relations: A Primer for Lay and Professional Helpers,* Vol. II: *Selection and Training.* New York: Holt, Rinehart, and Winston, 1969*b.*

Cartwright, C., and Zander, A. *Group Dynamics: Research and Theory.* New York: Harper and Row, 1968.

Dembroski, T.M., and MacDougall, J.M. Stress effects on affiliation preferences among subjects possessing the type A coronary prone behavior pattern. *Journal of Personality and Social Psychology* 36:23–33, 1978.

DeVellis, B.M., Wallston, B.S., and Wallston, K.A. Stereotyping: A threat to individualized patient care. In *Current Perspectives in Nursing: Social Issues and Trends,* ed. M.H. Miller and B. Flynn, Vol. II. St. Louis: Mosby, 1980.

Endler, N.S., and Magnusson, D. Toward an interactional psychology of personality. *Psychological Bulletin* 83:956–974, 1976.

Fenichel, O. *The Psychoanalytic Theory of Neurosis.* New York: Norton, 1945.

Fuller, G.D. *Biofeedback: Methods and Procedures in Clinical Practice.* San Francisco: Biofeedback Press, 1977.

Goldstein, M.J. Individual difference in response to stress. *American Journal of Community Psychology* 1:113–117, 1973.

Hall, C.S., and Lindzey, G. *Theories of Personality.* New York: Wiley, 1970.

Johnson, J.E. Stress reduction through sensation information. In *Stress and Anxiety,* ed. D.G. Sarason and C.D. Spielberger, Vol. II. Washington: Hemisphere Publishing Co., 1975.

Johnson, J.E., Morrissey, J.F., and Leventhal, H. Psychological preparation for an endoscopic examination. *Gastrointestinal Endoscopy* 19:180–183, 1973.

Lazarus, R.S. *Psychological Stress and the Coping Process.* New York: McGraw-Hill, 1966.

Lazarus, R.S., and Alfert, E. Short-circuiting of threat by experimentally altering cognitive appraisal. *Journal of Abnormal and Social Psychology* 69:195–205, 1964.

Lewinson, P.M., and Libet, J. Pleasant events, activity schedules, and depression. *Journal of Abnormal Psychology* 79:291–295, 1972.

MacPhillamy, D.J., and Lewinsohn, P.M. Depression as a function of levels of desired and obtained pleasure. *Journal of Abnormal Psychology* 83:651–657, 1974.

Rogers, C.R. The interpersonal relationship: The core of guidance. In *Person to Person: The Problem of Being Human,* ed. C.R. Rogers and B. Stevens, Lafayette, Calif.: Real People Press, 1967.

Rotter, J.B. *Social Learning and Clinical Psychology.* New York: Prentice-Hall, 1954.

Schaie, K.W. A general model for the study of developmental problems. *Psychological Bulletin* 64:92–108, 1965.

Seigler, I.C. Life span developmental psychology and clinical geropsychology. In *Geropsychology: A Model of Training and Clinical Service,* ed. W.D. Gentry, Cambridge, Mass.: Ballinger, 1977.

Seligman, M.E. *Helplessness: On Depression, Development, and Death.* San Francisco: Freeman, 1975.

Smith, R.A. The effects of sensation information, interpersonal support and coping style on the experience of persons undergoing endoscopy (George Peabody College, 1976). *Dissertation Abstracts International* 37:416B, 1977. (University Microfilms No. 77–3118.)

Speisman, J.C., Lazarus, R.S., Mordkoff, A., and Davison, L. Experimental reduction of stress bases on ego-defense theory. *Journal of Abnormal and Social Psychology* 68:367–380, 1964.

Wallston, K.A., and Wallston, B.S., eds. Locus of control and health. *Health Education Monographs* 6:107–117, 1978.

Wechsler, D. *The Measurement and Appraisal of Adult Intelligence.* Baltimore, Md.: Williams and Wilkins, 1958.

Wechsler, D. *The Measurement of Adult Intelligence.* Baltimore, Md.: Williams and Wilkins, 1944.

Wrightsman, L.S. *Social Psychology,* 2d ed. Monterey, Calif.: Brooks/Cole Publishing Co., 1972, 1977.

Part II
Delivery of Health-Care Services: Psychology's Role in Selected Aspects of Medical Practice

In the introduction to this book, we learned that one of the ways of viewing illness is as the outcome of a series of interactions among biological, social, and psychological factors. Not all these interactions need necessarily be directly mediated by the disease process itself. We are talking about an *interaction;* whenever we do that, it is difficult to separate and analyze or reduce any one interaction term without its losing much of its essential character. It therefore becomes apparent that when we talk about health and illness, we are talking about states that exist in a psychosocial context. In chapter 5, Wirt, recognizing the need for viewing health and illness contextually, shows how psychologists working among other health-care professionals can integrate observations of the environmental, social, and behavioral reinforcers of both adaptive and maladaptive behaviors in relation to what happens to people when they become patients. Because of their skills and training, psychologists also can provide an opportunity to view and evaluate relationships and functions in the health-care professions (including roles on both sides of the healing enterprise) from a larger systems perspective. So we are talking about relationships—*people* heal people. People who heal have functions, and it is sometimes easy, given the kind of social glorification with which our society tends to surround the healing professions, to forget that the person of the healer need not play a role that is secondary or unimportant in relation to the more easily identifiable technical functions that healers have. It feels like an insult to medicine to think of it as the technology of biology. What is missing in such a view is the personal element, one of the most important aspects of which is the development of listening skills.

Chapter 6 allows us, as the authors put it, to have a way of "listening beyond the words" of the patient. It is important to view a patient's illness within the context of the patient's whole life situation. We come across another challenge for the dualistic practitioner's view of the presenting symptoms and signs as possible indicators of emotional stress as well as organic illness. Ireton and Cassata present a very practical instrument, the Psychological Systems Review, for meeting this challenge, and in chapter 7, Hilliard shows how practitioners can broach the subject of discussing psychological etiology without making patients defensive. Much of what is dealt with in chapter 6 takes place in the relatively benign environment of a physician's office or in the less dramatic areas of a hospital or clinic. Chapter 8, on the other hand, lets us view some of the ways in which our thinking about emergency rooms can transcend the television-type drama to which even health-care professionals can be susceptible when we think about emergency rooms. The main point of chapter 9 is that psychological adjustment to illness is not of necessity to be viewed as psychopathological, that there is a breadth of functional capacity that people have, and that we can exhibit coping mechanisms even when we are children. Just how extraordinary these coping mechanisms can be is highlighted by Kellerman in chapter 10, when he writes about what we can do to facilitate coping in children stricken by cancer, as well as in their families. He deals with the multiplicity of roles faced by a psychologically sophisticated consultant in pediatric oncology and shows how psychological sensitivity in medical teamwork can rise to meet some extraordinary circumstances. In addition, he points out some excellent guidelines for effective consultation. Like Quast, Kellerman differentiates between stress-induced vulnerability and our more commonly held view of psychopathology. He also points out the uniqueness of every person, every patient, every family. Again, we are trying to avoid stereotyping. There is no such thing as "the typical cancer patient." Kellerman's psychosocial program in pediatric oncology is a fine example of an interdisciplinary team approach to handling every possible aspect of an illness that is almost invariably identified with death and that strikes terror in people's hearts and minds when they hear about it. Another area with a similar impact on people's feelings is spinal cord injury. Fazzari's clinical sensitivity is reflected in his discussion in chapter 11 of how to deal with our feelings and those of patients and families in handling with delicacy and tact the enormous loss and disruption of functioning that occurs in paraplegia and quadriplegia. Fazzari lets us know that we do not face loss and grief only in situations involving death and dying.

It is easy to become rather lost in a quagmire of psychological conceptual jargon unless we delineate rather carefully the parameters of the phenomenon with which we are dealing. Varni and Russo do just that in chapter 12 for the various dimensions of chronic disorders that are amenable to behavioral analysis. The interface between behavioral psychology and medicine, representing the new field of behavioral medicine, is clearly presented with very practical examples involving a specific illness, hemophilia. One of the characteristics of chapter 12 to which we would like to draw attention is the broad scope of intervention strategies in both preventive and treatment modalities, so that we learn something about treating diseases multidimensionally as well as about attending to risk factors involved in those diseases. The power of behavioral techniques explained by

Varni and Russo is taken up in chapter 13. Brockway shows how the field of pain control has progressed far beyond the prescription of analgesic substances and now involves a wide range of principles and techniques drawn from the behavioral psychologist's armamentarium. She shows how we can achieve significant pain control in ways hardly dreamed of before the skillful innovations of health-care professionals who were able to perceive and analyze the relationships between pain behavior and some of the results of modern experimental psychology. Her article makes it clear that pain is a complex, interactive biopsychological phenomenon.

In chapter 14, Lippman provides guidelines for obstetrics and gynecology which, if followed, would allow every physician to come close to the ideal of the benign healer, rather than the insensitively sadistic person about whom so many women complain when going through gynecological examination, which is commonly an experience that is an insult to their dignity. One would be well served by extrapolating a similarly high level of sensitivity and awareness for every medical specialty. Chapter 15 similarly points out ways in which even the most well-intentioned people can, out of mere lack of knowledge, sabotage their own efforts when working with older people in health delivery systems (and other systems too). We see a human, comprehensive view of older people as people with needs in many dimensions, and we get seven principles basic to more effective serving of older people.

We should not forget ourselves. In chapter 16, Smith lets us look at stress involved in our frequently taxing and demanding roles as health-care professionals. We frequently pay more attention to our patients' needs for rest and relaxation and lifestyle change than we do to our own. Smith provides us with a model for examining and treating stress in our own world as well as that of our patients. We know that many people seek relief from stress through the use and abuse of various substances. In chapter 17, Ersner-Hirshfield, Sobell, and Sobell provide an opportunity for us to examine the problems arising from abusing one of those substances: alcohol. We include their chapter because the attention they pay to the interaction of physical and psychological factors in alcoholism is another good illustration of a basic rejection of dualistic views of such problems.

5

Clinical Psychology and Health Psychology: The Application of Clinical Psychology to Health-Care Practice

Robert D. Wirt

There are important areas of knowledge, skills, and competencies in the traditions of clinical psychology that are relevant to the practice of health psychology. These relate especially to methods of assessment as well as to research; they generally relate rather less to strategies of intervention and prevention. Many current practitioners in health psychology were trained as clinical psychologists. While they found much of the training experience in clinical psychology to be useful for working in the health-care system, to become effective health psychologists, they found much had to be learned on the job and that some of the traditions of clinical psychology had to be replaced, most notably the emphasis in clinical psychology on illness rather than on health.

In replacing a model of psychopathology learned in psychiatric settings, there is risk of rejecting the whole of clinical practice for a model deriving from experimental psychobiology. There have been several advances in psychological science in the past two decades that have added important technology to the practice of health psychology. These have been in the renaissance of the clinical use of hypnosis, in biofeedback, and in behavioral management. All these are skills some clinical psychologists learn. All have potential utility for some patients. The pioneers in these fields have not been clinical psychologists; they have been experimental psychologists. Unhappily, too often the knowledge from these sources is applied in clinical settings by persons not properly trained in professional psychology. Proper training of clinical psychologists working in health-care settings will reduce the occurrence of, for example, using hypnosis with certain paranoid patients with somatic delusions who, as distinct from the patient suffering from conversion hysteria, might find the experience one of terrifying control and domination, or using biofeedback with patients not sufficiently assessed by relevant medical practitioners, or using aversive behavioral programs inappropriately. People being cared for in the health system are not subjects; they are patients, and it is the *professional* orientation of the sort imbued in good training programs in clinical psychology that is the most important personal quality the health psychologist can bring to the practice of this new profession.

Good practice is rooted in science as well as in the acquisition of a professional attitude. Psychology, as all sciences, begins with careful observation. The psychologist goes on to the construction of rational hypotheses, subjects the hypotheses to rigorous testing, revises the hypotheses, and tests further. In some sciences, these steps are based on theory, which guides the nature of the observations to be made, the form of the hypotheses, and the criteria by which hypotheses are tested. However, there are inductive theories that build as a result of observations that are subsequently linked. There are psychological theories of both origins, but none is universally accepted. In addition to a professional orientation, the good clinical psychologist will bring the disciplined curiosity of the scientist to the health-care setting.

Students of clinical psychology are taught to observe behavior indicative of psychopathology. Except for some behaviorists and, to a lesser extent, those engaged in work with families or social groups, the clinical psychologists' hypotheses emphasize the need for cognitive restructuring of the individual, guidance to improve reality testing, support to take interpersonal risks, reduction of neurotic anxiety and guilt, flexibility in the expression of feelings, encouragement to enhance enlightened self-interest, and similar strategies. The presumption is that insight on the part of the patient and instruction, persuasion, and approval from the therapist will generate or maximize behavior that develops pride in the individual and social reinforcement from the environment, and this, in turn, will lead to self-maintaining psychologically healthy behavior. Different theorists attach different language to these interactions between patient and therapist (interpretation, reflection, support, unconditional positive regard, rational-emotive, clarification of feelings, correcting of parataxic distortion, uncovering, and so forth). They have in common the belief that pathological behavior is learned, although it may involve strong genetic or biological determinants. In addition, they have in common the belief that with the therapist as guide, adaptive behavior can replace pathological behavior and thinking, sometimes with the assistance of biochemical agents.

Not infrequently, the health psychologist will encounter such problems and will find that the traditional modes of assessment and intervention of clinical psychology are useful. However, more often the health psychologist will not find these methods useful. The psychologist working in the health system should be looking instead at problems in the human ecology of the environment and for health behavior on the part of the individual. While training in clinical psychology is useful in helping the practitioner identify areas of weakness, traditional programs generally do not teach students to observe strengths, nor to maximize them.

There is some validity to the concept of the wisdom of the body—and of the mind. *Some* validity. Even inept medical practice is likely to seem to be effective because of the powerful influence of the placebo effect and the fact that for most conditions the organism can cure itself in time. If we think of health as optimal biopsychosocial functioning, the body is not always wise. The most obvious examples come from immunology, where we know that the body will often reject a transplanted organ which, if accepted, would improve bodily function, even arrest death of the body. The same body may not reject a metastasized carcinoma of its own making; thus sometimes the body attacks and kills itself. Nor is the mind always wise. We know, for example, that while sympathy and nurturance of dependency are helpful in dealing with normal grief, firmness and exhortation to independent behavior are more likely to be effective in treating clinical depression, which at first may appear to be simply normal grief. The competent clinical psychologist will know the difference, even if family and friends (including other health professionals) do not.

Clinical psychology has some contributions to make to an understanding of the components of unhealthy social systems. But health psychology has more to learn about human structures from social psychology, sociology, and industrial-organizational psychology. Social organizations are first of all self-serving, whatever their professed charter. The health-care system exists to promote health and to prevent and treat illness. In its operations it all too often loses sight of the patient. The emergency room logistics may provide for ascertaining who will pay for the analgesic before it is administered. The patient who becomes demanding of nursing time following visits from the family will find a sign on the door instructing "No Visitors." The patient with disturbed sleep, though not febrile, will be awakened at dawn for a "routine" check of temperature and pulse rate. Some clinics in hospitals schedule all patients for 8:00 A.M. That way there is always someone in the wings to keep the busy staff busy. It is a matter of luck for the patients and families who wait: at least one patient gets to wait with all those sick people until 5:00 P.M. Good training in clinical psychology can be of great help in these kinds of situations, if the clinical psychologist is seen as a credible consultant. It is useful for nurses to learn that giving attention to patients when they are behaving constructively is far more useful in shaping healthy behavior and a feeling of comfort than giving negative attention when the patient is behaving maladaptively. It is useful for physicians to discriminate between specifically needed data and data that are only sometimes needed. It is useful for all health professionals to learn that disgruntled patients recover more slowly than those who have pleasant experiences in the health-care system. While all this seems obvious, it is not at all obvious in the behavior of administration and health-care providers.

Social systems resist change. While it would seem from the millions of "How To . . ." books sold that individuals are eager to find ways to improve their own and their families' lives, organizations generally seek to maintain the status quo. Many health-care professionals have suffered through a college course in child psychology, but most know little of practical applications from developmental psychology. There are at least 100 books in print on how to be a constructive parent, but most people know very little about parenting, including most health professionals, except for the example they experienced in living with their own parents. So we find signs in most hospitals stating "No Visitors Under 16 Allowed." Such prohibitions have little to do with the wisdom concerning either patient care or developmental psychology. They have to do with the untested assumption that patients will be more comfortable if they escape having loud and restless children around. They have even more to do with another untested assumption that the staff will perform more efficiently if they are not distracted. In fact, where it has been tried judiciously, we find patients are more comfortable and more cooperative when they can see their children or children can see their siblings—and that reduces staff work. Similar rationalizations are used for the strange hours meals are served, visiting hours scheduled, and parents excluded from examining rooms. Flexibility in these rules creates minor initial inconveniences to staff, but these are far outweighed by the long-term improvement in staff morale because of patient comfort and visitor approval. There is much data that shows that when residents of nursing homes have some interesting things to do, they frequently can get out of bed and quit acting senile. Even so, many nursing-home administrators mistakenly do not provide such experiences, thinking they will be expensive. In fact, the addition is not only more humane, but cost-effective as well. Caring for bed patients is much more costly than caring for ambulatory patients.

The health psychologist is concerned with systems aspects of health care. Because of their focus on individual psychopathology, clinical psychologists are likely to attempt to modify the system either by changing the behavior of a troublesome patient or by altering a particular personal habit of a health professional or revising an administrative rule. This sometimes works, but more often it is met with frustration, anger, and failure. In such cases, the clinical psychologist is treating a system as if it were constructed of solid beams that can be changed to strengthen and improve the structure. The structure of systems, however, is more like a web than a solid. To pull at a strand of the web changes the shape of the whole system, thus warping the structure from the perspective of all its members. There are many examples outside the health-care system. One of the most risky assignments for the police is to answer a call concerning a domestic disturbance. In a fight between lovers, if a third party intervenes by forcefully attempting to modify the behavior of one of the belligerents, the anger of both is likely to be directed toward the stranger. Those trained in crisis intervention teach the police to treat the interpersonal relationship, not the individual comba-tants. The history of dictatorial regimes shows they often cement unity of their followers by raising the specter of an outside threat to the group. This appears to have been the psychology of the mass murder-suicide of the reli-gious cult in Guyana in the fall of 1978. Bringing a squabbling group to constructive cooperation has been shown experimentally by social psychol-ogists to succeed when the group members see an external danger to the group. Successful family therapists have learned these lessons. The clinical psychologist who tries to come between a schizophrenic patient and his or her mother will probably lose both. The health psychologist may wish, and frequently is asked, to consult in troublesome situations such as the man-agement of a dying child. To be effective, the skills of the clinical psycholo-gist come into play. The consultant is not a therapist in this situation, but the results one hopes for will be therapeutic. The skills of the therapist are needed: how to "read" interpersonal interactions, the manifestation of defense mechanisms, the ways to confront guilt, anxiety, anger, and despair. Multiple needs exist, including those of each parent and perhaps of siblings and even extended family, those of the staff—physician, resident, nursing assistant, nurse, occupational therapist, social worker, psycholo-gist, and often others—those of the dying child, and sometimes those of the chaplain or minister, the hospital administrator, the teacher, and the child's friends. It can be very complicated. All these people will have their own assumptions, expectations, and agenda based on their own experiences, per-ceptions, and needs. None will have expertise in multiple areas. Few will know much about child development, the nature of the disease process, a child's concept of death (or, in fact, even know what their own is), or understand the importance of their role in the total system; that is, how each one's behavior affects every other member whose responses in turn continually affect the total system in a dynamic way. The manifest content for each participant is the child's welfare (although the child may feel pro-tective of the parents). They will not understand how their own thinking and feelings affect each other through projections of guilt or anger, by ver-balization or other expression of anxiety, by rationalization, by the need for approval from others, by the need to do a good job, by evasion, and, of course, by grief. The skills of a clinical psychologist will assist the health psychologist in helping the group and its members meet each of the individ-ual's needs, including the patient's. The traditional clinical psychologist is likely to err in focusing too narrowly on perceived psychopathology in one or another member or on the child. The good health psychologist will be sensitive to these manifestations of psychopathology of everyday life and to potentially more serious psychological disturbances, as well as to the strengths, ego skills, and complex interrelationships.

As indicated, the health psychologist is not usually a therapist in the usual meaning of that term. Clinical skills are necessary, however. There are circumstances in which psychotherapy is indicated, and the health psychologist is the only staff person available to provide that care. So any graduate training program in health psychology should equip the student to engage in such practice. Those who wish a career as a psychotherapist, however, generally should consider postdoctoral training in clinical psychology. A more frequent occurrence is the situation in which the health professional consulting the health psychologist requires assistance in evaluating a patient's behavior with a possible view toward referral for psychological or psychiatric treatment. Here the assessment skills of the clinical psychologist become important. Knowledge of descriptive psychopathology, of techniques of interviewing, of psychometric evaluation, and of community mental health and special educational and counseling resources is essential. This means that the health psychologist must know how to evaluate such conditions as mental retardation, neurotic behavior (including "compensation" neurosis), learning disabilities, psychologically based sexual dysfunction, drug dependency, the psychoses, and mental deterioration, as well as how to distinguish when a patient showing symptoms can most optimally be helped by the referring person with further consultation and backup from the health psychologist, or when direct intervention by the health psychologist is necessary, or when referral to another resource is indicated.

Health and illness exist in a psychosocial context. In coming to understand that context and its impact on individual persons and the important others in their life space and communicating all that in a constructive way to relevant persons in the health-care system, the patient, the family, and sometimes school or agency personnel or employers, the health psychologist has a distinct professional role. For the most part, these other people are not skilled in integrating observations of that nature and, indeed, generally underestimate the importance of the psychosocial context.

There are whole areas of concern in promotion of health, prevention of illness, and early intervention that are of interest to health psychologists. Again, while training in clinical psychology can provide a desirable professional attitude and scientific orientation to such problems, only those few who have also studied community psychology will have the competencies to deal with the myriad problems in these areas. Public health education alone seems not to be a sufficient solution to the vast social and health problems associated with the fact that too many people eat too much, have unbalanced diets, smoke too much, drink too much, drive too fast, rest and play too little, cannot get pleasure from leisure or retirement, feel a lack of purpose in living, and so on. Nearly everyone knows that it is wise to get dental checkups. We all know tobacco and alcohol can be life-threatening. It is common knowledge that the automobile is a lethal device. Most people can cite the dangers of "all work and no play." While we might agree that these behaviors are, or potentially are, unhealthy, they are generally outside the sphere of interest of abnormal psychology. Treatment programs for eating disorders (for example, behavioral management of obesity) come too late, actually nearly always not at all, for most overweight people suffering from high blood pressure or cardiac insufficiency. There are vast and vexing research questions in these tragic human conditions. Popular responses include such reactions as dietary fads, mass jogging, and restrictive legislation on smoking in public accommodations. These reactions seem to be more in the research domain of applied social psychology or sociology than of clinical psychology. Some of the people caught up in these activities harm, rather than help, themselves.

Why do people behave—and encourage others to behave—in ways they know are harmful? We do not know the answer or answers. And this is an enormous challenge to the health psychologist. Some of these patterns have become socially tolerated, if not outright condoned and admired. Think of the "macho male" with cigarette, drink, and fast car. The "sophisticated female" is also pictured with cigarette, drink, and fast car. So part of the answer is social reinforecement. How do we change that? Perhaps, just recently, there has been some move toward aversive social reaction to these behaviors because of substantial mass media educational efforts. So health education does help some.

Part of the answer appears to be a better understanding of relatively normal reactions to stress. Many of these unhealthy behaviors clearly are stress-related. Alcohol is easily available, cheap, and effective. While the use of hard drugs has decreased among young people recently, the use of alcohol continues to increase. Another part of the answer, then, may be finding ways to relieve stress and/or to tolerate frustration which, while effective, do not have long-term destructive effects. Overeating or the use of drugs are destructive of health, but so is long-sustained, even low-level, distress. The answers must involve interdisciplinary research, and psychologists who are concerned with finding these answers must be those able to communicate and cooperate with these efforts. The expertise of the clinical psychologist in understanding twists in the human condition will be helpful; what is most needed, however, is knowledge of, and concern for, the population at large. This will require a public health orientation to the application of psychological knowledge to health promotion and the prevention of illness.

6

Interviewing and Psychological Screening in Medical Practice: The Psychological Systems Review

Harold R. Ireton
and *Donald M. Cassata*

Introduction

In the provision of primary care, constant demands are placed on the physician to assist patients and their families in coping with the impact of illness and with other problems in living. Physicians need a systematic method of obtaining psychosocial information to understand better this aspect of patient care. Physicians have some training in psychiatric syndromes, interviewing and mental status examination, and social history-taking, but how does the physician utilize this knowledge and experience in a specific encounter with a patient in order to obtain the necessary information, to develop rapport, and to understand the patient and his or her needs? Well-motivated physicians may find themselves at a loss regarding "What is the necessary information?" and "How do I proceed with the interview?" What may be needed is an interview guide for psychological screening that maps out the territory and provides suggestions about when and how to proceed. Depending on the results of this psychological survey, the physician may proceed to delve into certain areas, such as marital or sexual history, in a more specific fashion.

The Psychological Systems Review (PRS) was designed to provide physicians with a systematic method for evaluating patient's psychological status and for appreciating their life situations. It is basically an interview guide, geared to real-life presenting situations of patients and families in distress. The PSR identifies areas to be explored, critical observations to be made, and methods of interviewing. It is intended to be used as one element in a patient-care system that integrates organic and psychosocial factors. Through an appreciation of the social and environmental context in which the presenting complaints occurred, the PSR would help physicians to understand better their patients' distresses and to help them cope with their problems.

Analogous to the review of physical systems, the PSR reviews three main "systems" or areas: (1) emotional status, (2) life situation, and (3) personality (table 6-1). The three systems must be understood as three inter-related aspects of the whole person. From a problem-oriented perspective, the PSR facilitates recognition of emotional distress, identification of life stresses, and definition of personal maladjustments. Equally important, the PSR emphasizes definition of the patient's social support systems and personal coping resources. Overall, therefore, the PSR orientation is as much toward the person and his or her situation as toward the patient and his or her symptoms and problems.

The PSR assesses the patient's *present psychological status* and *life situation,* with extensions into history if indicated. The basic assumption is that to fully appreciate the patient's psychological status, the physician must understand how the person is feeling and functioning *in the present.*

Effective utilization of the PSR depends on the physician's willing-ness—at the outset—to consider the patient's presenting symptoms and signs as possible indicators of emotional distress as well as organic disease (Lipowski, 1969; McWhinney, 1972; Shochet, 1975). Simply by taking a good look at the patient's facial expression, physical appearance, posture, and gestures, the physician can begin to sense whether the person is experiencing emotional distress (Berger, 1977; Knapp, 1972). The patient's non-verbal behavior may be more revealing than his or her words. By listening "beyond the words" (for example, tone of voice) of the presenting complaints, the physician may discover the person's primary concerns and actual reason(s) for coming at this time. The PSR should be utilized when the patient manifests emotional distress and also may be included as part of a complete history and physical examination.

The physician's ability to recognize the patient's psychological state and to establish a supportive relationship sets the stage for conducting the review. Rapport and information gathering are facilitated by use of the following clinical interviewing techniques (Enelow and Swisher, 1972):

Ask general to specific questions that allow and assist the patient to tell his or her own story.

Communicate interest through eye contact, body posture, and tone of voice.

Listen well for feelings "beyond the words."

Use pauses and silences to facilitate disclosure.

Use feedback: reflect feelings and summarize issues.

Through these processes af attending, inquiring, listening, and providing

Table 6-1
Psychological Systems Review

General	Problems	Resources
Emotional status	Distress	—
Life situation	Stresses	Support systems
Personality	Conflict/maladjustment	Personal resources

Table 6-2
Emotional Status

Nature of feelings
    Comfortable, positive mood
    Depressed, "sad"
    Tense, anxious, fearful
    Angry, resentful
    Confused, "mixed up"
    Flat, affectless
    Masked distress
Intensity of feeling
    Subjective distress
    Interference with functioning
    Emotional control
Emotional outlook
Chronicity

feedback, the physician conveys concern and acceptance to the patient and establishes the basis for a therapeutic relationship (Balint, 1957).

Emotional Status—Distress

In assessing the patient's emotional status and possible distress, the physician should determine what *feelings* the patient is experiencing, their *intensity,* the patient's *emotional outlook,* and how *acute* or *chronic* they are (table 6-2).

The patient's emotional distress may be (1) suggested by his or her nonverbal behavior, (2) reported spontaneously, or (3) elicited by questioning. The physician may simply ask "Tell me how you are feeling," or comment, "You seem to be . . . upset, sad, very tense," and this is often sufficient to help the patient begin. As described earlier, nonverbal cues are very important to observe, especially for individuals who are suppressing negative feelings and using denial as a means of coping.

To judge the intensity of the patient's feelings, it is essential not only to appreciate subjective distress, but also to determine the extent to which distress is interfering with the patient's ability to function. Evidence of altered or disrupted functioning in areas such as the following should be investigated: the person's work, family relations, social and recreational activity, sleep, appetite, and sexual activity. Furthermore, loss of emotional control or inappropriate behavior warrant special consideration.

The patient's emotional outlook, that is, his or her positive or negative expectations about the outcome of his or her problem, is a measure of the depth of his or her discouragement. His or her hope or lack of hope is a key indicator of how well or how poorly he or she may cope. The patient's expectations are especially important to weigh in assessing suicidal risk. These considerations provide an overall estimate of severity of distress and need for help.

Finally, it is important to discriminate acute, reactive distress from long-standing, chronic depression or anxiety. Reactive distress related to life crises often requires immediate intervention on the physician's part. Emotional distress is most commonly related to current stresses in the patient's life.

Life Situation, Stresses, Support Systems

In understanding the patient's emotional distress, the physician must determine what the patient is concerned or upset about, the major stresses in the patient's life, and the patient's situation in general. Besides stresses related to illness and concerns about health, other stresses in the patient's work and personal life are also common bases for emotional distress. A patient's symptoms are often tied to an inability to cope with various situations or relationships which he or she considers critical for well-being. It is important to determine the nature of the person's situation and the status of key relationships in his or her life.

Individuals must confront and cope with six areas of adjustment: health, work, family relationships, friends, recreation, and religion (table 6-3). The physician should determine the patient's situation in each of these areas and inquire about the patient's concerns, frustrations, satisfactions, and functioning in each area. The following kinds of questions may be useful:

How worried are you about your symptoms? What do you think is wrong?

What's been happening in your life?

Tell me about your job. How is it going for you? How do you like it?

Who is in your family? (Diagram—names, ages, relationships.) How are things going at home? Tell me about your marriage. What do you like (dislike) about your marriage?

Another useful method of understanding the patient's world and how he or she operates in it is to ask the patient to describe briefly a typical day in his or her life. Feelings are obviously expressed in the telling.

Key factors to consider in assessing stresses in the patient's situation are *change, threat, loss,* and *conflict.* A myocardial infarction suffered by the breadwinner of a household results in a serious life change and fear or loss. The promotion of the husband or wife to a more demanding position results in a loss of time shared with the spouse, a change that may threaten the marriage. The birth of a child, the upheaval of adolescence, the conflict of divorce, the threat of retirement, the death of a loved one—all represent stresses and potential crises. (Holmes and Rahe, 1967). The impact of such events is determined by the personal meaning the individual gives them, namely, perceived threat or loss and consequent disappointment, resentment, or self-blame.

As stresses are indentified, the patient's support systems also must be identified. Sources of emotional support include the spouse, relatives, job, friends, religion, and importantly, the physician. The quality and extent of the patient's support systems are an important measure of his or her coping ability in times of stress (Caplan, 1974). The primary question for the patient here is "To whom can you talk when you need help?"

Table 6–3
Life Situation

Areas	Assessment Factors	Summary
Health	Concerns-problems	Life situation
Work	Frustration-satisfaction	
Family	Change	
Friends	Threat	Stresses
Recreation	Loss	
Religion	Conflict	
	Functioning-coping	Sources of support

The physician is able to appreciate the person in context by this inquiry: in the context of the patient's life situation, in the context of the patient's key relationships, and in the context of both stresses and support systems.

Personality, Conflict/Maladjustment, Personal Resources

Life stresses alone do not provide an adequate explanation of the patient's distress and dysfunction. The role of the patient's personality in contributing to his or her problems and methods of coping also must be understood in order to determine what kind of help he or she needs. Personality evaluation involves more than a symptomatic labeling of a patient as "neurotic," "psychopathic," or "schizophrenic" (Kahana and Bibring, 1964). Personality describes the individual's typical ways of adapting, based on the person's subjective view of himself or herself in relation to the environment (Dreikurs, 1967; Mosak, 1972). In other words, an individual's behavior expresses his or her personal perceptions and values. The physician's task is to look beyond symptoms and stresses in order to understand a unique person, including his or her characteristic ways of coping with life's demands as well as his or her personal outlook on life. It is important to identify problems, for example, maladjustment and internal conflict, and equally important to identify personal resources.

The physician can get a general sense of the patient's personality in terms of optimism or pessimism, sociability, expressiveness, independence, dominance, responsibility, competence, and self-worth (table 6-4). Personality information emerges as the patient tells of his or her distress, describes the stresses he or she is facing, and tells about how he or she is coping. The patient may display a pessimistic, fearful, or indecisive attitude or, present as domineering and dogmatic, or he or she may be defensive and manipulative or "smile until it hurts" although obviously in distress.

Beyond observing the patient's attitudes and behavior in the office, the physician must determine how the person is functioning in everyday life situations. A great deal can be learned about an individual by inquiring into the manner in which he or she handles key roles, such as work: Is the person inconsistent and irresponsible? Hard-working? Or superconscientious and driven, a "workaholic"?

The physician should also understand the patient's current ways of coping with problems. Is the patient denying or avoiding problems? Is he or she actively working or struggling toward solutions? Passively resigned to fate? Overwhelmed by problems? Distorting reality? Also, the patient's use of alcohol and drugs as a means of coping should be routinely investigated.

Recognizing that the patient's behavior is based on how events are interpreted, the physician also will inquire into the patient's outlook on life.

Table 6–4
Personality

Characteristics	Assessment Factors	Summary
Optimism	Ways of coping	Personality
Sociability	Outlook on life	
Expressiveness	Life	
Independence	People	Conflict/maladjustment
Dominance	Men-Women	
Responsibility	Work	
Competence	Self	
Self-worth		Personal resources

A person's outlook on life includes his or her view of life in general, of other people, of men and women, of work, and of himself or herself. One patient may view life as a source of opportunity, while another may see life as dangerous. One person may see people as a source of satisfaction, another as "no damn good." One individual may see himself or herself as capable and resourceful, while another may view himself or herself as inadequate and helpless.

A person's outlook consists of two basic elements: (1) *beliefs* or expectations regarding "the way things are," and (2) *values* and goals about "the way things should be." Most human conflicts are internal conflicts between an individual's beliefs and his or her ideals, or interpersonal conflicts between two individuals with differing expectations. Marital conflicts are a dramatic example of the latter. Considerable pain results from discrepancies between expectations and performance. Many patients presenting with emotional symptoms are individuals suffering from a sense of failure and diminished self-esteem.

In order to understand the patient's distress, the physician must appreciate specifically the individual's self-image and self-esteem: How does the patient see himself or herself, and how does he or she value himself or herself. In addition, the physician must find out how the person's self-esteem is affected by those events in his or her life which are considered critical to his or her well-being. The physician may ask such questions as

Tell me something about yourself. What sort of person are you?

What is most important to you?

How do you feel about yourself?

What would it take to make you feel o.k.?

As personality problems are identified, the patient's personal resources and coping skills also must be considered. The individual's competencies, for example, intelligence, special abilities, accomplishments, and resourcefulness under stress, should be well appreciated.

Within this framework, the physician gains a dual perspective on the individual's personality, including his or her characteristic ways of coping and his or her private perceptions of self and others. The physician can then portray the individual in terms of both personality problems and personal resources. This assessment gives the physician a sound basis for empathy, for developing doctor-patient rapport, for decision making, and for fostering cooperation with needed treatment (Gillum and Barsky, 1974).

Summary

The Psychological Systems Review (PSR) provides physicians with a systematic interview method of reviewing the patient's psychological status and personal circumstances. The combination of the physical examination and the results of the PSR regarding the patient's emotional status, life situation, and personality yields a comprehensive view of the person's functioning. The format of the review also serves as an outline for recording this psychosocial information in the patient's chart (figure 6–1).

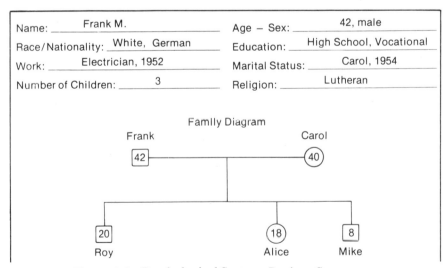

Figure 6–1. Psychological Systems Review: Summary

Presenting Complaints

"Tired, dizzy spells (2 weeks), need a check-up"

Emotional Status—(Distress)

Appears tense, reports difficulty relaxing, is mildly depressed.

Life Situation (Stresses, support systems)

Health: Hypertension, overweight, "worried about my heart"

Work: Dissatisfied, bored

Marriage: "Not going so good lately. Lot of arguing about kids, money."

Children: Oldest son recently engaged, daughter fighting with dad about independence

Support Systems: Has good friends, especially old army buddies (VFW), an uncle, strong religious commitment. Finances are good.

Personality (Problems, coping resources)

Capable, hardworking, somewhat rigid and compulsive, nonexpressive except for anger, independent. Sees life as a struggle; work as unrewarding, but a duty; himself as OK when productive and in charge of things. Gets angry when others do not see things his way. Coping techniques: routine of hard work, beer with the boys, overeating.

Patient Profile (Summary)

Mr. M. is a 42-year-old white, married male with three children. Frank has been an electrician for 23 years with adequate financial rewards. Basic attitude toward life is one of work and struggle to "get ahead" and maintain what one has. Frank is relatively nonexpressive except when he gets angry. He likes structure and conformity from others. Main supports are work, VFW friends, uncle, and Lutheran religion.

Problem List	Treatment Plan
1. Hypertension	1. Medication for hypertension
2. Overweight	2. Diet program
3. Mild depression	3. Exercise program
4. Work dissatisfaction	4. Periodic blood pressure checks.
5. Marital and family conflicts	5. Interview husband and wife together
6. Somewhat rigid, compulsive person	

Figure 6–1 continued

Typically, the full review takes about 20 minutes. Of course, this time will vary with the nature of the problem and the degree of emotional distress. Return visits may be scheduled to obtain a more complete assessment of the person and his or her situation. The PSR can be adapted to the needs of the situation and the physician's style of practice. For instance, the review could be abbreviated, for example, emotional status and health-work-family situation; other health professionals could gather these data; and questionnaires could be used to obtain some of the information.

Apart from the diagnostic information obtained, the process of identifying problems, needs, and resources with the patient is often therapeutic in itself. Further, it may provide a basis for engaging in further assessment or short-term supportive psychotherapy (Castelnuovo-Tedesco, 1965). A physician who feels that efforts at understanding the patient and his or her situation and at providing support are not productive should seek consultation and consider referral (Conroe, Cassata, and Racer, 1980). In any case, use of the PSR contributes to the development of trust and the patient's acceptance of some form of help.

References

Balint, M. *The Doctor, His Patient and the Illness.* New York: International Universities Press, 1957.

Berger, M.M. *Working with People Called Patients.* New York: Bronner/Mazel, 1977, p. 37.

Caplan, G. *Support Systems and Community Mental Health.* New York: Behavioral Publications, 1974.

Castelnuovo-Tedesco, P. *The Twenty-Minute Hour.* Boston: Little, Brown, 1965.

Conroe, R.M., Cassata, D.M., and Racer, H.J. A systematic approach to brief psychological intervention in the primary care setting. *Journal of Family Practice,* 1980.

Dreikurs, R. *Psychodynamics, Psychotherapy, and Counseling.* Chicago: Alfred Adler Institute, 1967.

Enelow, A.J., and Swisher, S.N. *Interviewing and Patient Care.* New York: Oxford Univ. Press, 1972.

Gillum, R.F., and Barsky, A.J. Diagnosis and management of patient non-compliance. *Journal of the American Medial Association* 228: 1563–1567, 1974.

Holmes, T.H., and Rahe, R.H. The social readjustment rating scale. *Journal of Psychosomatic Research* 11:213–218, 1967.

Kahana, R., and Bibring, G.L. Personality types in medical management. In *Psychiatry and Medical Practice in a General Hospital,* ed. Zinberg N.E. New York: International Universities Press, 1964.

Knapp, M.L. *Nonverbal Communication in Human Interaction.* New York: Holt, Rinehart and Winston, 1972.

Lipowski, Z.J. Psychosocial aspects of disease. *Annals of Internal Medicine* 71:1197–1206, 1969.

McWhinney, I.R. Beyond diagnosis: An approach to the integration of behavioral science and clinical medicine. *New England Journal of Medicine* 287:384–387, 1972.

Mosak, H. Life style assessment: A demonstration focused on family constellation. *Journal of Individual Psychology* 28:232–247, 1972.

Shochet, B.R. Psychological aspects of family practice. *Primary Care* 2:93–108, 1975.

7 Discussing Emotional Etiology for Illness with Medical Patients

Ronald D. Hilliard

Current surveys among practicing family physicians (for example, Werkman et al., 1976; Fisher et al., 1975) indicate that a substantial portion of the physician's time is spent in handling emotional and psychological problems. Often the patient is only vaguely aware of the contribution of emotional factors to his or her condition and comes to the doctor prepared to find a purely physical basis for his or her malady. Communication between doctor and patient often becomes strained (or even broken off) when the physician must share his or her belief with the patient that the latter's distress relates more directly to psychosocial than to physical events. Communication problems also occur when referral to a mental-health specialist is indicated. This chapter outlines productive ways of talking with patients about how their emotions may relate to current physical distress and also discusses considerations involved in referring patients to mental-health practitioners.

Discussing Psychogenic Etiology with Patients

It is important to keep in mind the expectations that the patient holds when consulting the physician. Commonly, the individual is experiencing physical distress for which he or she anticipates medication or definitive physical treatment. The physician typically begins to consider a hypothesis that the patient's illness has a psychogenic basis quite early in the diagnostic procedure. He or she must, at some point, convey this possibility to the patient.

The physician can arouse unnecessary defensiveness on the patient's part (1) by attempting to deny the reality of the symptom, thereby implying that the patient is lying about his or her distress; (2) by creating the impression that the patient's problem cannot be dealt with because the symptom is not discernible on physical examination or by means of laboratory tests; and (3) by using such phrases as, "It's all in your head," "You have a mental problem," or by prematurely suggesting referral to a mental-health practitioner.

Nothing can impede doctor-patient communication more quickly than for the participants to fight about the validity of the patient's complaint. The physician can delineate and clarify the patient's experience, but cannot deny it. It is imperative that the physician and the patient align themselves against the illness rather than allowing the patient and his or her symptoms to line up against the doctor. Exclusive willingness to deal only with the physical side of a patient's distress is at variance with the family-practice philosophy of comprehensive person care.

The following are recommendations for productive ways of discussing psychogenic etiology with patients. The physician typically has available substantial diagnostic information about the patient within the first few minutes of contact. Attention to the patient's style of verbalizing about his or her complaints as well as observation of his or her "body language" alert the physician to the possibility of a "medical psychological" problem. When the physician *begins* to suspect a psychogenic basis for the patient's complaint, he or she should start to lay some "preparatory groundwork" that will help the patient to understand that the physician intends to explore *all* possible contributions to the illness, not merely the physical. This conveys to the patient that he or she is receiving the best possible care and guards against the potentially traumatic introduction of the notion of a psychogenic etiology midway through the diagnostic process.

Empathy refers to the individual's ability and willingness to place himself or herself "in another's shoes" or to actively work at understanding the meaning of another person's communications. Empathy is conveyed by reflective statements (see, for example, Rogers, 1958; Egan, 1975), by means of which the listener restates what the speaker has said. Examples of reflective statements would be the following: "Are you saying that you don't believe your boss realizes how hard you worked on the project?" or "It sounds like you have some mixed feelings about your pregnancy."

Reflective statements on the part of the physician communicate an active interest in the patient's view of his or her situation and serve to assure the interviewer that the information gathered is truly valid. Studies of doctor-patient communication (for example, Korsch and Negrete, 1972) indicate that this rather fundamental aspect of help-intended communication is frequently missing in the medical interview. As a result, patient satisfaction and compliance, as well as the physician's sense of personal satisfaction, are compromised. Reflective physician statements guard against the possibility of the patient aligning himself or herself with his or her symptoms against the doctor.

In line with the idea of active listening is the concept of "reframing" the symptom. By this is meant encouraging the patient to view the symptom as a reflection of his or her body's inherent survival efforts and as a positive protective maneuver the body has mounted in an effort to aid the individual. Thus, rather than perceiving the pain as a loathsome source of irritation, the person can begin to respect his or her body's attempt to signal that "all's not well." Physician statements illustrating the reframing technique are of the following sort:

> "Your body has a sort of primitive alerting system that serves to let you know when something is going on that is not in your best interest. I am glad that you are paying attention to this signal and that we have been able to talk about it. Since your headache starts when you are on your way home each evening, I wonder if it is signaling you that something is going on at home that is upsetting you."

> "Your body seems to recognize a source of stress that you may or may not yet be aware of. I would like to suggest that you think of your rash as a sort of natural signal from your body that something is wrong— your body works in your own best interest and seems to be telling you that something is making you uncomfortable right now. I would like for you to think about what message your body is sending and we can talk about it next week."

Some educative comments also may be helpful concerning individual bodily differences in channeling stress. An inherent part of the reframing technique is to credit the patient for paying attention to bodily cues and knowing when to seek help.

The physician's sharing a personal experience with tension-related somatic distress also may be helpful in this regard. For example, "I recall when I was preparing for my Board Certification Examination, I had a cold that lasted for two months! I was miserable! And immediately after finishing the exams my cold disappeared."

Another important consideration in conveying the idea of psychogenic etiology has to do with timing: avoid introducing too much information too soon. In patients with "medical psychological problems," it is sensible to carry out diagnostic efforts over a period of several visits, so as to allow the patient (once he or she has the idea of psychogenic cause) to reflect on the specific aspects of his or her life that may be stressful. The physician can gradually move from a diagnostic to a supportive counseling approach with the patient once the underlying sources of stress are understood by the patient.

Occasionally, patients will attribute their illness to "nerves" or will request antianxiety medication in order to alleviate distress. The physician can err by too readily assuming that the illness is exclusively referable to psychogenic factors, thereby failing to diagnose an underlying disease process. This caveat simply reiterates the *comprehensive* nature of the family physician's diagnostic efforts.

Considerations in Referring Patients to Mental-Health Practitioners

Although the recognition of psychogenic etiology is not an automatic indicator for referral, the physician may believe that a particular patient could profit from the assistance of a psychologist, psychiatrist, or social worker. Referrals to mental-health practitioners for psychotherapy are similar to those involving other specialists, and depend on the following principles for their success.

The patient's utmost fear in being referred to another practitioner is that his or her family doctor is thereby abandoning him or her. Thus it is imperative that the family physician convey to the patient that his or her interest in and concern for the patient will continue. Such continuity can be signaled by the physician's request to contact the psychotherapist to "introduce" the patient and also to inquire at periodic intervals as to the progress the patient is making in the therapeutic process.

Mental-health practitioners, like other specialists, differ in terms of their personality styles, fee structure, and preferred approach to problems. Thus, for example, psychotherapists differ according to personal characteristics (namely, age, sex, religious preference, race), theoretical approach (for example, client-centered, hypnosis, Gestalt therapy, and so forth), and preferred treatment modality (for example, family therapy, group therapy, biofeedback). In addition, community agencies perform distinct mental-health functions. In view of such diversity, it behooves the family practitioner to establish good working relationships with likely referral resources so that the "match" between patient and referral agent is optimal. Often it is helpful to discuss with the patient what characteristics he or she feels are important in a therapist and attempt to respect these wishes in making the referral.

In order to bridge the referral successfully, the patient must know such basic data as where the therapist's office or agency is located, how fees are structured, and some description of the therapeutic process itself. The attitude of the physician regarding the potential helpfulness of a mental-health specialist is inevitably conveyed to the patient. Research studies of the determinants of "successful" psychotherapy (Frank, 1961; Abroms, 1968) have shown rather clearly that patient expectations regarding the potential value of psychotherapy affect resultant outcomes. The patient will detect a desire on the physician's part to "dump the turkey" and understandably abort the referral. Similarly, such indirect messages as "It probably won't do any good, but . . ." are quickly sensed and weaken the referral endeavor. Since the patient typically respects his or her doctor's opinion, it is valuable for the physician to offer the referral in a genuine sense of hopefulness and optimism, as this will enhance the patient's expectations of the psychotherapeutic process.

References

Abroms, G.M. Persuasion in psychotherapy. *American Journal of Psychiatry* 124: 1214, 1968.

Egan, G. *The Skilled Helper.* Monterey, Calif.: Brooks/Cole, 1975.

Fisher, J.V. Mason, R.L., and Fisher, J.C., Emotional illness and the family physician. *Psychosomatics* 16: 55, 1975.

Frank, J.D. *Persuasion and Healing. A Comparative Study of Psychotherapy.* Baltimore, Md.: Johns Hopkins Press, 1961.

Korsch, B.M., and Negrete, V.F. Doctor-patient communication. *Scientific American* 227: 66, 1972.

Rogers, C.R. The characteristics of a helping relationship. *Personnel and Guidance Journal* 37: 6, 1958.

Werkman, S.L., Mallory, L., and Harris, J. The common psychiatric problems in family practice. *Psychosomatics* 17:119, 1972.

8 Psychological Factors in Emergency Medical Services

Elaine Wustman

One need only sit in an emergency room for a matter of minutes to sense the degree to which stress and tension prevail for all involved. Patients and family, generally attempting to cope with anxiety and fear of illness, injury, or any of a number of crisis situations are faced with long waits, hospital red tape, and a staff whose primary goal is rapid diagnosis, treatment, and discharge. The result is patient hostility and regression.

Staff, however, often able to cope with the most critical of medical and traumatic crises, become agitated at the first signs of rage, grief, or hysteria. These responses require time and energy from a staff already pressured by the number of patients waiting, the limited number of available rooms and personnel, and the continual unpredictability of the arrival of the next critical case. Therefore, such responses, although normal, interfere with emergency room operations and frustrate staff in meeting their goal.

Additionally, patient anger and resentment are frequently manifested by attacks on the staff's self-esteem and dignity. Although intellectually staff may be able to recognize that patient hostility is not directed at them personally, anxieties and fears about their own image of themselves as competent controlled professionals are often unrecognized and unaccepted. Thus they respond as angry parents to the demanding regressed patient and the process is then perpetuated. This result is compounded when both patient and staff carry this unresolved anger and hostility into subsequent interactions. At times one senses throughout the emergency room that a war is being waged between staff and patients.

The fact that this process is avoidable is evidenced by the dramatic and calming effect achieved when patients or family are provided with a suitable place and a calm, concerned individual whereby they are able to ventilate feelings, explore their origin, and consider alternatives. Mutual staff support and reassurance are also required. However, often they are unavailable owing to busy work schedules and interpersonal problems among personnel. There is an apparent need for regularly scheduled staff groups wherein feelings can be explored and recognized, support given, and problems worked through. This too is difficult given the unpredictable nature of the emergency room.

The role of psychological factors in emergency medical services take on even greater significance when one examines the involvement of emergency departments in current and changing trends of health-care delivery. Originally emergency rooms were primarily "accident" rooms treating only physical trauma and acute medical illness. Thus they were designed to implement such services and often administrated by surgeons. However, within the last three decades, visits to emergency rooms have increased dramatically [1-6, 9], as demonstrated in Figure 8-1 [7]. In addition, this increase is several times that of inpatient or outpatient medical services [8]. The trend for community utilization of the emergency room and its staff as primary deliverers of health and social services is apparent. This is reflected in the facts that even those patients having private physicians tend to bypass their services and come to emergency rooms instead [9, 10, 14], and approximately half of emergency visits are for objectively nonurgent problems [8, 11-13].

Given the disadvantages of emergency room use for ambulatory care, that is, inconsistent and unfamiliar doctors without knowledge of a patient's background, unavailability of records with concomitant excessive use of laboratory and radiological studies, impersonal care, long waiting times, and little to no follow-up, one questions the motivation behind emergency room utilization. Low socioeconomic status, security of the hospital setting, and inaccessibility or perceived inaccessibility of private physicians are part of the picture [7, 14].

However, the more central issue appears to be the presence of and need for assistance with psychosocial problems. Although only a minority of patients (between 2 and 10 percent) initially verbalize such concerns, upon further exploration it has been found that as many as two-thirds come not for primary treatment of physical problems, but as a result of psychological stress [14, 15]. These patients tend to have multiple and vague chief complaints not limited to one body system, and in fact, the severity and nature of the patient's complaint has been found to be unrelated to the decision to seek medical care [14, 16, 17]. More specifically, studies investigating emergency unit patients' perceptions of recent stressful life events and their relationship to presenting symptomotology not only validate recent stressors as the major predictor of the presenting picture in the emergency room, but also indicate a significant relationship between the degree to which an individual is adapting to stressful life events and his or her perception of the severity of his or her medical problems [14, 18]. The degree of adaptation is a function of both severity of a stress and the total number of stresses. It should be noted that any life change, regardless of its desirability, evokes an adaptation response. Furthermore, no relationship was found between life-change unit scores and physician's perceptions of the severity of the presenting problem [18]. These data, then, account for the enormous discrepancy between emergency room physician and patient perceptions of illness. Thus a decision to seek emergency medical care is frequently the result of a

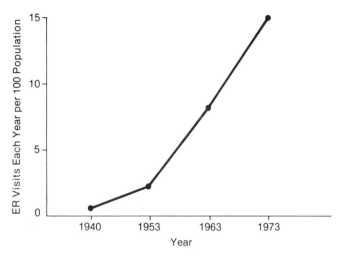

Figure 8–1. Rise in Emergency Room Use, Southside Hospital, Bay Shore, New York, 1940–1973

crisis situation that by nature requires urgent action. As well as a direct result of stress, the high incidence of physical complaints associated with psychiatric problems also may be due to a deterioration in self-maintenance habits, such as diet and sleep, secondary to the presence of stress. An additional explanation lies in the perception of the public that only through physical illness can one make entry into the health-care system.

In fact, this perception may be well founded. For although community utilization of emergency rooms has evolved to demand a greater provision of psychological services and expertise, emergency room operations and personnel do not reflect the same evolution and thus are unequipped to meet such demands.

The attitude of emergency medical staff is rooted in the antiquated concept of the emergency room, whereby their professional commitment lies in providing emergency medical care to the critically ill and injured. In response to definable medical emergencies, they are oriented to action of an overt kind, which produces immediate observable results. It is in such situations that medical personnel come to see their finest hour. In fact, emergency medicine, when compared with other specialties and as characterized by emergency physicians, was found to be most like surgery and least like psychiatry [19].

Additionally, provision of emergency care to critical patients demands a continual preparedness for the next unannounced emergency that may "roll" in. This requires an available reserve of time and energy and an attempt to provide quick yet comprehensive care so that patients can be moved through rapidly. Furthermore, this emphasis on rapid assessment is facilitated by the emergent nature of critical cases. Therefore, the more exploratory approach required in relation to psychological problems necessitates a marked change of pace. Families of patients must be included in the process as well, since they are considered a hindrance to treatment by taking up staff time with continual questions and requests and manipulation to remain with the patient, as well as other "nonessential" demands.

This discrepancy between public and staff perceptions of roles has a significant effect on both groups. Frustration and resultant hostility are generated in the staff, who view such patients as either ignorant, in not realizing the true purpose of an emergency room, or self-indulgent, in using the emergency room as a means of avoiding clinic waiting lines or private physicians, thus glutting the emergency unit with inappropriate cases. In response, personnel tend to dismiss such cases as "crocks," or if they deal with at all, perfunctorily refer them to a mental-health facility. This reflects a further complication of dealing with mixed physical and emotional problems in an emergency room.

There is a tendency to dichotomize patients, whereby once a patient is labeled "psych," physical complaints are ignored as being nonurgent or false or, as is more often the case, little attention is paid to emotional factors involved in medical illness. The result is not only failure to meet the patient's needs, but a dangerous interference with the patient's ability to obtain necessary treatment. In this regard, patients with psychiatric histories are at greatest risk [20].

Incidents of acute medical crises or traumatic injury, in themselves, create particular psychological stress for patients, for their families, and although consistent with their values and role perceptions, for staff.

Strain [21] describes seven categories of psychological stress to which anxiety in the acutely ill patient may be attributed:

1. A threat to narcissistic integrity.
2. A fear of strangers.
3. Separation anxiety.
4. Fear of loss of love and approval.
5. Fear of loss of control of bodily functions and emotions.
6. Fear of loss of, or injury to, body parts.
7. Feelings of guilt and shame with fears of retaliation for past mistakes.

It is not difficult to realize how such stresses may be evoked by the emergency room experience. As the patient rolls in strapped to a gurney, he or she is announced not by name, but by the nature and severity of his or her physical problems. He or she is abruptly separated from family or friends and placed in a totally alien and frantically fast-paced environment, where he or she is poked, prodded, and questioned, if able to communicate, by numerous strangers. Additionally, severe pain, which often cannot be relieved by medication until a diagnosis is determined (since analgesics mask symptoms), decreases his or her ability to cope with other stresses. However, the degree of pain a patient perceives is also directly affected by his or her ability to maintain adequate defenses against the other stresses operating.

Of course, the ultimate fear of such patients is that of impending death and the unknown dimension which that represents. There is one certainty— no matter who is around, he or she will ultimately experience it alone. This may be the first time in his or her life that he or she has truly been confronted with the reality of mortality. Thus in a matter of minutes or hours the patient must go from being functional and feeling well to being critically ill and facing the possibility of death or long-term residual effects.

The primary objectives of psychological intervention for both patient and family, who have experienced or anticipate a major loss, is the facilitation of expression of grief and reduction of anxiety produced by other stresses. Initiation of the process of grief and mourning and proper management of grief reactions in the emergency room lay the groundwork for a healthy mourning process later on. *Grief* consists of a series of emotional responses that typically follow the realization or anticipation of the loss of a valued object. *Mourning* refers to the psychological processes necessary to overcome the objective state of grief that usually leads to a giving up of the object. Loss of a valued object applies to any situation in which the valued object is rendered inaccessible to the person or is altered in such a way that it no longer has certain qualities that were valued. Grief is not a negative response to be resisted or avoided, but a normal mechanism of release and restoration.

Acute grief will be evidenced over a period of several months. However, the initial reaction of shock, disbelief, and denial will be expressed in the emergency department, if that is where the person's first realization occurs. Characteristically, this stage of grief and mourning consists of a stunned numbness and a refusal to accept or comprehend what has happened. A common example is the acute trauma victim's refusal of treatment as he or she continually attempts to climb off the gurney to go home. Moreover, the patient or relative may accept the situation intellectually while denying emotional impact in an attempt to protect himself or herself from overwhelming feelings. A family member may busily make arrangements, attempt to comfort others, and appear to be managing everything appropriately. This is accompanied by the presence of somatic sensations, such as tightness in the throat, an empty feeling in the abdomen, loss of appetite, and loss of strength. These symptoms may last from 20 minutes to an hour at a time. The sensorium is also altered, whereby there is at least a slight sense of unreality and increased emotional distance from people. In addition, there is an associated feeling of guilt. Patients ask themselves "Why me?" and frequently arrive at the answer of retribution for past wrongs. Families search for evidence of failure to do right by the loved one, for example, not having provided appropriate prehospital treatment, not being present at the time of death, not having reconciled old feelings of anger. Current anger may be expressed by their perception of the senselessness and unfairness of the injury, illness, or death.

For the patient, a realization of loss may not occur in the emergency room, but later on, owing to a disturbance in thought processes from the physical condition or from analgesic medication. Additionally, many of the stresses described earlier cannot be relieved because of the realities of the emergency room and the priority for diagnosis and immediate initiation of life-saving measures. However, since the patient's primary support system, his or her significant others, is unavailable to him or her, medical staff must provide the necessary support and reassurance. Continual explanation of procedures and protection of the patient's dignity are critical. In addition, an available person to function as a link or message carrier between family and patient can help to relieve anxiety from separation and fear of loss of love. Arrangements to have the family rejoin the patient should be made as soon as major medical procedures are completed.

The focus of psychological intervention in a medical-crisis situation is on the patient's family, and it begins as soon as the patient arrives in the emergency room. If family have not accompanied the patient, it is probable that they will have to be notified. In accident cases in which the police have been involved, notification of the family is usually performed by the police, who go to the family's home and provide transportation to the hospital when indicated. In all other situations, this is the responsibility of the staff member providing psychological management of the case. Telephone notification begins with the staff member identifying himself or herself and the institution slowly and distinctly, followed by a verification of the person's relationship to the patient. A brief explanation of the situation is given without voluntary announcement of death, if that is the case. It is preferable to postpone notification of death until the family is in the secure, supportive hospital setting, particularly for elderly significant others and those alone and without immediate supports. Emphasis on the importance of caution in coming to the hospital, is helpful since everything possible is being done to help their relative and their being there will not affect that. The relative will already be in a degree of shock at this point; therefore, assistance in problem solving or making arrangements with transportation, directions, and accompaniment may be necessary.

Whether the situation is death, trauma, or serious medical illness, families are faced with the loss of a loved one as he or she existed prior to this incident. Of course, the severity of the medical crisis, that is, the degree to which the patient risks death or will suffer resultant deficits, affects the degree of coping required. Therefore, clear, accurate, and comprehensive communication with the family regarding the patient's condition, procedures being employed, and medical plans and alternatives is critical. As is always the case, communication should be geared to the family's assessed level of medical sophistication. Families who are left alone and not given such information have only their fantasies (for example, "Maybe he's dying," "Maybe its really nothing and he'll be able to go home"), thereby increasing anxiety and helplessness and delaying their process of coping with realistic possibilities. It is also important to obtain information from the family and to relay it to medical personnel for assistance in diagnosis and treatment. This includes recent and past medical problems, current medications, allergies, and an eyewitness description of the onset or injury.

The location of the family is another significant issue. They require a quiet private room, out of visual range of the trauma or treatment area, to be able to talk and express feelings freely. In addition, access to a private telephone is necessary, and families should be encouraged to call significant others in order to mobilize their support system.

In dealing with the family's response, attention should be given to the presence of denial. Denial should not be confronted directly, since it is a normal reaction to the shock from loss and may be the only or best coping mechanism available to that family member at the time. Careful repetition of the reality of the situation does not encourage denial, but makes the information available for the person to accept at a rate tolerable to him or her. An overly fearful response should be explored for its origin. Frequently, such responses reflect unfinished or unresolved feelings related to some past experience. A discussion of the family member's past may uncover such an experience, and this provides an opportunity for clarifying and distinguishing the past events from the present situation.

In general, encouragement to express feelings of grief in their own way without judgment is the important factor. Asking questions about what their relative was like prior to the incident may help to initiate grieving and may provide information from which to determine the extent to which their lifestyle will be forced to change and thus the degree of loss and adaptation with which they will have to cope. Cultural background and the value system of the family also will affect their responses and should be respected. However, in cases where those values are a burden to the family and frustrate grieving rather than being a support in finding meaning in the event, a more therapeutic interpretation should be offered. There is a tendency, particularly for those in the medical professions, to want to ease the pain of acute grief with medication. This impulse should be resisted, since only when the pain is fully experienced will the individual be able to move through the mourning process to resolution. Therefore, sedation only serves to postpone the grief reaction, not relieve it. However, when the reaction is one of hysteria that does not subside with intervention, medication may be used to decrease the disorganization and confusion, so the individual can proceed consciously and thoughtfully to deal with the issues of the loss involved.

It is important that the treating physician talk with the family. If this does not occur, the family may have lingering unspoken doubts about the quality of care that was given their relative or if a physician was present at all. In cases of death, relatives frequently have questions for the person present at the time of death, such as, "Did he say anything?" and "Was he in pain?" A discussion with the physician prior to contact with the family both prepares him or her for the situation he or she is to encounter and assists him or her in making the transition from the hectic pace of the medical setting to the calm concerned atmosphere necessary. The physician should be informed of what relatives and friends are present, their current understanding and response thus far, and any clarification or reassurance needed. Laypeople are often intimidated when talking with physicians, so they may need encouragement to ask any questions they may have or may need to be reminded of questions asked earlier.

Medical personnel frequently have difficulty explaining death to relatives for reasons that will be discussed later. As a result, their interaction with the family may be quick and blunt, leaving the relatives confused and angry. Excessive apologies, however, may be interpreted by the bereaved as apologies for the care given rather than the occurance itself. This approach also has a tendency to elicit sympathy and support from the family, who need it themselves. The most helpful approach appears to be a gentle but factual description of the events in chronological order. It should be slow, clear, and unambiguous, including the words *dead* or *died* in order to prevent perpetuation of denial.

Hospital rituals may serve to confirm the reality of death as well. The question of autopsy and the involvement of the coroner (when there is no recently seen private physician to confirm cause of death), the collection and release and the deceased's personal belongings, notification of the other family members, and the decision of a funeral home will all have to be confronted. Bereaved families may request, or should be offered, the option of viewing the body, again as confirmation of reality. They may feel it for heat, listen to the chest for a heartbeat, or look for movement. However, this should be solely their decision based on their needs, feelings, and value system. Intervention includes only a discussion of the possible consequences of viewing or not viewing, and they should not be swayed in either direction. The body should be prepared for viewing by removal of tubes and equipment, cleansing of blood, and draping of badly mutilated areas. However, it may be left in the room to indicate medical care was provided. Privacy at that time is important; therefore, accompanying them while remaining at a distance is appropriate.

Family members of patients admitted to the hospital following emergency treatment require information regarding future medical plans and events to anticipate. Concrete problem solving and planning for the next 24 to 48 hours may be necessary, since there is a tendency to ignore personal needs such as food, sleep, or private time to reconstitute. Deprivation of basic needs will eventually result in a decreased capacity for coping. Additionally, outside stresses and obligations create a further expenditure of energy and therefore should be discussed and means to decrease them explored.

Although acute medical crises are considered by emergency room personnel to be legitimate and consistent with their perception of an emergency department and of their professional role, such incidents create often ignored stress reactions in all personnel involved.

Clerks are faced with the initial contact with the family members, who are requesting information the clerks do not have and are not permitted to provide. Furthermore, it is their responsibility to ask highly stressed families routine and seemingly irrelevant questions. They are aware that they may be compounding the family's stress and feel helpless in the face of the family's fear and pain. To defend against this, they often maintain a high degree of detachment and objectivity, which may be perceived as cold, insensitive, and uncaring.

Doctors and nurses, as mentioned previously, are forced to be prepared for the event of a medical crisis at all times, no matter how busy or tired they are. Stresses of routine emergency room practice, that is, rapid diagnosis and treatment without a medical history and full knowledge of the patient, become intensified. They must work closely together as a team in which errors in judgment and interpersonal conflicts can have disastrous effects.

Strain [21] describes stresses to which personnel are vulnerable as similar to those experienced by the patient, although often defended against by unconscious feelings of omnipotence. The patient whose condition does not improve may threaten the staff's sense of narcissistic integrity. Continual contact with unfamiliar patients and families, from whom they wish love and admiration, may revive a fear of strangers. Identification with patients who must undergo mutilating procedures or death may evoke in a staff member feelings of guilt, shame, and fear of his or her own death. If the critical caregiver does not possess the self-knowledge necessary to recognize and cope with such stresses, feelings may find expression in an image of himself or herself as a powerful healer, an indestructible force, and/or destructive force. Thus he or she may continually feel that he or she has not done enough and either overtreat the patient or blame other staff members for a patient's deterioration. As identification becomes more intense (with similarity in age, ethnicity, and so forth), judgment becomes less objective, and the ability to deal directly with the family and patient decreases. Included in omnipotence is the power to destroy. Such feelings result in failure to institute appropriate aggressive medical treatment or reluctance to talk with the patient or family for fear of harmful effects. The inappropriate approaches to families mentioned earlier are examples of the expression of such problems.

It is apparent that whether psychological stress is the underlying causative factor in a perceived medical emergency or actual acute physical illness, injury, or death is resultant in severe psychological stress, the majority of patients in the emergency room are in need of psychological intervention. However, owing to numerous factors, including time constraints and a lack of psychological sophistication, health-care practitioners are unequipped to meet such needs. An exploration of the theory and practice of crisis intervention evidences that these patients are, in fact, in a state of crisis and that crisis intervention is an appropriate model for treatment in an emergency room.

Caplan [22] postulates that in the face of an emotional hazard, there are adaptive and maladaptive methods of attempting to cope with the problem that have a major influence on later adjustment and ability to cope. An *emotional hazard* is defined as a loss or threatened loss of a significant relationship, introduction of new individuals into one's social sphere, or transition in social status or role relationships. *Crisis* is a person's internal reaction to an external hazard and is characterized by disequilibrium, increased anxiety, and depression, with disorganized and fluctuating coping mechanisms.

Everyone is on a mental-health continuum and typically in a state of relative equilibrium. When in crisis, an individual is not quite as healthy on the continuum because he or she is in an unstable state. When the crisis is resolved, equilibrium may be reestablished at a lower or higher point on the mental-health continuum. The individual who successfully resolves a crisis is likely to emerge healthier than before, and vice versa. Therefore, crisis is both a danger and an opportunity for growth.

Individuals encounter hazardous situations with relative frequency in their everyday lives, and they are typically solved by means of previously learned coping techniques. However, a crisis develops when either the problem is greater than experienced previously, when it corresponds significantly to a problem area within the individual, or when previous problem-solving mechanisms are unsuitable. Additionally, between the perceived effects of a stressful situation and resolution of the problem there are three balancing factors that determine the state of equilibrium. These are a realistic perception of the event, adequate situational supports, and adequate coping mechanisms. When any one or more of these factors are absent, a crisis will ensue.

There are four phases in a crisis that typically will resolve positively or negatively within 4 to 6 weeks. The first is the impact of the stimulus or hazard, which is characterized by tension, an unpleasant affect, and disorganization of behavior. In the first phase, the individual calls forth habitual problem-solving techniques in an attempt to regain the previous state of equilibrium. In the second phase, a lack of success in phase 1 results in continuation of the stimulus and thus a further rise in tension. In the third phase, tension reaches a point where it mobilizes additional internal and external resources and a use of emergency problem-solving techniques. In this stage, the problem may abate in intensity, it may be defined in different ways, or certain goals may be given up as unattainable. If the problem continues and cannot be solved by need satisfaction or avoided by giving up goals or perceptual distortion, the individual moves into stage 4—major disorganization.

There are a number of key implications arising out of this theory. First, the person in crisis is ripe for change in a relatively short time because of his or her disequilibrium and the extreme tension he or she is experiencing. Therefore, a minimal amount of force exerted by a family member, therapist, or care-giving agent can govern the outcome of the crisis to a significant degree. Second, a crisis repeats important features of a person's emotional struggles, but the outcome is not determined by this, and current psychological forces play a large role. Third, equilibrium following a crisis may be reestablished at a lower or a higher point in the mental-health continuum. A crisis may have widespread results in the adjustment and coping capacity of the individual in future crises and in his or her overall adjustment to life. Factors affecting the outcome include physical health, choices made on significant variables, chance, and availability of resources. Also of influence are personal factors, such as the extent to which the crisis situation is dynamically linked to parallel problems of the past, cultural influences, and others [23].

Crisis intervention is extremely short term, since time is at a premium. It is directed to resolution of the problem only and does not deal with material not directly related to the crisis. The caregiver takes an active, but not a directive, role, and the goal is explicit—return of the individual's level of functioning to a precrisis or better than precrisis level. The steps or phases of intervention are as follows.

1. Assessment of the individual and the problem. The individual is initially assessed for suicidal or homocidal potential, and when this is present,

he or she is referred directly to a psychiatrist for hospitalization. The caregiver actively explores the current situation in order to identify the precipitating event and the resulting crisis. Little attention is paid to the case history not directly related. Ask the following: What is the most recent threat, challenge, or loss that has caused the present disequilibrium? What is new in your ongoing situation? When did you begin to feel worse or acutely upset? Who is the significant person or persons involved in the crisis? What is the immediate problem, as differentiated from the basic problem?

2. Planned therapeutic intervention. The caregiver determines the degree of disruption in the individual's life and the effects it has on others in his or her social orbit. He or she assesses the strengths the individual possesses, support persons available, and coping mechanisms used in the past that are not presently useful. He or she also examines alternative coping mechanisms available. The caregiver listens for mention of situations in the person's past even symbolically analogous to the current predicament. Ask about similar problems encountered earlier in life. What is the impasse brought about by the new element? Why can the patient not handle the present problem by previously used mechanisms, for example, regression, denial, withdrawal, or projection. The caregiver formulates the dynamics of the current situation as thoroughly as possible.

3. Intervention that is flexible and creative. The goal is helping the individual gain intellectual understanding of his or her crisis and the relationship between the hazardous situation and his or her discomfort. The caregiver describes the crisis and its relationship to events in the person's life. The person is assisted to bring into the open present feelings to which he or she may not have access, for example, denial of angry feelings toward a lost object. The caregiver may suggest alternative coping mechanisms, but he or she never directs the person, since that must be the person's choice.

4. Anticipatory planning. If the last intervention has been successful, the patient will show a marked increase in his or her ability to cope and thus a decrease in anxiety and depression. Lend appropriate support to the patient's new efforts at solving his or her now defined problem.

The caregiver should be prepared to find that in many instances the patient does not desire or require further professional help after equilibrium is restored. For others, consider referral for further treatment, looking for evidence of long-standing problems together with clear motivation and goals, as well as available community resources.

Crisis intervention is a form of primary psychiatric prevention whereby individuals who would not normally require or accept psychiatric treatment can deal with a crisis situation before frank psychopathology results. The emergency room is an ideal location for such measures, since, as we have seen, the crisis often originates there and it is a commonly utilized emergency coping mechanism. Furthermore, the techniques do not require extensive knowledge of psychodynamics; therefore, they can be employed in a short time by a health-care practitioner with a knowledge of specific situational and maturational crises.

For example, in the case of loss or threatened loss of a loved one, it is necessary to know that an expression of grief is necessary for resolution and that feelings of guilt and anger are associated with loss. Exploration of previous losses and coping mechanisms used were discussed earlier. Anticipatory planning includes recalling past losses that were successfully dealt with, an explanation of the process of grief and mourning, and open discussion of the effects of the loss on one's life. In those cases in which the only presenting complaint is physical symptoms, identification of the precipitating event will be necessary. However, through crisis-intervention techniques the individual will gain an understanding of the origin of those symptoms and how they relate to the crisis situation. Furthermore, one must consider application of crisis-intervention principles in relation to other cases in the emergency room, such as suicide attempts, abortions, rape, and so forth.

There are other emergency room patients for whom the term *crisis* does not apply. However, a description of psychological factors in emergency medical services would be incomplete without discussing them. These patients are particularly difficult for staff to deal with because they bring forth a sense of frustration and futility. They are characterized by chronicity and an apparent lack of motivation to follow through on referrals and thereby help themselves. Thus these patients tend to evoke social and moral judgments on the part of doctors and nurses. Furthermore, the severe management problem they often present to the emergency room is significant since this creates disruption of the routine flow of patient care.

Chronic alcoholics and drug abusers meet all the preceding criteria. Attitudes of emergency room personnel toward alcoholics and drug abusers are well described in the literature [24, 25]. Their passive-dependent personality styles and tendencies toward manipulation make them the antithesis of what emergency room personnel consider a "good patient." Furthermore, their behavior is extremely disruptive, since they are uncooperative, abusive, and, at times, physically dangerous, thus requiring security personnel and physical restraints. Again, the most significant factor is the amount of staff time they consume. Because they are unpredictable and unsafe, personnel are required to remain with them constantly, which is often unpleasant, since they are frequently unkempt, malodorous, and difficult to be reasoned with. All procedures and treatments seem to take twice as long with these patients as with others.

Furthermore, the clinical picture of these cases is unclear, since their change in mental status prevents them from giving an adequate medical history and their drugged state tends to mask other symptoms. Knowing that these patients frequently have multiple medical problems, the physician is left with the dilemma of whether or not to obtain extensive laboratory and radiological studies, which are expensive (since few of these patients are able to pay for their medical care) and time-consuming. Since the staff's need to remove these patients from the emergency room as quickly as possible is even greater than with others, the physician's decision becomes one of determining the need for hospitalization and thus immediate transfer to an inpatient unit (preferably to another facility) or home. Patients who are not hospitalized become difficult disposition problems owing to their poor social system and lack of money.

The degree of psychological problems, particularly the incidence of suicide, in these patients is high, although rarely addressed by staff. Even if concerns are present, few emergency rooms are equipped with space and staff to keep such patients long enough to mentally clear so that a psychiatric evaluation can be provided.

Another group of problem patients is the "repeaters" or "regulars." Every emergency room has its own list of patients who "abuse" the emergency room by using it as their primary social system, as other people use bars, restaurants, neighborhood drug stores, or friends. These people appear to find the hospital setting and the emergency room staff a source of security, support, and relief from the loneliness of their world. However, few are able to verbalize this. Because their attachments are to a medical facility, most have a standard set of physical complaints with which they present to make entry, although some vary from visit to visit. Nevertheless, on physical examination all such complaints are consistently medically unfounded. The problem exists in the refusal of these patients to accept any psychological help or to even admit that this is a possible contributing factor to their regular and frequent visits. Referrals to mental-health facilities are futile and, in fact, often evoke intense anger and frustration. Referrals to private medical physicians are accepted, but never followed through.

Included in this category is a group of psychiatric patients, who, as part of their pathology, find it difficult to follow through on referrals or to maintain contact with one therapist for any length of time. Consequently, they use the emergency room to provide treatment. As with medical patients, the inconsistency and variability of emergency room physicians can provide only substandard care and does nothing to help these patients with their problems in maintaining intimate relationships. Thus their loneliness and detachment continue. However, in the majority of cases, these patients do not meet the criteria for involuntary hospitalization and therefore cannot be forced to obtain appropriate treatment.

Because of the basic reason why these people come to the emergency room, as described earlier, they tend to demand a great deal of attention.

Their waiting time is grueling for other patients and family as well as for staff owing to the disruption caused and continual requests made. In addition to being uncooperative, these patients are usually unappreciative as well, since neither their psychological needs nor their perceived medical needs are ever met.

Needless to say, the frustration evoked in staff is enormous. To deal with this frustration and in an attempt to communicate to the patient the inappropriateness of his or her emergency room visits, personnel resort to verbal abuse and frequently are forced to have the patient escorted out of the emergency room by security personnel. This treatment does not appear to affect these patients, since they continue to return. It seems that negative attention is better than none at all. These cases are particularly difficult, since personnel can truly provide nothing for them without reinforcing their behavior. Furthermore, although staff members are aware that there is no basis to the physical complaints of these people, there is a legal issue involved in refusing them medical evaluation. This problem is compounded when the patient has a medical history consistent with his or her complaints, for example, the patient with heart disease who complains of chest pain. The result is an exorbitant expenditure of wasted staff time and energy. The situation is somewhat improved when the doctor treating the patient knows the case from previous visits. However, this is usually not the case, since emergency room physicians rotate so frequently. The patient's past medical record can be ordered, although it is usually voluminous and physicians are forced to wade through a series of emergency room visit reports in order to comprehend the situation and feel comfortable not doing an extensive workup.

The best solution appears to be the formulation of an emergency room "repeater file," wherein each of these patients has a chart containing a general summary of the case, a list of previous visits with dates, chief complaint, findings, and treatment, and most important, a treatment plan. The treatment plan must be agreed on by both physicians and nurses, with a detailed description of the minimal amount of medical care legally and ethically accepted, with a primary emphasis on psychological treatment. Psychiatric consultation in developing that portion of the plan is appropriate. As with any long-term patient, the treatment plan should be regularly evaluated and updated. This approach has a number of positive effects. It simplifies and decreases the time medical personnel must spend with the patient, provides optimal and consistent treatment, and decreases personnel frustration, since they now have something very specific they can do to help the patient. In addition, since these patients often use more than one emergency room, treatment plans can be communicated to other facilities, thus providing communitywide coordination and consistency.

However, there are potential risks to this approach that must be cautiously guarded against. For example, the fact that these patients are "repeaters" does not preclude their developing actual serious medical problems or exacerbation of their present minor ones. In an effort to strictly comply with the designed plan of approach, such problems may be overlooked or ignored. Therefore, the treatment plan regarding evaluation must reflect this consideration. Furthermore, there are patients who, after initial treatment in the emergency room, return numerous times owing to inadequate assessment and/or treatment or inappropriate referral. Personnel not willing to look at possible deficiencies in previously given care become frustrated. Because a repeater file exists, they are quick to refer such patients after only a few frequent visits. This is particularly the case with patients for whom medical personnel have neglected to assess the psychological problems underlying the medical complaints. However, when assessed and referred appropriately to mental-health facilities, these patients follow through with the referral and are not seen in the emergency room again. This illustrates the importance of a thorough evaluation of the patient and his or her history and treatment over a period of time prior to entry into the repeater file.

It is interesting that even in the emergency room setting, with its strong adherance to an arbitrary professional definition of its purpose and goals, patients' and families' priorities of needs show through. Supposedly, societal values dictate health-care practices; however, emergency medicine appears slow to respond to the clearly communicated psychological needs of the community. Until there is a structural reorganization whereby the hospital setting can provide 24-hour-a-day availability of an alternative to the trauma and acute-care facility, emergency rooms are faced with providing extensive psychological services.

Accordingly, emergency-medicine physicians and nurses are faced with a redefinition of their professional roles. The likely place to begin is academia. Medical and nursing schools are going to have to discard their compartmentalized concept of human beings and begin to view them as a whole—mind and body. More specifically, emergency-medical and nursing education must reflect as its goal the creation of professionals particularly skilled in psychological assessment and crisis intervention as well as having the necessary tolerance for the psychological stresses mentioned earlier. In this way, professionals unequipped for or uninterested in such areas of practice may appropriately choose other specialties, thus reducing the presently existing resistances to these changes.

Emergency room administration also has a responsibility in promoting a philosophy of care and enforcing expectations of staff to provide comprehensive assessment and treatment. Staffing patterns must be such that doctors and nurses are permitted the time necessary for psychological intervention. Furthermore, the physical plan of the emergency room must reflect attention to psychological needs by providing quiet rooms for the patient or family to comfortably talk with staff and a padded safe room for patients requiring seclusion and/or restraints. There is a further need to employ personnel trained in other than just emergency medicine, for example, psychologists, psychiatrists, social workers, psychiatric nurses, and clergy. These are extensive and seemingly expensive revisions. However, when one considers the resultant increase in efficiency and quality of emergency medical services, the value is apparent.

References

1. Alpert, J.J., et al. The types of families that use an emergency clinic. *Medical Care* 7: 55–61, 1969.

2. Jacobs, A.R., Govett, J.W., and Wersinger, R. Emergency department utilization in an urban community. *Journal of the American Medical Association* 216: 307–312, 1971.

3. Kluge, D.N., Wegryn, R.L., and Lemley, B.R. The expanding emergency department. *Journal of the American Medical Association* 216: 301–305, 1965.

4. Weinerman, E.R., et al. Yale studies in ambulatory medical care: Determinants of use of hospital emergency services. *American Journal of Public Health* 56: 1037–1056, 1966.

5. Vaughn, H.F., and Domester, C.E. Why patients use hospital emergency departments. *Hospitals* 40: 59–62, 1966.

6. Roth, J.A. Utilization of the hospital emergency department. *Journal of Health and Social Behavior* 12: 312–320, 1971.

7. Caplan, C. Emergency room use by patients from a family practice. *Journal of Family Practice* 2: 271–275, 1975.

8. Silver, M., Manegold, R., and Gortland, J. The emergency department problem. *Journal of the American Medical Association* 198: 380, 1966.

9. Coleman, J.V., and Errera, P. The general hospital emergency room and its psychiatric problems. *American Journal of Public Health* 53: 1294–1301, 1963.

10. Shortliffe, E.C., Hamilton, T.S., and Noroian, E.H. The emergency room and the changing pattern of medical care. *New England Journal of Medicine* 258: 20–25, 1958.

11. McCarroll, J.R., and Skudder, P.A. Conflicting concepts function shown in a survey. *Hospitals* 24: 35–38, 1960.

12. Lee, S., Salon, J., and Sheps, C. How new patterns of medical care affect the emergency unit. *Modern Hospital* 94: 97, 1960.

13. Hyman, S. The Cook County Hospital Emergency Department. *Postgraduate Medicine* 40: 375, 1966.

14. Satin, D.G. Help: The hospital emergency unit patient and his presenting posture. *Medical Care* 11: 328–337, 1973.

15. Nigro, S.A. A psychiatrist's experience in general practice in a hospital emergency room. *Journal of the American Medical Association* 214: 1657–1660, 1970.

16. Ludwig, E.G., and Gibson, G. Self perception of sickness and the seeking of medical care. *Journal of Heath and Social Behavior* 10: 125–133, 1969.

17. Staeckle, J.D., Zola, J.K., and Davidson, G.E. On going to the doctor, the contributions of the patient to the decision to seek medical aid. *Journal of Chronic Disease* 16: 975–989, 1963.

18. Andersen, M.D., and Pleticha, J.M. Emergency unit patients' perceptions of stressful life events. *Nursing Research* 23: 378–383, 1974.

19. Zimny, G., Iserson, K., and Shepard, C. A characterization of emergency medicine. *JACEP* 8: 147–149, 1979.

20. Leemon, C. Diagnostic errors in emergency room medicine: Physical illness in patients labeled "psychiatric" and vice versa. *International Journal of Psychiatric Medicine* 5: 533–540, 1975.

21. Strain, J. Psychological reactions to acute medical illness and critical care. *Critical Care Medicine* 6: 39–44, 1978.

22. Caplan, G. *An Approach to Community Mental Health.* New York: Grune and Stratton, 1961.

23. Marley, W. Theory of crisis intervention. Reprint from *Pastoral Psychology,* April 1970.

24. Abram, H., and McCourt, W. Interaction of physicians with emergency ward alcoholic patients. *Quarterly Journal of Studies of Alcohol* 25: 679, 1964.

25. Schwarz, L., and Fjeld, S. The alcoholic patient in the psychiatric hospital emergency room. *Quarterly Journal of Studies of Alcohol* 30: 104, 1969.

9

The Pediatric Health Psychologist, the Pediatrician, and Other Caregivers

Wentworth Quast

In 1545, Thomas Phaire wrote not only the first book on pediatrics written by an Englishman, but also one of the first medical books in English. In the preface to *The Boke of Chyldren* he states, "But my purpose is here to do them good that have moste nede, that is to saye, chyldren." Today a significant part of this "nede" in the daily practice of pediatricians involves their responding (both in office visits and by telephone) to the needs of parents with regard to information and guidance about problems of behavior. A questionnaire sent to a sample of practicing pediatricians (Toister and Worley, 1976) indicated that all respondents recommended formal training in child behavior and development in medical school, especially because their past education had been inconsistent and relatively inadequate given their role in consultation on problems of behavioral development.

In an attempt to respond to this lack of training, the federal government established the Health Professionals Educational Assistance Act (PL 94–484) in 1976 to alter the balance between specialty and primary-care physicians by requiring that an eventual 50 percent of all resident slots be in primary-care specialties. Training requirements for psychiatrists now include a first-year rotation in a primary-care setting. Similarly, mental-health training is being *mandated* for primary-care residents to prepare them *to provide mental-health care* and to help them appreciate the special skills of core mental-health practitioners. Governmental plans included an allocation of $17 million in fiscal year 1978 for mental-health training of generic health providers. Twenty-seven million dollars is allocated for continuation of current training for core mental-health practitioners (a 10 percent reduction), with the stipulation that these programs be phased out by 1982.

It is not surprising that the government has concluded that the first-contact, family-oriented provider is best suited to respond to the nation's mental-health needs.

At the time of the last comprehensive survey of ambulatory care in the United States [1969], 78 percent of all outpatient visits to physicians occurred in private office practice settings. Hospital emergency rooms accounted for 7 percent, outpatient departments of mental health centers

103

for 11 percent, health maintenance organizations for 4 percent, and neighborhood health centers for less than 1 percent. Although these percentages may have changed slightly over the last few years, and could change more with the advent of national health insurance, health care will probably continue to be centered in the offices of private practitioners.

Further, 59 percent of all patient visits in which there is a classifiable mental disorder already are accounted for by nonpsychiatric physicians, and nonpsychiatric physicians now account for 46 percent of all visits in which psychotherapy or *therapeutic listening treatment* is provided. National Center for Health Statistics data show that approximately 5 million persons per year receive such services from psychiatrists, while an additional 5 million obtain them from nonpsychiatric physicians. In all, another 10 million or more people may require these services but do not receive them.

In addition to treating patients with clearly defined mental disorders, primary health care providers now are required under the new law to give support and guidance to patients with a wide range of emotionally related "problems of living." Beyond that, pediatricians are required to attend to problems of childrearing, normal biological and psychological development, impact of sociocultural forces on the child, and effects of severe illness on the child and his or her family.

Finally, the trend toward deinstitutionalizing patients with mental retardation, juvenile behavioral disorders, and severe emotional disturbances forces these individuals to rely on primary care physicians for general medical treatment, psychotropic drug therapy, and family counseling [Wright, 1978].

In my view, as comprehensive and problem-directed as this sounds, it will not work.

The Association of American Medical Colleges (AAMC) has published—the Longitudinal Study of Medical Students of the Class of 1960—essentially a 15-year follow-up of 2,821 medical students from twenty-eight U.S. medical schools (D'Costa and Yancik, 1974). In these voluminous materials, there is no reference, let alone any data, to indicate that as freshmen medical students, or now as physicians in practice, these people showed, or show, any interest, aptitude, skills, or *time* to provide guidance and support to patients with "a wide range of emotionally related problems of living."

The widely recognized gaps in health-care delivery can hardly be solved by governmental mandate regardless of how well-intentioned that mandate may be. To order a particular health-care provider—in the case in point, the pediatrician—to become all things to all patients is to confer on that hapless professional a Godlike status he or she has neither sought nor is likely to fulfill. The skills required to effectively carry out the mandate are those of the physician, biologist, developmental psychologist, social worker, sociologist, economist, and philosopher all rolled into one—in short, the magician. It would seem the government is getting into "Peter Pan Land" with its Health Professional Assistance Act, to wit, mandate mental-health training, and presto, a latterday version of Solomon himself is magically produced and magically equipped to solve the medical and emotional ills of society.

As Schofield (1975) so clearly states,

> It is a paradox that psychologists typically have a better appreciation of man's physiology and its import for psychological health than the physician has of man's psychology and its import for his bodily functions. In recent years, responding in part to growing public dissatisfaction with the quality of medical practice, medical educators have been concerned with training physicians to have a persisting orientation to the diagnosis and treatment of the whole person. This concern has been reflected in some medical schools by efforts to make a place for psychological studies (behavioral science) among the basic sciences of the medical curriculum. The student comes to medical school to learn about anatomy, not anxiety; to study the nervous system, not neuroses. His general attitudinal bias toward the so-called "soft" sciences has proven frustratingly resistant to a variety of endeavors to prepare primary care physicians with a continuous awareness of the holistic organism, which is their patient.

Even though some progress has been made by some medical schools to educate their students in human behavior, especially in courses on human behavior taught often in the first 2 years of training, in my view the rewards for most pediatricians, regardless of course offerings, lie not in their treating psychosocial or developmental behavior problems, but in their involvement in strictly medical problems and often very special problems at that. Some years ago, a pediatric resident friend stated that "there were not pellets given [at least at this school] for being a good clinician" and that he was going to be an expert in one cell—and he did just that. Even in the so-called team approach, the pediatrician is quite ready to give over problems of behavior to the pediatric psychologist, child psychiatrist, or social worker, and like many parents, he or she hopes that these professionals will "take over or make over" the child. This may well be appropriate, especially with the increased emphasis on specialization within pediatrics. In addition, especially at medical centers, there is an increasing addition of child psychologists who are specialists in the psychological components of the many specialty areas, such as neurology, neurosurgery, physical medicine and rehabilitation, oncology, speech, language and hearing, family practice, chronic diseases, transplants, mental retardation, and special learning disabilities (whatever they are), to name some. Relative to the last, the concept of learning disabilities is based on a confusion of ideas and understanding, and it is often difficult to identify myths and unfounded concepts from realities (Cruickshank, 1977). It is unfortunate that some pediatric specialists, psychiatrists, and medical psychologists have become involved in this area when educational psychologists are confused enough. Louise Bate Ames, (1977) has written an excellent editorial, the title of which is also the punchline: "Learning Disabilities: Time to Check Our Roadmaps?"

Pediatric Psychologists: A Collaborative Model

Much has been written about the multiple roles of the pediatric psychologist in *Pediatric Psychology,* a publication of the Society of Pediatric Psychology. Most of these roles are extremely important in the total health care of children—in prevention, early diagnosis, treatment, and aftercare or continuity of care. These roles are usually carried out in large university medical centers or private children's hospitals. In my view, looking at the future and the great need for education in the self-help of children and families, the pediatric psychologist, with his or her comprehensive knowledge of medical psychology, can contribute significantly as a public health-care psychologist. Early in my own professional career, I stopped working predominantly with psychiatrists and moved toward a prophylactic stance that involved direct consultation with the primary providers of care. To be most effective, and in the best interest of the consumer, the role of the consulting pediatric psychologist is in working with a variety of caregivers. The role is one of liaison with caregivers in the community—educators, counselors, public health nurses, nurse practitioners, a variety of welfare and other social service workers, court personnel, and others.

Before health-care professionals can work effectively with children or collaboratively with one another, a thorough understanding of developmental psychology is crucial. Many typical developmental deviations, while admittedly disturbing to others, are actually within normal limits. In recent research on the adult outcome of over 1,000 former adolescent psychiatric and pediatric patients, the results indicate that the majority of disturbed teenagers did not continue to be notably disturbed in adult life (Shea, Hafner, Quast, and Hetler, 1980). Since precious little information on outcome predictors exists, one of the primary aims of this research was to construct simple, straightforward, predictive combinations of characteristics that various caregivers can use to predict which adolescents will continue to have problems in specific areas and which will have few problems in adulthood (Shea, Hafner, Quast, and Hetler, 1980).

Along with the need for accurate predictors of emotional disturbance in adulthood, health-care professionals need to understand the meaning of "dysfunctional behavior" in the context in which it occurs. In presenting the concept of functional disintegration, Dabrowski's (1964) basic tenet was that many behaviors that professionals and laypeople alike consider maladaptive are in fact very functional. A common example is depression or, in a child in lesser form, moodiness, withdrawal, loss of motivation, and so forth. Today the minute a person shows such symptoms, everybody gets themselves upset—off to the physician and down goes the Elavil. Mood swings are often functional, even necessary, for growth, since such growth is by nature saltatory—one has to back up in order to gain strength and momentum to go forward. It is in this way that psychic tension promotes creative inner development. Dabrowski (1964) states, "One must clearly understand that, for an individual and for the society he belongs to, only such development is positive which takes into account the creative aspects of the difficulties of everyday life, pain, dissatisfaction, and discontinuities in the—superficially desirable—uniform process of growing up."

In 30 years of experience working with pediatricians, it is my view that the most productive role for the pediatric health-care psychologist is to serve *not* in the training of pediatricians to be "junior psychiatrists," but as a consultant in primary prevention, as well as to work *with* the pediatrician in helping him or her know when and to whom to turn in early intervention and parent education. This is not to say that the role should be one of exclusively working with systems and leaving the responsibility with him or her or other primary caregivers, but to continue to work one-to-one with children and families as demonstration of how he or she and others can exploit resources in the community. Thus there is a double purpose: to help solve the immediate problem through consultation, and to educate the practitioner at the same time.

It is important to be supportive of pediatricians, whether they are operating out of a large hospital, inpatient or outpatient, or in community practice, since they are in very strategic positions to solve problems of behavior. Often they are the first person parents will contact, even if the parents have had prior contact with a number of other agencies, such as schools or social agencies. In an attempt to communicate with the physician, a parent will frequently choose a somatic problem of a child that is patently false or inconsequential. For a long time I have been impressed with the poor correlation between the presenting complaint and final diagnosis.

In a study that has now gone on for over 15 years at a large health maintenance organization in California, 60 percent of all patients coming to see a physician were suffering from problems that were emotional and not physical in nature. The researchers found that when patients are systematically referred for attention to the emotional problem, there was a dramatic reduction in utilization of medical services which continued over an 8-year period (Follette and Cummings, 1967).

Parents also will seek out the pediatrician for the very important reason of protecting their anonymity. While we might hope otherwise, there still exists a strong reluctance to be identified as "mental" (to borrow the label the kids themselves use). The success of the solution of a problem often lies in the delicate manner in which the pediatrician makes a referral and to whom.

As a child and parent advocate, the pediatrician need not immediately wisk the patient and parents off to a mental-health center if he or she has a comprehensive knowledge of resources that can help acknowledge this need for anonymity. While on a sabbatical leave, I was working in a rural area of northern Wisconsin, where I attempted to convince pediatricians and other physicians, social workers, and teachers of the efficiency of making home visits as a team. We were able to address many chronic problems (in some cases, where whole families were problem-ridden) because we were dealing with them on their own turf and not asking them to sit in waiting rooms and be identified as "mentally something or other."

It was important in relating with these people to make the professionalism of the consultant as "low key" as possible. Both families and the consultee were more comfortable when help was given on an egalitarian and nonauthoritarian basis.

I have heard arguments that home visits could not be cost-efficient. However, when one sees the number of office visits to the physician, to welfare workers, to courts, and to guidance clinics with little or no change in the family patterns, I am confident that home visits will be seen as effective and can be justified economically. In many instances, this is the only way the father can be reached, and in my view, the father has for years been a missing piece of the puzzle in trying to solve the behavior problems of a child. Professionals have fostered "father's" nonparticipation by their own behavior—often not even asking for his participation, but more important, passively accepting the father's excuse that he cannot arrange the time. In my practice I am absolutely uncompromising in this regard and will not accept a child unless both parents are willing to participate. This holds for assessment as well—parents as well as the child are given personality tests. Some colleagues have questioned this practice on the grounds that parents would be reluctant to expose their own psyches when it is "clearly" the child's problem. In my total experience, I have had only two parents who at first refused to be evaluated; both later recognized that they were significant, if not etiologic, agents in their child's problem. I abhor the frequently heard "show me a disturbed child and I will show you a disturbed parent." It is not my purpose to blame or fault parents, but rather to recognize that there are many irrational ideas and false beliefs that we as parents often idiosyncratically and unwittingly project onto our children.

Relative to assessment and intervention strategies, I think there is now and has been for some time a tendency on the part of many psychologists to overtest. The cost of assessment also can be reduced by the use of psychometrists. It still amazes me to see the numbers of highly paid Ph.D.'s that are employed by school districts as test-givers, when the use of psychometrists would not only be appreciably cheaper, but would free up the school psychologists to do things for which they are trained that would be of significant benefit. As a pediatric psychology consultant to a school district, I rely a great deal on the use of screening devices. Instruments such as the MMPI, sentence completion tests, the Goodenough Draw-a-Man, the Minnesota Child Development Inventory, and the Personality Inventory for Children have been most helpful to have in hand before interviewing the child. The art of the practitioner reaches its highest form in the expertise with which an interview is conducted. John Benjamin Murphy, an early American surgeon, in lectures to his students had advice we might well heed. He said, "Listen, listen to the patient's story! He is telling you the diagnosis." This is especially true when one is interviewing the triad of mother, father, and child. In the initial interview, I have made it a regular practice to always interview all three together, regardless of the age or mental abilities of the child.

It goes without saying that the pediatric health psychologist necessarily needs a strong foundation in child development as a knowledge of psychopathology and medicine. Since psychologists are called upon to deal with a tremendous range of problems, often fraught with considerable ambiguity, they must first be generalists. They are also called upon to be knowledgeable about a wide range of resources not only in their local community, but also in the state and nation. Only with this information will the psychologist be able to know how to explore resources with community workers who may appear to be at a loss in how to handle the many effects of physical illness on development.

Rational-Behavior Training: A Self-Help Intervention Strategy

Relative to intervention strategies, effort should be made to encourage self-help strategies by parents and children. The method of rational self-counseling is an offshoot of Albert Ellis's rational emotive therapy developed by Maxie C. Maultsby and entitled *Rational Behavior Training (RBT)* (Maultsby, 1975). There has been very little application of RBT to children, although Hauck (1967) has written an excellent book for parents on the rational management of children, and Knaus (1974) has a manual for elementary school teachers on rational emotive education. Critics have stated that these rational approaches are highly semantic and are not readily applicable for children. In my clinical practice, I have not found this to be true. Children are basically very rational until we adults introduce them to our irrationality. Children can readily grasp the basic theory of self-counseling, that what people think determines what they feel, or that "people are disturbed not by things, but by the views which they take of them" (Epictetus, 1st Century A.D.). Children, parents, and caretakers can be taught rational alternatives to some of their false beliefs, as well as to learn they can disturb themselves less. The youngest child to learn the rational behavior principles was a 5-year-old gifted and talented girl who was in tears when she failed ceiling items on an intelligence test.

In clinical practice, I spend as much time teaching cognitive behavior-modification (CBM) strategies to parents, teachers, and other caregivers as teaching children, since the real question is whether the children are disturbed or disturbing. Workshops are held in schools, where administrators as well as teachers and supportive staff are given didactic lectures with practical homework assignments regarding specific situations with children they perceive as disturbing. A similar format is used with children in the classroom. Parents are given books instructive in the rational management of children (Hauck, 1967). Children are introduced to RBT and CBM using materials particularly from Waters (1979), Spivack and Shure (1974, 1976, 1978, and Meichenbaum (1977). In addition, both parents and children are given homework assignments dealing with real-life everyday problems that were discussed in treatment sessions. Human fallibility and perfectionism are two subjects frequently discussed by parents and children. Other common topics include the difference between facts and opinions, the necessity of making assumptions and why people make unsound assumptions, the notion of the imperfect person in an imperfect world, and that making mistakes is a necessary and usual part of the learning process.

There is some efficacy in working with both parents and children at the same time on homework assignments having to do with daily practice of RBT. Recently, a mother came with her daughter to an appointment and opened the session by stating that she (the mother) had unnecessarily upset herself and her 8-year-old daughter had calmly offered her rational alternatives to her behavior that the mother accepted graciously. The situation resulted in bringing the two closer, when the presenting complaint had been their difficulty getting along with each other.

In this chapter, the broad role of the pediatric health psychologist as consultant to a variety of helping professionals has been highlighted. Research and current clinical practice have emphasized self-help education of parents and children, with rational-behavior training being an easily grasped intervention strategy. Much is happening in this area. Obviously, much remains to be done, but an important starting point is the acknowledgment of the pragmatic role that the pediatric health psychologist can play in maintaining children's well-being.

References

Ames, L.B. Learning disabilities: Time to check our roadmaps? *Journal of Learning Disabilities* 10:328–330, 1977.

Caplan, G. *Principles of Preventive Psychiatry*. New York: Basic Books, 1964.

Cruickshank, W.M. Myths and realities in learning disabilities. *Journal of Learning Disabilities* 10:51–58, 1977.

Dabrowski, K. *Positive Disintegration*. Boston: Little, Brown, 1964.

D'Costa, A., and Yancik, R. *A Follow-Up Study 1974–1979. The Longitudinal Study of Medical Students of the Class of 1960*. Association of American Medical Colleges, 1974.

Follette, W., and Cummings, N.A. Psychiatric services and medical utilization in a prepaid health plan setting. *Medical Care* 5:25–35, 1967.

Hauck, P.A. *The Rational Management of Children*. New York: Libra, 1967.

Knaus, W.J. *Rational Emotive Education. A Manual for Elementary School Teachers*. New York: Institute for Rational Living, 1974.

Maultsby, M.C. *Help Yourself to Happiness Through Rational Self Counseling*. Boston: Marlborough-Herman, 1975.

Meichenbaum, D.H. *Cognitive-Behavior Modification: An Integrative Approach*. New York: Plenum, 1977.

Toister, R.P., and Worley, L.M. Behavioral aspects of pediatric practice: A survey of practitioners. *Journal of Medical Education* 51:(12):1019–1020, 1976.

Schofield, W. The psychologist as a health care professional. *Intellect* 103:255–258, 1975.

Shea, M.J., Hafner, A.J., Quast, W., and Hetler, J.H. Outcome of adolescent psychiatric disorders: A long term follow-up study. In *The Child and His Family: The Vulnerable Child*. Yearbook of the International Association for Child Psychiatry and Allied Professions. Vol. IV. ed. E. James Anthony and Cyrille Koupernik, New York: Wiley, 1980.

Spivack, G., and Shure, M.B. *Social Adjustment of Young Children: A Cognitive Approach to Solving Real-Life Problems*. San Francisco: Jossey-Bass, 1973. (Includes program script for teachers of four-year-olds.)

Spivack, G., Platt, J.J., and Shure, M.B. *The Problem Solving Approach to Adjustment: A Guide to Research and Intervention.* San Francisco: Jossey-Bass, 1976.

Shure, M.B., and Spivack, G. *Problem Solving Techniques in Childrearing.* San Franciso: Jossey-Bass, 1978 (Includes program script for parents of young children.)

Waters, V. Institute for Rational-Emotive Therapy, New York. Personal communication, 1979.

Wright, L. Primary health care physicians to assume expanded role. *Feelings and Their Medical Significance* 20(1):1–4, 1978.

10 Psychological Interventions in Pediatric Oncology

Jonathan Kellerman

The practice of medical psychology is inextricably linked with the dynamic nature of contemporary medical care. An excellent example of this is the area of pediatric oncology, where treatment advances have brought about major changes in the nature of the illnesses and have created growing challenges to the behavioral sciences. Three decades ago, the majority of childhood cancers were incurable, untreatable, and rapidly fatal. It is not surprising, therefore, that early references regarding psychological support for children with malignant diseases addressed themselves, mainly, to issues of death, dying, and terminal care. Owing to the recent renaissance of interest in death and the growth of thanatology as a specialized area of inquiry, such studies have not diminished.

Simultaneously, however, the recognition of increased life expectancy in children with many types of cancer, notably, acute lymphoblastic leukemia, Hodgkin's disease, and Wilm's tumor, has led many authors to consider the utility of viewing pediatric cancer from the conceptual viewpoint of chronic disease (Koch et al., 1974; Lanksy and Lowman, 1974; Holmes and Holmes, 1975; Katz et al., 1977; Kagen-Goodheart, 1977; Kellerman, 1979). This has led to an increased awareness of the importance of identifying problems of adaptation and of developing clinical approaches that help patient and family achieve optimal rehabilitation.

Since 1975, I have been involved in the psychosocial care of children treated for a variety of malignant diseases at Childrens Hospital of Los Angeles (CHLA). The bulk of that time has been spent in developing and directing a comprehensive, multidisciplinary psychosocial program that functions as part of the hospital's hematology-oncology division. Detailed descriptions of that program can be found in a recent volume on the psychological aspects of pediatric cancer (Kellerman, 1979). In the course of conceiving, carrying, delivering, and nurturing a new system of clinical care, there has been much gratification and some pain. Lessons have been learned, often through trial and error. It is my feeling that there exist certain important organizational and methodological issues that should be considered by the mental-health professional working with this patient population

113

in order for maximal clinical success to take place. Discussion of these is the focus of the remainder of this chapter.

The Practitioner's Role

In recent articles, Lewis (1978) and Peebles and O'Malley (1978) have outlined some of the problems encountered by the mental-health professional who serves as a consultant in a medical setting. These stem, basically, from perceptions on the part of medical and nursing personnel of the psychologist, psychiatrist, social worker, and so forth as outsiders who can never fully empathize with and understand the relevant issues at hand. This can be particularly true when dealing with diseases, such as cancer, where emotional loading is high, often causing medical personnel to adopt a stance of defensive stoicism.

In addition, calling in a consultant may be viewed as evidence of failure on the part of physicians and nurses and may thus be postponed until problems have escalated to a point where treatment efficacy is seriously impaired, or it may be neglected entirely.

The mental-health consultant may contribute to these problems by entering the treatment setting with an incomplete or inaccurate understanding of the medical issues or by adopting an attitude of superiority and omnipotence—a posture I prefer to label the "Cosmic Mr. Fixit."

While Lewis (1978) and Peebles and O'Malley (1978) offer much in the way of useful suggestions for the consultant, it is my position that the consultant role itself is inherently fraught with problems that stem from its imposition of an insider-outsider system upon the consultant and those to whom he or she consults. This may not be of much consequence when the consultant expects to have a transitory or short-term relationship with the consultee, as is true in many industrial or organizational settings. When, however, extended contact with patients is desired, it can be destructive.

It is therefore advisable that the medical psychologist working with pediatric cancer patients be as closely affiliated with the hematology-oncology division as possible. When it is realistic, this should take place in the form of an appointment within the cancer division. The neophyte practitioner also should expect there to be an initiation process, during which he or she maintains a low profile, concentrates on learning as much as possible about the diseases and treatments encountered by the patients he or she will be seeing, and adopts an empirical approach toward the nature of psychological problems experienced by these children rather than entering the treatment setting with fully developed preconceptions and prefabricated clinical notions.

It is a fact of life that he psychosocial practitioner must have the support of the medical staff in order to be successful. An understanding of the primary responsibility borne by the physician in the conventional medical setting is essential. The psychologist must strive to avoid becoming a patient advocate, interceding on behalf of patients rights while placing medical staff in the "bad guy" role. There will be times when the mental-health professional will observe behavior on the part of medical staff that he or she feels is inappropriate. Once again, this is most likely in circumstances where the issues are highly emotionally charged. Moreover, there will be times when criticism will be appropriate and in the best interests of the patient. Such criticism must be delivered with the same clinical sensitivity that is adopted when working with patients, however, and will be effective only if there is an atmosphere of mutual trust between psychosocial and medical personnel.

In line with maintaining such an atmosphere, it is important that the psychologist be clear about treatment goals and techniques. There may be much hocus-pocus associated with psychotherapy, in the minds of medical staff some of it justified. The steps the psychosocial practitioner can take to remedy this include minimal use of jargon and obfuscative language, spelling out of perceived problems in operations, maximally behavioral terms, and careful recording of all clinical activities in the medical chart.

With regard to the last point, it should be noted that there will be material that arises in the course of psychological interviewing that is not appropriate for inclusion in a general medical chart. Detailed accounts of such information are not necessary. The alternative, however, is not a blank page, but rather, a general process description. The important issue to bear in mind is the need for the physician to be familiar with what is happening to his or her patient. He or she need not know that the patient has discussed the gory details of a recent parental altercation at home, but he or she should be aware that stress exists.

Psychosocial notes should not end with a description of findings, but should include recommendations for treatment. There will be times when specific recommendations are not feasible, but this too should be explicitly noted. There are few things more frustrating to medical personnel than to receive detailed, elaborate evaluative data without accompanying suggestions of what to do with such information.

The preceding suggestions have focused on contextual strategies that can help strengthen the psychologist's ability to function in a health-care setting. In the final evaluation, however, mutually supportive working relationships between psychosocial and medical practitioners grow out of clinically effective collaboration. And if a bit of teleologic thinking may be permitted, good patient care is the desired end result of effective collaboration. Before such care can be accomplished, an understanding of the nature and incidence of psychological problems experienced by children with cancer is necessary.

Children with Malignant Disease: A Mentally Healthy Population

In contrast with work done in traditional mental-health or psychiatric settings, psychosocial care in a pediatric oncology setting addresses itself to a group of children and families who are psychologically representative of the general population. While assertions have been made concerning the "cancer personality" and the relationship between the development of malignant disease and psychopathology (Bahnson and Bahnson, 1966), there is nothing that even approaches valid data to back these up, especially with regard to children.

The psychiatric patient or consumer of services at a community mental-health center enters the treatment situation because of a primary behavioral dysfunction. Such is not the case with the children with leukemia or osteogenic sarcoma who encounter a psychologist in the course of their treatment. They come for medical amelioration of a medical condition and will need an appropriate explanation of why mental-health services are being offered.

Receiving news of a diagnosis of cancer in their child is one of the most stressful events that can occur for parents. If, soon after, they are approached by a psychosocial practitioner without careful explanation, the level of stress can be raised. It is not uncommon for parents to worry if somebody has judged them "crazy," "weird," "neurotic," or otherwise psychologically inappropriate, when they lack a full understanding of the psychologist's role. Thus, rather than lower distress, the psychosocial professional can, inadvertently, increase it.

In order to prevent such confusion, it is important to offer parents and child an explicit statement to the effect that nobody in the hospital feels they are mentally unsound. On the contrary, the psychologist might add, they are normal individuals undergoing stress, and it has been found that stress can make people more vulnerable to such things as anxiety and depression. I have found most families to be very receptive to the notion of stress-induced vulnerability and to psychosocial support when it is presented in this context. The Childrens Hospital Psychosocial Program sees over 150 newly diagnosed patients each year, and refusal of services occurs in only one or two instances and is usually related to refusal of general oncologic care.

In addition, the psychologist can further dispel the stigma attached to psychosocial care by familiarizing himself or herself with *normal* situational reactions to stress and communicating their normalcy to patient and family. Thus a mother whose 12-year-old daughter is depressed following a diagnosis of lymphoma may worry less after hearing that such depression is common during the initial postdiagnostic period, often lasting for 1 or 2 weeks, and that it is transitory. Similarly, the psychosocial practitioner can validate the feelings of guilt, anger, and despair that are virtually ubiquitous in parents and patients. By informing them that such feelings are normal, common, and even useful, he or she can open the way for freer expression and communication of affect. It is quite enough to experience depression without having to worry if such feelings are "okay."

A strong recommendation is made here for routine psychological contact with all patients within a cancer division rather than a singling out of those who are perceived to be pathological. The reasons for this have been discussed in detail elsewhere (Kellerman, 1979) and include the lack of validity of initial evaluations of pathology and the ubiquitous nature of stress reactions in this patient population. Virtually all children with cancer become depressed and anxious at one time or another and can benefit from psychosocial support. In addition, routine care aids further in destigmatizing the nature of intervention.

In a recent study (Kellerman et al., 1978), inquiry was made into the nature and incidence of psychological problems of pediatric cancer patients. A sample of 147 children, representing all psychological referrals at Childrens Hospital over a 16-month period, was studied. From this, a treatment sample of 101 patients seen past the point of initial evaluation was obtained, and presenting problems were analyzed.

The single largest reason for referral was conditioned anxiety related to multiple medical procedures. It is a singular irony that treatment for childhood cancer often brings about more physical discomfort than do the diseases themselves. The child experiences bone-marrow aspirations, lumbar punctures, intravenous and intramuscular injections of chemotherapeutic agents, blood transfusions, exploratory surgery, and radiotherapy. Pain may result from the intrusive nature of the administration of chemical agents or from the chemical activity of the agents themselves. Other side effects of treatment include nausea, vomiting, alopecia, weight loss, and skin discoloration.

It is not surprising, then, that over 35 percent of the treatment sample presented with anxiety reactions relating to treatment-induced distress. Such anxiety was anticipatory, occurring at varying times prior to the administration of procedures. Some children reported feelings of discomfort for several days before a scheduled medical appointment; others began to vomit as they entered the hospital parking lot. Symptoms included nausea, emesis, muscle tension, insomnia, nightmares, depression, and withdrawal. Such anxiety is best viewed as classically conditioned with the unconditioned stimulus (UCS) being the medical procedure itself and the conditioned stimuli (CS) consisting of any of a number of stimulus characteristics of the hospital setting, both spatial and temporal.

Other major problems included behavioral difficulties at home (oppositional behavior), sibling and peer conflicts, prolonged depression most often associated with relapse of disease, and difficulties returning to school after prolonged absence (Katz et al., 1977; Lansky, 1974).

In contrast with the adult oncology population, chronic pain was not common, and when it did occur, it was most often related to atypical pediatric tumors such as nasopharyngeal carcinoma. Likewise, psychotic or psychotic-like behavior was rare and could almost always be attributed to the psychoactive effects of drugs such as methotrexate and vincristine. This is in concordance with data reported by Holland (1971; 1977) that emphasized the lack of severe psychopathology in adult cancer patients even while undergoing restrictive isolation and with similar studies of children (Kellerman et al., 1976; 1977).

The general picture created by this information is of a sample of psychologically intact youngsters and families faced with life-threatening disease. Of course, psychological disturbances do exist in some children prior to diagnosis, but there is no reason to believe that the rate of such problems exceeds that of the general population.

Because of this, it is felt that the adoption of a psychiatric orientation that assumes pathology and orients itself to long-term, interpretive, intensive psychotherapy is inappropriate. Put in the vernacular of everyday life, the key to successful work with physically ill patients is not to be too "shrinky," but to approach both child and parents as a caring person whose goal is to foster maximal self-help and mastery.

The following sections attempt to outline some of the specific approaches to optimal psychosocial care of pediatric cancer patients and their families.

Recognition of the Interactional Bases of Behavior

Much evidence has accumulated that points to the importance of considering behavior in an interactional context (Endler and Magnusson, 1976). In this scheme, both personological and situational factors are considered. This consideration of both personological and situational factors is extremely important when working with serious disease, because there is an extreme degree of environmental stress imposed on the individual by the treatment system and the disease process itself.

For example, a naive evaluator, upon viewing extreme fidgeting, short attention span, and disruptive behavior on the part of a 9-year-old boy, might conclude that the youngster is hyperkinetic. A more complete knowledge of situational variables, however, might alter this perception. Such knowledge might include the awareness that 10 minutes before, the child had just experienced a bone-marrow aspiration and a lumbar puncture in quick succession or found that his disease was in relapse. If this appears to be a simple-minded example, it represents one that the author has observed occurring more than once. Attributions of pathology and affixing of labels are less than useful and can lead to self-fulfilling prophecies that alter the course of staff response to the patient over a prolonged period.

Psychologists must be acutely aware that when they encounter a hospitalized child, and especially a youngster diagnosed with malignant disease, they are unlikely to be viewing typical behavior. Conclusions should be based on repeated observations and should take into account the reality stresses encountered by the patient.

The interactional approach is important, additionally, because it channels attention toward *psychosocial care*. The term correctly implies a certain dualism: both psychological and social factors must be evaluated and dealt with. All the psychotherapy in the world may not aid the family who needs help in obtaining transportation to the oncology clinic or whose friends have withdrawn because of fears of contagion or increased anxiety about how to treat someone with cancer. However, individuals will vary in the coping styles they utilize in dealing with environmental stress. It seems clear, then, that no single health professional is equipped to single-handedly care for the child with cancer and his or her family. The skills of social workers, psychologists or psychiatrists, and patient-activity specialists can all be used to maximize the quality of care offered by the pediatric oncologist.

Respect of Premorbid Family Functioning

It is not useful for the pediatric psychologist to concentrate his or her efforts on modifying long-standing patterns of behavior that predated the child's diagnosis. A far more realistic and helpful approach is to aid the child and family in returning to doing things the way they did before the child became ill. This implies the importance of a healthy respect for the virtually infinite nature of human coping. I have encountered parents who, in a psychiatric setting, might have received a diagnosis of "borderline psychotic" or "low functioning" and who, given psychological support, have coped with a diagnosis of malignancy with few or no serious psychological problems.

Similarly, care must be taken to be aware and respectful of cultural and ethnic factors that families bring with them into the treatment setting. For example, the CHLA hematology-oncology patient population includes a 20 percent sample of children who are primarily Spanish-speaking. The families of these patients, mostly Mexican-American, often are highly reluctant to "let their children know" about their disease. Rather than approach this issue from a combative stance, we have found it useful to employ the services of a Spanish-speaking social work assistant who is able to operate from a shared cultural background. This enables her to gain entry into the family communication system, develop optimal trust, and work from within the system in order to improve the quality and quantity of disease-related information given to the patient. A similar approach is used when dealing with issues of folk medicine and home cures.

There are, of course, exceptions to the laissez-faire acceptance of premorbid family styles, such as when the psychologist becomes aware of long-standing behavior patterns that endanger the well-being of the child, as in cases of abuse, deprivation, and neglect. In addition, there will be times when a family member with a premorbid psychological problem is obviously requesting help. The most appropriate way to deal with these is through assignment of referrals to those professionals who specialize in the necessary service. In the case of child abuse, practitioners must operate within prescribed legal and clinical boundaries to ensure the safety of their patients. Prolonged treatment, however, is best left up to others, so that maximal attention can be paid to ameliorating the behavioral problems that accrue from the diagnosis of cancer.

Therapeutic Techniques

There is ample data supporting the common-sense notion that individuals are better able to cope with stressful experiences that they have been prepared for (Cassell, 1965; Janis, 1958; Bandura and Menlove, 1968; Melamed and Siegel, 1975). With regard to the child with cancer, preparation can take several forms.

First, care must be taken to provide the child with age-appropriate and accurate information about his or her illness and its treatment. The question of "Do you tell them what they have?" is basically a false issue and one that has been abandoned by experienced clinicians for several reasons. Spinetta (1973) showed that children with leukemia had an understanding of the severity and life-threatening nature of their diagnosis even if they had not been formally told about it. The practitioner who has spent an appreciable amount of time in a hospital will know that it is virtually impossible to keep secrets on a medical ward. As Vernick and Karon (1965) have pointed out, policies of secrecy have often been the result of anxiety on the part of staff members and not the result of an accurate reading of patient needs.

Apart from the lack of feasibility of withholding disease-related information from the child, there is little doubt that approaches that foster incomplete communication are harmful for the patient. The mind abhors an informational vacuum. When information is not provided, the mind will conjure up fantasies which are often more disturbing than actual reality. When this is combined with the concrete nature of children's thinking, the results can be detrimental. For example, consider the 7-year-old boy diagnosed with Hodgkin's disease who asks his mother what he has and is told "You have a bug." This particular child construed this to mean that there were, literally, insects teeming inside of him. His response was one of terror. When this came to light in a therapeutic session, he was provided with accurate information about his disease, asked several questions, and exhibited noticeably lower levels of anxiety throughout follow-up.

It is also important for children to understand what is going on in, and with, their bodies so that they can achieve mastery over feelings of dependency and helplessness and in order for them to cooperate with medical procedures. In the CHLA program, patients are encouraged to participate in laboratory tours, where they can view microscopic slides of their blood and tissue and receive explanations for the reason behind venipunctures, lumbar punctures, and bone-marrow aspirations.

Patients are further prepared through the use of preprocedural play therapy, during which they can behaviorally rehearse medical procedures using bona fide medical apparatus and surrogates such as dolls and puppets. In addition, through the use of hospital playrooms, the children are offered the opportunity to express feelings related to disease, treatment, and hospitalization through structured and unstructured play. The specifics of a play therapy preparation approach to pediatric oncology patients has been detailed by McCue (1979).

Preparation of parents is accomplished using individual and group counseling, specialized hospital tours oriented specifically to the pediatric cancer patient, and written orientation booklets. There must be a recognition, on the part of the clinician, that a diagnosis of cancer in a child creates an intensive bond between family and hospital. The treatment setting can become a home away from home, particularly during periods of high emotional stress (initial diagnosis, relapses, medical crises), and families need support in coping with the intricacies of a hospital bureaucracy. We have found it useful to provide such support after a treatment plan has been determined and the initial shock of the diagnosis is somewhat reduced. This usually takes place toward the second week after diagnosis.

Owing to the high levels of anxiety generated by repeated medical procedures, it will be useful for the practitioner to be familiar and skillful with those techniques which help in ameliorating such distress. In particular, a recommendation is made for use of autogenic methods of relaxation training, such as desensitization, guided imagery, and self-hypnosis. These modalities are beneficial owing both to their efficacy in reducing anxiety and to their encouragement of self-help and mastery.

Several authors have presented substantial evidence of superior hypnotic susceptibility of children when compared with adults (London, 1962; London and Cooper, 1969; Morgan and Hilgard, 1973). This is especially true of children between the ages of 6 and 14 and appears to be due to a well-developed sense of fantasy and imagination in young patients. Other authors (Crasilneck and Hall, 1973; Cullen, 1958; Jacobs, 1962) have reported working successfully with preschool children, including patients with cancer. La Baw et al. (1975) have reported on the successful use of group hypnotic training for pediatric cancer patients, and both Gardner (1976) and Dash (1979) provide more recent accounts of individual hypnotic work with this patient population.

Training in self-hypnosis appears to be preferable to more structured approaches, such as systematic desensitization, when working with children with cancer because it is quicker and offers more flexibility. My experience is that establishment of hierarchies and careful progression along graded steps is not necessary and that, particularly when the images employed are tailored to the individual needs of the patient, successful hypnotically induced relaxation can take place in one session.

Because anxious behavior is often operantly maintained both at home and in the hospital, familiarity with reinforcement strategies is also recommended. There will be times when the line between organically and psychologically induced distress is impossible to draw, as in instances of nausea and vomiting, which can result from administration of chemotherapeutic and radiotherapeutic agents, the disease process itself, classically conditioned anxiety, and operantly maintained avoidance. Therefore, the psychologist may find that he or she is successful in reducing the frequency or intensity of the symptom, but not in eliminating it completely.

An example of this is the case of an 11-year-old boy with acute lymphoblastic leukemia referred because of high levels of nausea and emesis that appeared, to his attending oncologist, to exceed those symptoms expected to result from the particular chemotherapeutic agents he was receiving. Pretreatment behavioral analysis revealed an incidence of 35 to 40 times per day and a pattern of social reinforcement of vomiting in which the child's mother would rush to his side with an emesis basin as soon as he began to make gagging sounds. Withdrawal of this attention combined with encouraging the patient to hold the basin for himself resulted in the rate of emesis being cut in half. Subsequent hypnotically induced relaxation further reduced frequency of vomiting to 3 to 6 times a day where it remained.

We have observed children who are sufficiently motivated and skillful at self-hypnosis to be able to achieve limb anesthesia during medical procedures, and we have seen patients who achieve no benefit at all. The majority of patients fall somewhere in between, with most children reporting at least minimal increases in relaxation.

Hypnosis, like any therapeutic modality, must be used by a fully trained clinician who is aware of the psychological and medical context within which the patient is functioning. There will be times when patients do not wish to experience relaxation, or even to work on anxiety reduction, because these are not primary issues for them. Depression related to relapse or downward disease course can overshadow attempts to reduce situational distress, and what may be called for in such a situation is nondirective, supportive counseling. There will exist families whose patterns of interrelationships do not encourage successful hypnotic induction. An example of this is the parent who becomes overly enthusiastic about the use of hynosis for the child and who, by overselling it or adopting an authoritarian stance, channels the child's rebellion toward nonsusceptibility.

Nondirective therapeutic techniques are helpful in aiding the patient express feelings regarding the state of his or her disease and its treatment. In younger children, play therapy is often the preferred modality, while verbal methods are more suitable for the patient above the age of 8 or 9. There will be instances, however, where the stress of disease and treatment will bring about periodic regression, and the psychologist may find it useful to offer the older child opportunities to engage in play therapy and other symbolic activities. For example, it has been helpful for adolescent patients to behaviorally rehearse medical procedures using dolls and apparatus. These older youngsters are surprisingly enthusiastic about participating in preparation when it is not presented to them in a demeaning or patronizing manner.

Client-centered counseling has played an important role in dealing with the issue of noncompliance. It is not unusual for patients, most often adolescents, to suddenly refuse to undergo further treatment. This may arise during periods of relapse or treatment failure, and there may be times when discontinuation of treatment is a sensible alternative. More commonly, however, noncompliance is more closely related to the adolescent's feelings of loss of control and need not be tied in with medical realities. We have seen patients undergoing treatment that was producing marked results suddenly decide to discontinue therapy.

A nondirective approach to the noncompliant patient can help him or her focus on feelings of reduced mastery and loss of control and can aid in facilitating expression of this distress. Most often when such counseling is combined with genuine attempts to increase the adolescent's sense of mastery (that is making minor modifications in scheduling to accommodate the patient's calendar of events, working with staff and family to avoid the infantilization that is inherent in the typical hospitalization experience, teaching the patient self-help methods of pain control), there will be renewed decision to resume treatment (Moore et al., 1969; Kellerman and Katz, 1977). The fact that an explicit decision has been made by the adolescent often ensures greater commitment to future treatment.

The psychologist working with pediatric oncology patients must have at his or her disposal the full range of therapeutic modalities. Recognition of the impact of cancer on the family is important, along with skills in family therapy and systems approaches to behavior change. In general I have found long-term interpretive techniques that concentrate on acquisition of insight and resolution of intrapsychic conflict less useful than the short-term modalities that take into account the situational reality stresses brought about by serious disease and its treatment and offer the patient specific, concrete skills in the mastery of anxiety and helplessness. Such methods include, but are not limited to, crisis counseling, time-limited psychotherapy, behavior therapy, hypnosis, and group therapy, particularly group therapy that aids patients and parents in acquiring relevant information and exposes them to others undergoing similar experiences as well as behavioral preparation.

Research Issues

As therapy for pediatric cancer becomes increasingly complex and intensive, there will be a corresponding need for behavioral scientists to monitor the psychological effects of treatment.

The use of protective isolation offers an example of this scientific interplay. The fact that many patients with cancer die of infection spurred several researchers to examine the utility of gnotobiotic (germ-free) environments in reducing the risk of bacterial infection (Preisler and Bjornsson, 1975; Bodey et al., 1971; Levine et al., 1973). Such research was particularly important subsequent to the development of powerful chemotherapeutic agents that temporarily reduced or destroyed patients' immunologic integrity. In most instances, protective isolation was accomplished through the use of restrictive modular units (laminar-airflow rooms) in which patients were placed for periods of up to 6 months. Prior data on the psychological effects of sensory deprivation and social isolation, however, dictated that the behavioral ramifications of isolation treatment be investigated. Several such studies were conducted with both adult and pediatric patients (Kohle et al., 1971; Holland et al., 1977; Kellerman et al., 1976), and results indicated that laminar-airflow treatment was possible without producing debilitating psychopathology if proper support was offered to patients during the course of their therapy. Although the medical utility of protective isolation during chemotherapy is equivocal, there is increased probability of its usage in the future as part of bone-marrow transplantation procedures. Thus the psychological information produced by the laminar-airflow studies may transcend the medical studies with which they were associated.

Another important area of psychological inquiry is the effect of cranial radiation on the central nervous system, particularly as it impinges on intellectual performance. Such radiation is often given prophylactically to children with acute lymphoblastic leukemia to reduce the risk of CNS leukemic infiltration. There is evidence from the literature (Meadows and Evans, 1976; Eiser and Lansdown, 1977; Eiser, 1978) that children who have experienced CNS radiation show decrements as measured by standardized I.Q. tests. These data, however, are limited by the retrospective nature of the studies, leaving it open to questions of confounding owing to impact illness, lack of baseline data, and varying courses of treatment. Prospective studies will play a major role in controlling for many of these variables and in providing new information regarding the long-term effects of treatment.

There are those who will question the value of this research, viewing CNS radiation as inevitable and wondering whether producing information indicating that treatment reduces intellectual functioning will serve any purpose other than to raise parental anxiety. There is a twofold response to such an objection.

First, as treatment protocols become increasingly sophisticated, there is a strong likelihood that medically equivalent treatments employing varying degrees of radiation will be developed. Psychometric data would then be important to consider when choosing among protocols.

Second, psychometric data may be able to pinpoint the nature of radiation-induced decrement and thus aid in developing prophylactic and ameliorative special-education techniques that mediate the effects of treatment.

In addition to monitoring the effects of treatment, the behavioral sciences have a major investigative role in exploring the incidence and frequency of psychological disturbances that are related to a diagnosis of cancer in children, in predicting high-risk factors that predispose families to difficulties, and in refining therapeutic modalities. As pediatric patients continue to live longer, they will face new challenges of adaptation. Issues such as sexual functioning and job discrimination will take on new importance, as will the long-term effects of serious disease on family stability.

A cooperative approach combining the skills of medical and social science will accomplish much in raising the quality, as well as the duration, of life for the seriously ill child. Pediatric psychology, in particular, can be expected to play an increasingly important role in this expanding and vital area.

References

Bandura, A., and Menlove, F.L. Factors determining vicarious extinction of avoidance behavior through symbolic modeling. *Journal of Personality and Social Psychology* 8:99, 1968.

Bahnson, C.B., and Bahnson, M.B. Role of the ego defenses: Denial and repression in the etiology of malignant neoplasms. *Annals of the New York Academy of Science* 125:827, 1966.

Bodey, G.P., Gehan, E.A., Reireich, E.J., and Frei, E. Protected environment: Prophylactic antibiotic program in the chemotherapy of acute leukemia. *American Journal of Medical Science* 262:138, 1971.

Cassell, S. Effects of brief puppet therapy upon the emotional responses of children undergoing cardiac catheterization. *Journal of Consulting Psychology* 29:1, 1965.

Crasilneck, H.B., and Hall, J.A. Clinical hypnosis in problems of pain. *American Journal of Clinical Hypnosis* 15:153, 1973.

Cullen, S.C. Hypno-induction techniques in pediatric anesthesia: *Anesthesiology* 19:279, 1958.

Dash, J. Hypnosis with pediatric cancer patients. In *Psychological Aspects of Childhood Cancer,* ed. J. Kellerman, Springfield, Ill.: Thomas, 1980.

Endler, N.S., and Magnusson, D., eds. *Interactional Psychology and Personality*. New York: Wiley, 1976.

Gardner, G.G. Childhood, death and human dignity: Hypnosis for David. *International Journal of Clinical and Experimental Hypnosis.* 24:122, 1976.

Eiser, C. Intellectual abilities among survivors of childhood leukemia as a function of CNS irradiation. *Archives of the Diseases of Children* 53:391, 1978.

Eiser, C., and Lansdown, R. Retrospective study of intellectual development in children treated for acute lymphoblastic leukemia. *Archives of the Diseases of Children* 52:525, 1977.

Holland, J. Acute Leukemia: Psychological aspects of treatment. In *Cancer Chemotherapy,* eds. F. Elkerbout et al., Leyden: Leyden Univ. Press, 1971.

Holland, J., Plumb, M., Yates, J., and Harris, S. Psychological response of patients with acute leukemia to germ-free environments. *Cancer* 40:871, 1977.

Holmes, H.A., and Holmes, F.F. After ten years, what are the handicaps and lifestyles of children treated for cancer? *Clinical Pediatrics* 14:819, 1975.

Jacobs, L. Hypnosis in clinical pediatrics. *New York State Journal of Medicine* 62:3781, 1962.

Janis, I. *Psychological Stress* New York: Wiley, 1958.

Kagen-Goodheart, L. Re-entry: Living with childhood cancer. *American Journal of Orthopsychiatry* 47:651, 1977.

Katz, E.R., Kellerman, J., Rigler, D., et al. School intervention with pediatric cancer patients. *Journal of Pediatric Psychology* 2:72, 1977.

Kellerman, J. (Ed.). *Psychological Aspects of Childhood Cancer.* Springfield, Ill.: Thomas, 1980.

Kellerman, J., and Katz, E.R. The adolescent with cancer: Theoretical, clinical and research issues. *Journal of Pediatric Psychology* 2:127, 1977.

Kellerman, J., Katz, E.R., and Siegel, S.E. Psychological problems of children with cancer. Unpublished manuscript, 1978.

Kellerman, J., Rigler, D., Siegel, S.E., et al. Psychological evaluation and management of pediatric oncology patients in protected environments. *Medical and Pediatric Oncology* 2:353, 1976.

Koch, C.R., Hermann, J., and Donaldson, M.H. Supportive care of the child with cancer and his family. *Semiars in Oncology* 1:81, 1974.

Kohle, K., Simons, C., and Weidlich, S. Psychological aspects in the treatment of leukemia patients in the isolated-bed system "life island." *Psychotherapy and Psychosomatics* 19:85, 1971.

La Baw, W., Holton, C., Tewell, K., and Eccles, D. The use of selfhypnosis by children with cancer. *American Journal of Clinical Hypnosis* 17:233, 1975.

Lansky, S.B., and Lowman, J.T. Childhood malignancy: A comprehensive approach. *Journal of the Kansas Medical Society* 75:91–94, 1974.

Levine, A.S., Siegel, S.E., Schreiber, A.D., et al. Protected environments and prophylactic antibiotics. *New England Journal of Medicine* 288:477, 1973.

Lewis, S. Considerations in setting up psychological consultation to a pediatric hemotology-oncology team. *Journal of Clinical Child Psychology* 7:21, 1978.

London, P. Hypnosis in children: An experimental approach. *International Journal of Clinical and Experimental Hypnosis* 10:79, 1962.

London, P., and Cooper, L.M. Norms of hypnotic susceptibility in children. *Developmental Psychology* 1:113, 1969.

McCue, K. Preparing children for medical procedures. In *Psychological Aspects of Childhood Cancer,* ed. J. Kellerman, Springfield, Ill.: Thomas, 1980.

Meadows, A.T., and Evans, A.E. Effects of chemotherapy on the central nervous system. A study of parenteral methotrexate in long-term survivors of leukemia and lymphoma in childhood. *Cancer* 37:1079, 1976.

Melamed, B.G., and Siegel, L.J. Reduction of anxiety in children facing hospitalization and surgery by use of filmed modeling. *Journal of Consulting and Clinical Psychology* 43:511, 1975.

Moore, D.C., Holton, C.P., and Marten, G.W. Psychological problems in the management of adolescents with malignancy. *Clinical Pediatrics* 8:464, 1969.

Morgan, A.H., and Hilgard, E.R. Age differences in susceptibility to hypnosis. *International Journal of Clinical and Experimental Hypnosis* 21:78, 1973.

Peebles, J.J., and O'Malley, F. Problems in mental health consultations facing the professional in training. *Journal of Clinical Child Psychology* 7:68, 1978.

Preisler, H.D., and Bjornsson, S. Protected environment units in the treatment of acute leukemia. *Seminars in Oncology.* 2:377, 1975.

Spinetta, J.J., Rigler, D., and Karon, M. Anxiety in the dying child. *Pediatrics* 52:841, 1973.

Vernick, J., and Karon, M. Who's afraid of death on a leukemia ward? *American Journal of Diseases of Children* 109:393, 1965.

11 Psychological Aspects of Loss and Grief in Spinal-Cord and Other Chronically Disabling Injuries

Patrick J. Fazzari

Grief is a process, a movement, a transition. It is real, but often ignored or left unrecognized, because it seems to require the participation of those who dare to deal with it in a clinical setting. This can be an uncomfortable challenge.

How does one write of loss and grief in chronic disabling injuries in order to provide a guide for those who wish to deal with or understand this process? It cannot be done in a cook book or a "how-to-do-it" fashion, since this is not possible or even desirable. One method would be to provide an overview of an injury and to demonstrate that grief over loss is such a fundamental aspect of the ensuing disability that to ignore it would be to render treatment of the disability woefully incomplete. Such is the case with spinal cord injury, which exemplifies the permeating effects of an injury that remains for life. To comprehend the loss, one must understand the disability. But here patient care is the essential ingredient, a care that is persistent as well as consistent, a care that is supported by a team approach.

The concepts of loss, grief, and mourning are similar for most tragic situations in human existence. For example, the stages outlined by Dr. Elizabeth Kübler-Ross (1969) for a patient approaching death (denial, anger, bargaining, depression, acceptance) also can be used as a guide for physical loss, whether it be for loss of a limb or loss of the ability to move. It is therefore essential to understand the nature of the disability as the matrix in which the process of mourning is analyzed. This understanding must be fortified by a knowledge of the patient's preinjury personality dynamics. It should be remembered that the ability to cope need not be determined by the severity of the injury, since a seemingly minor trauma may totally incapacitate an individual, while an injury of devastating proportions may be met with a surprising perseverance.

Loss can be artificially analyzed separately in a physical handicap, but the injury colors its meaning nonetheless. Likewise, dealing with the patient's altered physiology alone excludes the "person" while it ignores the fact that as time passes it is the adjustment to a disability that is of greater significance than the nature of the disability itself.

Team Challenge

For the health-care team, the challenge in providing comprehensive, individualized care for a person with a persisting disability is to find an operational, unifying concept that gives special meaning to a management approach that can be both emotionally and physically draining. In a sense, the team's quest for this meaning reflects a similar process within the patient. A knowledge of the spinal-cord-injured patient's disordered physiology will unite the team on one level only, the physical data base. However, the team's special unity derives from the patient being a member of the team, from a mutual trust, from a belief in the value of communication, and from a willingness to express the difficulties encountered in patient care as solutions are sought and goals are established.

The team should recognize that for a child or adult with a long-term disability, it is not only the sum or coordination of the efforts of the surgical specialties, nursing, medicine, pediatrics, psychology, occupational therapy, and physical therapy that makes up the rehabilitation of such individuals, but also an understanding of the dynamics of growth and development for adults as well as children. For the young child, it may be necessary to grasp the ramifications of the mother-child relationship or the factors that enhance or hinder maternal attachment. The goals and aspirations of adolescence and adulthood also must be understood in a developmental framework. Management too, and not just diagnosis, requires expertise, an expertise that is not merely a matter of coping with an unending series of acute episodes or surgical procedures seemingly unrelated to and occurring over an undercurrent of "chronic disease." Dealing with the acute, physical episodes alone can give the false sense of security that the disability is being managed. Such thinking ignores the profound impact that trauma and disability have on an individual and his or her family. What I am saying is that as we attempt to foster a resolution of loss and grief within the patient, we must be assured that each team member understands the process and his or her reaction to it individually and as a team member. For the health-care practitioners who deal with such patients, it is the continuing nature of the problems—the "disability continuum"—that represents the overriding challenge. Loss, grief, and mourning are just parts of it.

Spinal-Cord Injury

Spinal-cord injury is the very definition of disability. Using it as an example allows us to examine patient management when loss of function, as in quadriplegia, is practically complete.

Injury to the contents of the spinal canal may result from a momentary force, but the ramifications of such a blow continue for a lifetime. The brain's function as modulator is disrupted in complete high-cord lesions because essentially it is separated from that part of the cord remaining below the lesion. The distal, surviving cord continues as a mediator of reflexes. This concept may be simplified, but it allows us to understand the pathology that ensues.

No system or function in the human body is spared the effects of spinal cord injury. The individual cannot move at will; bowel and bladder are lost to voluntary control. Metabolism is disrupted, and the automatic nervous system may respond with exaggeration to what in the past would have been perceived as pain or discomfort. Muscle mass decreases, and sensory input from the periphery is abnormal. What should be evident, then, is that the pathology of spinal-cord injury develops from a loss of functional control, a loss of homeostasis. Comprehensive care of such an individual then becomes fundamentally a matter of preventing complications as a new homeostasis is awaited, a homeostasis that is not only physiologically balanced, but also psychologically at equilibrium.

Equilibrium becomes the last stage in the process of physical adjustment and also the last step in the mourning of a profound loss. This parallelism should force us to pursue the psychological "system" along with the other disrupted systems in the patient. The pursuit of equilibrium is process-oriented, just as rehabilitation itself is a process and not a product. Again, this continuum of management is placed within the context of the patient's own process or continuum of human development, now greatly influenced by chronic disability.

Such principles also can be applied to recovery from head injury and coma. System disruption may not be the same, but loss of control may be complicated by disordered perception, reduced ability to learn, and altered receptive and/or expressive language. Parallelism is necessary here also, but extra time may be spent determining what the patient comprehends.

Loss and Mourning

It was stated that spinal cord injury results in an absence of functional control. In actuality, this is a definition of loss. We then can expect grief and mourning as natural consequences.

It is here that the health-care practitioner must understand the patient's preaccident personality and prior way of life. What were the patterns of response to stress and frustration? Was there any socially deviant behavior? How would one characterize the patient's "life plan" prior to the trauma?

If the patient is a child or adolescent, was psychosocial development proceeding normally prior to the injury? Such questions must be asked because each individual lives within the environment that is himself or herself and the environment that includes spouse, family, and friends. Not only does the patient mourn, but parents, spouse, and other family members mourn too. Old defenses may fail, and those personality characteristics, such as dependency, so diligently defended against before the accident may become fully expressed.

What must be guarded against (and this is the difficult part) is judging a patient in his or her loss by those standards and characteristics we would expect in ourselves if we were confronted by such a loss. This merely points up the need for the practitioner to thoroughly understand his or her own possible reaction to a similar loss within himself or herself and why the patient's reaction may differ significantly.

Nemiah (1961) speaks of loss and depression as acutely painful human experiences. If we ponder the loss of a loved one through death and consider its depressing effects, we may take some comfort in the fact that in the normal course of events we can look forward to a resolution of this grief, an acceptance of the loss. In the normal course of events of spinal cord injury, there is also a resolution. However, "equilibrium" should replace "acceptance" as a final stage of the process, since, in many instances, the process of mourning seems to reappear as patients confront repeated reminders of their disability during their lifetime, for example, decubiti, urinary tract infections, marriage dissolution. In addition, a chronic disability may isolate an individual from people and constrict a person's sense of self. This is why we emphasize the *persistence* of the disability.

For the parents of children and adolescents with brain injury, mourning may be manifested as a refusal to accept medical opinion concerning the finality of the disability, while they seek repeated consultations to verify the diagnosis. Rather than being personally affronted, the practitioner should suggest and offer guidance in seeking a second opinion, recognizing this parental reaction to loss and the need for an advocate during the turmoil. While they reflect, parents need a listener who will allow them to speak of the future as well as of the present.

A person's body or a parent's child is at the very center of his or her system of valuables. Trauma that produces persistent disability can constrict a person's sense of self while isolating that individual from other people. The depression following this loss is an extremely painful human experience. This may be preceded by denial and anger, as well as an effort at diligent cooperation with hopes that therapy and time will return most, if not all, as it once was.

Through all this the team must be the center of care, asking such questions as

What does the patient understand about the cause of the injury?

What does the patient comprehend about the nature of the disability?

What do the parents, spouse, and family understand?

What is the knowledge base of each health-care practitioner on the team?

Is the patient suffering too much?

Would it have been better if the patient had died?

How would each practitioner react with a similar injury?

Is caring for such a person too emotionally draining?

Does the team understand the stages and purposes of mourning?

Does the team express its *feelings* about the patient?

Does each practitioner understand the value of nondirective listening?

The Child

Caring for a child with a long-term disability requires that the parents be included as essential members of the health-care team. The child cannot be treated apart from the family, and it is wise for the practitioner to consider the parents and child as a unit. A handicapped child does not have the insight into loss of function to project the impact of that loss into the future. Parents do this. The process of loss and mourning occurs with them, for it is the loss of the once-normal child they mourn.

If the child's injury occurs during birth, as in cerebral palsy, the mother is then confronted with the dual task of mourning for the hoped-for normal child and developing a maternal attachment to the child who is in fact not lost (Solnit and Stark, 1961). This significant task of working through two processes requires frequent, trusting contact with a team member identified by the team as capable of listening and allowing the parents, especially the mother, to express the frustration, the anger, and the hope as the child goes through the inevitable evaluations and procedures—events that repeatedly serve to remind the parents of their child's disability and vulnerability. It cannot be overemphasized that the attitude of the parents toward their child and his or her disability and their continued acceptance of him or her as a person in large measure determine how that child eventually arrives at an equilibrium with his or her lot in life and how he or she weathers the developmental crises common to all children.

Availability is the key to working with parents experiencing the difficult work of mourning. Such availability means being present at the bedside when the parents visit as well as being available by telephone when the child is home. Such presence admits to the evolutionary process involved with loss, while a friendly, attentive, nonthreatening attitude on the part of the practitioner legitimizes feelings that may be not only new to the parent, but also frightening.

Second, the parents need significant participation in the decision making concerning the medical care and rehabilitation of their child. After all, they will manage the child long after we have finished. Tokenism, paternalism, and a patronizing 'Now now, don't worry" attitude heightens parental frustration and serves only to feed anger. The result may be the iatrogenic so-called noncooperative or troublesome parent. Active participation neutralizes this possibility.

Mothers must be given the opportunity to touch their children and to participate in their care. For a child in a coma, parents often fear that they will not be recognized when their child awakens. Opportunities for touching, reassurance, and listening help keep grief from becoming overwhelming.

Although he or she may not possess a total awareness of his or her disability's impact for the future, and although he or she may lack a typical expression of grief, the older child must be given an opportunity for age-appropriate communication of feelings. This may be provided through play or when nursing care is nonthreatening. Fantasy may play a large part in a child's attempts to come to grips with what has befallen him or her. Acting out destructive behavior may be one manifestation of situational depression owing to the confinement imposed by the disability or the frustration of being unable to move. Again, the opportunity to express fears and fantasies to a nonthreatening, sympathetic listener helps return the order and control most handicapped children need in their lives.

The Adolescent

What was stated earlier concerning parental participation in the care of a young child applies equally when the patient is an adolescent. However, by adolescence, ego development and self-awareness have developed to a point where the health-care team is now confronted with the process of mourning in an emerging adult.

Self-control, self-determination, and independence are major developmental issues during adolescence. Relating these issues to the loss of functional control in spinal cord injury emphasizes how an adolescent's self-image as a social being is severely threatened and how the comfort usually possible in a temporary surrender of autonomy in order to return to health is not possible. It becomes particularly important when dealing with the grieving adolescent to understand or enter the world of his or her perspective. One enters the adolescent's own world by learning as much as possible about interests, ambitions, fears, and family perspective. Personality styles of adolescents remain relatively unchanged despite drastic changes in life situations following trauma. We then deal with *that* person *with* quadriplegia, *that* person who is grieving. Psychopathology before will be psychopathology after, with a totally new dimension—a persisting disability.

When dealing with a grieving adolescent, the team must be careful not to exclude the patient on the false premise that "he or she is not ready to hear what has to be said." This may be legitimate early in the course of management, but if this policy continues, the team becomes less productive. Such a personal process as mourning can only be *observed* by a team and rarely *influenced* by it if the mourner cannot participate in the approach to his or her physical and emotional support. Adolescents are acutely aware of team meetings and resent being excluded. They wish to sort out their options and come to an understanding of their body's disordered function, including sexual function. The well-adjusted adolescent will pass through a "well-adjusted" grief process, while the disturbed adolescent will have a disturbed passage. What distinctly helps both is the parallel team process of including the adolescent in understanding that over which he or she grieves. This is the first step in overcoming disability.

No discussion of injury and loss is complete without a mention of their impact on the adolescent's sexuality. Sexuality is based on an individual's concept of himself or herself as a person capable of intimacy and worthy of giving and receiving love. A successful passage through adolescence helps a person achieve these feelings. When an injury is profound enough to drastically alter bodily functions permanently, these feelings of self are threatened. No wonder, then, that the spinal-cord-injured adolescent often asks (if given the opportunity) if he or she can have children, if he or she is sterile. It is not unusual for an adolescent incapacitated by spastic quadriparesis from a brain stem injury, for example, to flirt with staff or ask for a date. Sexuality is essential to "personhood," and if the goal of dealing with loss and mourning is to arrive at a person at peace with his or her lot in life, then health professionals will not hesitate to deal with the issues of sexuality and disordered genital function in the chronically disabled before the patient gets up the courage to ask first. Let us not forget that often handicapped adolescents lead isolated, lonely lives with little peer interaction and less chance of testing their sexuality, and that most people, including their parents, come to think of them as asexual.

The Adult

This heading includes a broad age spectrum: the young adult at the peak of ability, the mother with children, the father supporting a family, or the aging grandmother. The fundamental mourning process is the same; *who* has the disability must again be clarified by the team with the inclusion of spouse and/or family. As grieving continues long after discharge from a rehabilitation facility, availability and listening must be maintained, with the ultimate goals being the prevention of further functional decline, the continuation of the ability to choose, and the preservation of personal dignity.

Summary

Mourning is an acutely painful process. When it occurs as a result of severe functional loss owing to trauma, it is not enough to attempt to understand the psychological process of grieving. One must also thoroughly comprehend the physical implications of the resulting disability. We say this because in mourning of death, the loss is eventually completed, but in chronic disability, the loss persists for the rest of the person's life. Mourning is resolved when the individual reaches a state of equilibrium with the disability.

If the persisting disability is present in a child, growth and development will seem to modify its expression, and mourning, perhaps not experienced at the time of injury, may occur during predictable times of crisis, such as adolescence. The need, then, is for persistent, process-oriented team management for a persistent disability.

Grief and mourning occur within the context of a social being. Understanding how an injury changes a person's concept of self becomes essential for understanding the total meaning of grief.

For the health-care practitioner managing a grieving patient, it is necessary to understand that

1. Grief over loss is a process.
2. This process is related to developmental stage and personality.
3. Grief cannot be understood apart from the nature of the injury and disability.
4. With persisting disability, mourning may be repeated as new crises appear.
5. Caring for a patient with a persisting disability is difficult and cannot be done by one individual apart from a team.

6. Patient participation in the team is essential.
7. The foundation for team success is communication.

References

Cunning, J.E. Emotional aspects of head trauma in children. *Rehabilitation Literature* 37:335, 1976.

Hohmann, G.W. Psychological aspects of treatment and rehabilitation of the spinal cord injured person. *Clinical Orthopaedics and Related Research* 112: 81, 1975.

Kübler-Ross, E. *On Death and Dying.* New York: Macmillan, 1969.

Lundholm, J., Jepsen, B.N., and Thornval, G. The late neurological, psychological, and social aspects of severe traumatic coma. *Scandinavian Journal of Rehabilitation Medicine* 7:97, 1975.

Mattsson, E.I. Psychological aspects of severe physical injury and its treatment. *Journal of Trauma* 15: 217, 1975.

Nemiah, J.C. *Foundations of Psychopathology.* New York: Oxford Univ. Press, 1961.

Parkes, C.M. Psycho-social transitions: Comparison between reactions to loss of limb and loss of a spouse. *British Journal of Psychiatry* 127: 204, 1975.

Robson, K.S., and Moss, H.A. Patterns and determinants of maternal attachment. *Journal of Pediatrics* 77: 976, 1970.

Solnit, A.J., and Stark, M.H. Mourning and the birth of a defective child. In *The Psychoanalytic Study of the Child,* Vol. 16. New York: International Universities Press, 1961.

Steiner, H., and Clark, W.R., Jr. Psychiatric complications of burned adults: A classification. *Journal of Trauma* 17: 134, 1977.

Stewart, T.D. Spinal cord injury: A role for the psychiatrist. *American Journal of Psychiatry* 134: 538, 1977.

Weller, D.J., and Miller, P.M. Emotional reactions of patient, family, and staff in acute-care period of spinal cord injury, Part 1. *Social Work in Health Care* 2: 369, 1977.

12 Behavioral-Medicine Approach to Health Care: Hemophilia as an Exemplary Model

James W. Varni
and *Dennis C. Russo*

Behavioral-Medicine Approach to Health Care

A rather recent development in health management has been the application of the principles of behavioral psychology toward the enhancement of patient care, hospital services, and treatment delivery. Through the principles derived from previous research efforts with other clinical populations and problems, the techniques of behavior therapy and behavior modification are beginning to be applied and evaluated as a component in the comprehensive treatment of medical disorders. This interface between behavioral psychology and medicine has been termed *behavioral medicine* (Birk, 1973; Schwartz and Weiss, 1978). As an emerging field, behavioral medicine is concerned with both the role of contributory psychological factors in health status and the development of treatment strategies in the prevention (Masek et al., 1980) and treatment (Cataldo et al., 1980b) of disease states. Work in behavioral medicine is based on the assumption that through the discovery of causal links between disease and the environmental factors that contribute to its development, maintenance, and/or exacerbation, treatments can be developed resulting in improved health care. While in the past, behavioral approaches have been applied to a myriad of "psychiatric" disorders, such as obsessive-compulsive neurosis (Marks, 1973), phobias (Wolpe and Lazarus, 1966), psychosis (Liberman et al., 1973; Varni et al., 1979), anorexia nervosa (Agras et al., 1974), and sexual disorders (Barlow et al., 1973; Rekers and Varni, 1977a), the field of behavioral medicine represents an independent area of inquiry. The 1977 Yale Conference on Behavioral Medicine proposed that "behavioral medicine is the field concerned with the development of behavioral science knowledge and techniques relevant to the understanding of physical health and illness and the application

This work was supported by Grant No. MC-B-060001-02-0 from the Bureau of Community Health Services, Department of Health, Education and Welfare, and Grant No. 917 from the Maternal and Child Health Service, Department of Health, Education and Welfare. The authors would like to thank Shelby Dietrich, M.D., Edward Gomperts, M.D., and Carol Hyman, M.D. for providing valuable feedback during the preparation of this chapter.

139

of this knowledge and these techniques to prevention, diagnosis, treatment and rehabilitation. Psychosis, neurosis, and substance abuse are included only so far as they contribute to physical disorders as an end point" (Schwartz and Weiss, 1978).

As the authors point out, this definition provides a number of specific restrictions in behavioral-medicine practice and implies a number of directions appropriate to the development of the field. Perhaps most important, behavioral medicine is to be considered an interdisciplinary endeavor, with its contributions provided within the framework of existing disciplines of medicine, the allied health professions (for example, epidemiology and physiology), and the behavioral sciences (for example, psychology, psychiatry, and sociology). In the long run and following the empirical tradition of behavioral approaches, behavioral medicine will be judged not on this preliminary definition, but rather on the basis of its accomplishments in and value to the health-care sector.

General Dimensions of Behavioral Medicine

The proper conceptualization of behavioral-medicine inquiry is still a subject of much debate (Cataldo et al., 1980b; Schwartz and Weiss, 1978). However, much as the Yale conference has attempted an initial definition of behavioral medicine as a field, it is perhaps appropriate to attempt to define some dimensions that are likely to characterize the *practice* of behavioral medicine, so as to differentiate it procedurally from other psychologically based approaches. Similarly, it is vital to consider that the dimensions presented in subsequent paragraphs represent initial starting points based on present conceptualizations. If and when the combined skills of all disciplines in health care functionally define the field of behavioral medicine, its parameters could be quite different. In this chapter, we have chosen to focus on the behavioral health psychologist and the basis for this inquiry.

Focus on Behavior. Many of the symptoms of disease appear as overt physical behaviors. Other symptoms may be biomeasurable through either invasive or noninvasive measuring instruments. In either case, symptoms are definable as discrete events or as interval-based measures of some physiological function (for example, muscle-produced electrical activity or EMG). A number of behaviors also may be defined which, although not symptoms of a disease state, may be correlated with its development, its maintenance, or the presentation of symptoms. The focus on behavior as a locus of treatment and determinate of outcome represents a primary dimension of behavioral medicine. Similarly, the behaviors of others in the patient environment, such as physicians, other health personnel, and the patient's family and friends, also serve as events that may influence the behavioral approach.

Reliance on Measurement. The behavioral psychologist in the health-care setting has access to methods for the assessment, measurement, and delineation of behaviors and their causal effects developed in other settings with non-health-related problems (Hersen and Bellack, 1976). The application of this methodology provides a starting point for behavioral-medicine research to determine the efficacy of treatment and its effects on the patient and his or her environment. Reliable measurement of change may further be useful in biomedical research in which correlation of behavioral and physiological/biochemical states may provide clues to the mechanism of disease (Bird and Cataldo, 1978).

Understanding the Environmental Correlates of Disease. Physical disease occurs within the context of the social and physical environment of the patient. While such relationships have long been recognized, the focus on behavior and its measurement by the behaviorally oriented practitioner may help to better elucidate the causal relationships between environmental events and the development, maintenance, and exacerbation of disease. Particularly important in this regard may be the study of the behaviors of the patient with chronic illness and the response of the patient's caretakers (Cataldo et al., 1980*b*).

Behavioral Medicine Intervention Strategies

Behavioral procedures for the change of health behavior are noncontextual. That is, they specify how to change behavior rather than which behaviors to change or the environment in which the change is to occur. Under these circumstances, most chronic diseases and service settings provide a virtually unlimited potential for assessment and intervention. The procedures developed for behavioral assessment (see Hersen and Bellack, 1976) and environmental modification (Cataldo and Risley, 1974) are well documented. Their application to disease, medical procedures, and medical-service settings represents a new area for their utilization. To illustrate this point, the application of behavioral procedures to four areas will be considered: (1) disease and disability prevention, (2) disease and disability treatment, (3) adjunctive treatments, and (4) health-care delivery. For example, prevention can be illustrated by the example of coronary heart disease, where behavioral procedures may be implemented to reduce the risk of coronary heart disease through the modification of such risk factors as hypercholesterolemia, hypertension, cigarette smoking, obesity, and physical inactivity (Margolis,

1977). The control of hypertension through relaxation therapy (Jacob et al., 1977), and the management of migraine headaches through biofeedback (Friar and Beatty, 1976) provide examples of treatment problems. The application of behavioral procedures in medicine compliance (Epstein and Masek, 1978) and drug-effectiveness evaluation (Varni et al., 1978) are illustrative health-care delivery strategies. These intervention categories are presented below in further detail.

Prevention. Prevention of disease represents a major priority for national health care in the coming decade (Breslow, 1978; Lalonde, 1975). With this shift in emphasis, an increasing role is likely for the behavioral sciences (Hamburg and Brown, 1978; Schwartz and Weiss, 1978). Prevention programs focused on the reduction of risks for development of chronic disease through research on risk-factors identification, the study of events maintaining these risks, and the development of procedures to train alternative healthful behaviors (Masek et al., 1980). Research on cardiovascular disease (Williams et al., 1977; Boyer, 1975; Meyer and Henderson, 1974), liver disease (Goldstein et al., 1976), cancer detection (Fink et al., 1968), and kidney disease (Barnes, 1976) has already begun to demonstrate the efficacy of behaviorally based prevention programs in primary and secondary (Breslow, 1978) as well as tertiary prevention programs (Cataldo et al., 1980b). A review of behavioral approaches to prevention is provided by Masek et al (1980).

Treatment of Disease. Behavioral intervention in the reduction of active disease also represents an area of current research and potential. Since the presentation of symptoms in many diseases may be exacerbated by environmental events, their evaluation may provide the key to their treatment. Programs for the reduction of asthmatic attacks (Renne and Creer, 1976), epileptic seizures (Cataldo et al., 1980a; Zlutnick et al., 1975), and dermatological conditions (Cataldo et al., 1980c) provide direct evidence for the efficacy of behavioral treatment of disease states. Similarly, the potential use of biofeedback and conditioning approaches has been demonstrated in the reduction of symptoms associated with neuromuscular disease (Bird and Cataldo, 1978), cardiac arrythmias (Weiss and Engel, 1971; Scott et al., 1973), fecal incontinence (Engel et al., 1974; Kohlenberg, 1973), and Raynaud's disease (Surwit, 1973).

While these initial studies have demonstrated laboratory and short-term benefits, careful study of long-term management and maintenance factors remains to be conducted (Bird and Cataldo, 1978; Cataldo et al., 1980b). Until such outcome research is undertaken, the applicability of behavioral procedures as a viable procedure to disease management remains to be determined.

Adjunctive Services. In addition to direct treatment of disease, behavioral treatments have been applied as adjunctive procedures to traditional medical therapies. The primary application has been the provision of treatment for the psychological side effects of chronic disease.

Patients with long-term illness must adjust to the altered life situations and interpersonal relationships that are likely to develop as a result of disease-imposed limitations. Under these circumstances, the patient may learn strategies to provide immediate relief or obtain sympathy from others, which may be counter to his or her long-term recovery (Cataldo et al., 1980b; Fordyce, 1976). The patient may become depressed (Lewinsohn et al., 1976), helpless (Seligman, 1975), and evidence exaggerated physical symptoms such as pain (Fordyce, 1976; Varni et al., 1980). Behavioral procedures such as relaxation (Benson, 1975), thought stopping and competing response training (Cataldo et al., 1978), or assertiveness training (Bower and Bower, 1976) may facilitate the development of skills better enabling the individual to cope with his or her disease.

Health-Care Delivery. Medicine is practiced within the context of a number of settings, such as hospitals, clinics, and physicians' offices. The design of these environments and their procedures is an appropriate subject for behavioral research. For example, Cataldo et al. (1980a) studied the behavior of children on a pediatric intensive care unit (PICU). They found that a large percentage of the children were awake and alert while hospitalized, despite their serious medical conditions. Through the use of simple procedures and instructions to staff, improvements were seen in the affect, contact with play materials, and social behaviors of these children. This study suggests that behavioral procedures may be helpful in relieving at least some of the fear and concern often exhibited by patients, particularly young children. Utilizing methodologies similar to those outlined in this study, programs to increase clinic staff performance (Cataldo et al., 1978) or to minimize the negative effects of hospitalization may be designed to improve general health-care services.

Behavioral procedures also may be of value in developing and maintaining patient participation in the compliance with medical procedures. Procedures to increase compliance to oral medication regimens (Epstein and Masek, 1978) and dietary restrictions in patients undergoing hemodialysis (Magrab and Papadopoulou, 1977; Barnes, 1976) provide examples of behavioral procedures designed to maximize the outcome of medical treatments.

While initial studies have suggested that behavioral programs may be of value in several areas, more research clearly needs to be undertaken to fully understand the proper place of these programs within medicine. Particularly, the applicability of behavioral intervention in chronic disease may be an area in which initial studies will show immediate impact. Hemophilia represents one disease that may provide a base for this research.

Medical Aspects of Hemophilia: A Brief Overview

Hemophilia represents a congenital, hereditary disorder of blood coagulation, transmitted by a female carrier to her male offspring. This life-long, chronic disorder is often characterized by recurrent, unpredictable bleeding episodes affecting any body part, especially the joints and the extremities. The severity of the disorder varies among individuals, with the failure to produce one of the plasma proteins required to form a blood clot being the identifying characteristic. The incidence of hemophilia is estimated to be 1 in 10,000 of the male population, with the most common variety named *hemophilia A* (or classical hemophilia), represented by a plasma protein factor VIII deficiency; *hemophilia B* (or Christmas disease) is the next most common, with a factor IX deficiency in the coagulation chain (Hilgartner, 1976). There are other blood-clotting disorders (for example, von Willebrand's disease), many of which are considerably rarer.

Since one of the clotting proteins is lacking, a blood clot takes a substantially longer period of time to form, and it may not be an effective clot for the ruptured vessel (Kasper, 1976). Small external cuts on the skin can usually be treated by pressure bandages; however, internal bleeding (typically indicated by pain, loss of motion, and/or swelling) may be quite prolonged. Although internal bleeding episodes can occur as a result of physical trauma, many bleeding episodes occur spontaneously, that is, without clear precipitating cause (Agle, 1977). Spontaneous bleeding episodes are typical in severe hemophiliacs (that is, those individuals with extremely limited available blood-clotting proteins), whereas moderate to mild hemophiliacs may experience excessive bleeding only as a result of obvious physical injury. Repeated bleeding into the joint areas (hemarthrosis) eventually results in a form of arthritis, accompanied by chronic pain (Dietrich, 1976). Acute episodes of pain also are caused by muscle bleeds (hemotomas) owing to hydraulic pressure on sensitive nerves. Typical of any chronic medical disorders where pain is an outstanding and recurrent symptom, analgesic drug misuse and/or addiction are of constant concern (Varni, 1979; 1980*a*). As medical treatment has improved, a larger population of adult hemophiliac survivors has appeared, with an increased incidence of degenerative arthritic-induced chronic pain. An estimated 75 percent of adult hemophiliacs have one or more affected joints, with the most frequently affected being the knee, then the elbow, ankle, shoulder, and hip, respectively (Dietrich, 1976).

A major breakthrough in the medical care and management of hemophilia came less than 15 years ago with the discovery and separation of the essential clotting factors from the plasma of normal blood. Freeze-dried concentrates of the clotting-factor proteins made from pooled plasma are now available and are reconstituted with sterile water. Dosage of factor-deficiency replacement is calculated on the basis of the patient's weight, the assumed plasma volume, and the severity of the bleeding episodes. The intravenous infusion of the concentrate temporarily replaces the missing clotting factor and converts the clotting status to normal, allowing a functional blood clot to form. As a result of home-based administration and self-infusion of concentrate, early treatment is now possible, consequently reducing the severity of bleeding episodes. Since prolonged bleeding into the joints often results in crippling arthritis and prolonged bleeding in the neck, throat, head, and retroperitoneal areas is potentially life-threatening, the benefits of prompt treatment become evident. The hereditary nature of the disease and the additional fact that it may occur as a result of one of the most frequent mutations known in medicine suggest that the incidence in our society will increase rather than decrease (Boone, 1968). Further information on the medical aspects of hemophilia may be found in several recent texts (Boone, 1976; Hilgartner, 1976).

Behavioral-Medicine Approach to Hemophilia

Behavioral-medicine intervention strategies in the comprehensive management of hemophilia consist of prevention, treatment, and health-care delivery. The specifics of each area of intervention as applied to hemophilia are now presented.

Prevention

The fact that hemophilia is genetically transmitted precludes the more traditional approach of identifying and modifying risk factors in the individual so as to prevent the development of a chronic disorder (such as chronic heart disease). However, an alternative primary prevention strategy involves the screening of females at risk of being genetic carriers of the disease, as indicated by their relationship to a hemophilic male (Merrit and Conneally, 1976). Through a regional registry of families with a history of hemophilia, individuals can be identified and advised on the probabilities of producing an affected child, thereby allowing the potential parents prior time for a rational and thoughtful decision regarding having children and its subsequent risks (Childs, 1975). Further, a secondary prevention strategy, through early education programs for all hemophilic children and their parents, would stress the importance of immediate concentrate infusion and the selection of reasonable physical activities in an attempt to prevent the severe orthopedic disabilities and accompanying chronic pain that result from repeated hemorrhage into the joints, causing progressive arthritic deterioration.

Typical of chronic medical disorders with an inherently unstable clinical course, hemophilia is often accompanied by secondary emotional dysfunction; that is, the hemophiliac tends to be at risk for demonstrating psychological adjustment difficulties (Agle, 1977). From this perspective, a tertiary prevention strategy would be directed toward the early identification of the familial and individual risk factors (such as unassertiveness or social-skills deficits) of emotional dysfunction. Specific techniques to modify these risk factors are described in the next section.

Treatment

Behavioral-medicine treatment techniques may be classified as either bio-feedback procedures or nonbiofeedback behavioral procedures (Blanchard, 1977). In general, clinical biofeedback involves the direct modification of aberrant physiological states through the use of instrument-produced feedback. This feedback may be in the form of an auditory tone or a digital or graphic display of the monitored physiological response, for example, electromyographic (EMG), skin temperature, electroencephalographic (EEG), electrodermal (GSR), blood, or heart rate (Kamiya et al., 1977). Through the use of feedback and cognitive strategies, the patient attempts to modify the abnormal physiological condition (Fuller, 1978; Gaarder and Montgomery, 1977). Nonbiofeedback behavioral procedures are designed to change the antecedent stimulus conditions that precede, or the consequent events that follow, the symptoms of the disorder and may potentially influence its course. Often, biofeedback and nonbiofeedback procedures are combined in a treatment package for certain disorders, such as chronic pain.

In the behavioral-medicine approach to hemophilia, a number of specific problem areas are outstanding. The most common of these will be discussed in subsequent paragraphs, with illustrations of the various behavioral techniques utilized as part of their comprehensive management.

Chronic Pain. As a result of repeated hemorrhages into the joints over time, an arthritic condition develops with accompanying incidents of chronic pain. Pain has been conceptualized as containing both physical and psychological components, with their relative contribution to perceived pain varying according to the individual (Ince, 1976). Thus pain perception involves not only sensing painful stimuli, but also behavioral and cognitive components that may intensify or lessen the pain experience (Varni, 1979). Whereas acute pain is clearly elicited either by disease or physical injury (for example, pain associated with a specific bleeding episode), chronic pain represents a sustained condition over an extended period of time (for example, arthritic pain), often without clear precipitating cause. Merskey (1970) cites evidence that particular pain patterns are learned through the interaction of the individual and his or her social environment, with statements of pain and its intensity appearing to have "psychological concomitants," even though the initial insult was physical trauma or illness (Epstein and Harris, 1978). Therefore, chronic pain experiences may best be viewed as an interaction between an initial trauma or precipitating factor and social-environmental influences (Varni et al., 1980).

A number of medical approaches for the potential amelioration of chronic pain are available, including pharmacological agents (Halpern, 1974), anesthetic nerve blocks (Black, 1974), electrical stimulation (Ebersold et al., 1975), and surgical procedures (Stravino, 1970). Unfortunately, the effectiveness of these procedures has been inconsistent (Black, 1975; Swanson et al., 1976). Pain management from a behavioral-medicine perspective involves electromyographic and/or skin-temperature biofeedback, as well as stimulus-consequent events assessment and modification (see figure 12-1 for an example of a pain-analysis data sheet). Biofeedback application to chronic pain is still a relatively new area, with the current major focus being the reduction of tension and anxiety associated with pain experiences. In this model, pain has been suggested to be both an antecedent to and a response of physical stress (Gentry and Bernal, 1977). Gentry and Bernal propose a pain-tension-pain cycle whereby the physiological response to pain involves the immediate tensing of muscles surrounding the afflicted area, which may then increase the subjective experience of pain, leading to further tension in adjacent muscle groups, resulting in eventual immobilization of the affected area. Such immobilization may result in shortened muscle fibers or contractures over time, eventually causing even more pain. Both temperature and EMG biofeedback for chronic pain attempt to induce a more relaxed state and, as such, break the pain-tension-pain-cycle. Recent work using imagery and thermal biofeedback techniques in the management of chronic arthritic pain in hemophilia has been very encouraging (Varni, 1979a; 1980a).

The nonbiofeedback behavioral assessment and modification of chronic pain focuses on the external accompaniments of an assumed internal pain state (Fabrega and Tyma, 1976). External manifestations include the absence of "well" behaviors and the emission of pain behaviors, that is, verbal reports of pain and such nonverbal expressions as facial grimaces, compensatory posturing, restricted movement, and limping (Fordyce, 1976). Well-behavior deficits include decreased activity levels and restricted interpersonal contacts associated with depression. Assessment of the poten-

Date	Time		Type	Intensity Scale	Antecedents	Location	Medication	Pain Reduction	Tension Scale
	Start	Stop							

Code: Type = Arthritic pain (A)
Bleeding pain (B)
Other pain (O)

Location = for example, left
elbow, right knee.

Antecedents = for example, physical trauma,
interpersonal stress, unknown.

Intensity = 1 (mild) to 10 (severe).

Medication = analgesic or concentrate;
type and amount.

Pain reduction = 1 (not effective) to
10 (100% effective)

Daily tension = 1 (relaxed) to
10 (stressed).

Figure 12–1. Self-Report Pain and Hemorrhage Data Sheet Utilized in Assessment and Management of Pain and Bleeding Episodes

tial environmental influences on pain and well behaviors can often delineate which stimulus-consequent events are candidates for change. Since Fordyce's original publication in this area over 10 years ago (Fordyce et al., 1968), an increasing amount of attention has been paid to the behavioral management of adult chronic pain (Weissenberg, 1977). However, little empirical evidence exists of the efficacy of behavioral procedures in the management of pediatric chronic pain.

In order to illustrate a behavioral approach to pediatric chronic pain, a single-subject investigation is presented (Varni et al., 1980). A salient point of this study involves the rationale developed for the treatment program, which was important not only for considerations of scientific understanding and advancing good clinical practice, but also in presenting the program to medical and professional staffs managing the child and enlisting their aid in conducting the program. The rationale involves the proposition that attending to pain complaints in attempts to comfort the child may not always be in the child's long-term best interest, but demonstrations of affection, concern, and comfort may be rescheduled to maximize rehabilitation and improve the child's psychological status.

The patient was a 3-year-old female who had been hospitalized for 10 months for treatment of second and third degree burns to her buttocks, legs, and perineum as a result of immersion in hot water. Circumstances surrounding the burn incident indicated the possibility of child abuse. Scar contractures and subsequent decreased range of motion in both knees necessitated the wearing of Jobst stockings and knee-extension splints. At the time of the initiation of the program, the patient was exhibiting an array of chronic pain behaviors that interfered significantly with her rehabilitation and constructive patient-caretaker interactions. Furthermore, these pain responses appeared to increase in both intensity and frequency in attention-seeking and demand situations. Data were obtained in three different settings: (1) clinic room, where the patient wore the knee-extension splints in a contrived setting; (2) bedroom, where the patient wore the splints in a natural hospital environment; and (3) physical-therapy situation, during which the physical therapist focused on improved range of motion and independent ambulation (figures 12–2 and 12–3).

Three categories of pain behaviors were recorded: crying, which ranged in intensity from sobbing to screaming; verbal pain behaviors, which consisted of such statements as "My leg/ankle/foot/stomach hurts," "Ouch," or "I can't stand up"; and nonverbal pain behaviors, consisting of any gestural response expressing pain or discomfort, such as facial grimaces, rubbing the legs or buttocks, or not standing. In addition, an activity measure, number of steps descended, was measured in physical therapy, since it was important for the child's range of motion and independent ambulation. In the baseline assessment, it became evident that the child's pain behaviors were a function of adult attention and demand situations. In the absence of

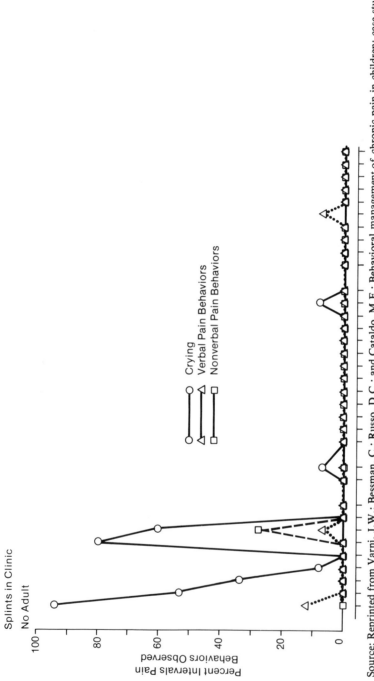

Source: Reprinted from Varni, J.W.; Bessman, C.; Russo, D.C.; and Cataldo, M.F.; Behavioral management of chronic pain in children: case study, *Archives of Physical Medicine and Rehabilitation*, 1980. Reprinted with permission.

Note: The vertical broken line indicates when treatment (reinforcement for nonpain behaviors) or a return to baseline was intitiated. The date abscissa indicates the distribution of sessions across days.

Figure 12-2. Percent of Observation Intervals per Session in which Pain Behaviors Were Noted in Each of Three Settings.

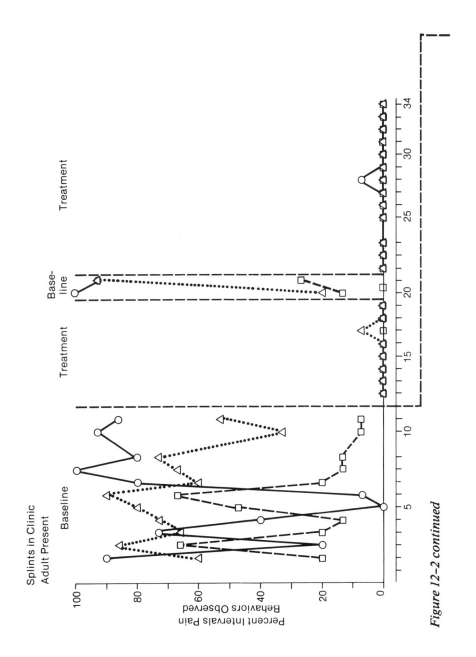

Figure 12–2 continued

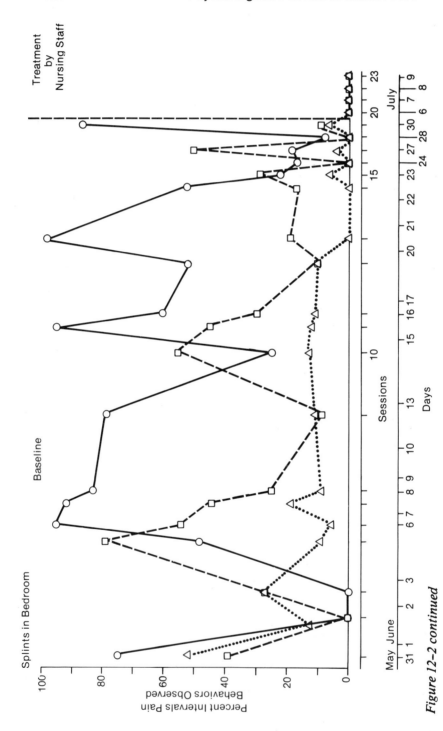

Figure 12–2 continued

adult presence, chronic pain behaviors were noticeably infrequent. Perhaps more important, it was observed that when the child was engaged in interesting activities with accompanying staff attention for these appropriate behaviors, pain complaints were reciprocally low.

Since the baseline assessment suggested that the pain behaviors were influenced by environmental factors, treatment consisted of rearranging the existing contingencies. Thus, both in the clinic and in the bedroom settings where the child wore her knee-extension splints, attention and tangible reinforcers (for example, ice cream) were made contingent upon such "well" behaviors as helping to put on the splints, positive verbalizations, smiling, and the like. Once the techniques were shown to be effective in decreasing pain patterns in the clinic, both the rationale and a demonstration were presented to other staff managers, along with a review of data-collection procedures. The nursing personnel were then taught how to carry out the procedures in the hospital environment. In the physical-therapy setting, since the child was required to descend a number of steps as part of the therapeutic exercise, treatment consisted of the therapist rewarding the child for descending the steps and ignoring pain responses. Reliable behavioral data on pain and appropriate well behaviors obtained throughout baseline and treatment conditions indicated a successful program (see, for example, figures 12-2 and 12-3).

In summary, a functional analysis indicated that the child's chronic pain behaviors were under social-environmental influences. Reinforcement of well behaviors and the removal of attention from chronic-pain behaviors resulted in substantial decreases of pain responses and increases in rehabilitative behaviors. While it was not possible to determine whether the patient actually felt pain or simply displayed the associated behaviors, in the present case, no further pain displays were observed with the onset of the behavioral intervention. Fordyce (1976) suggests that in certain circumstances, patients, through learning, may actually come to experience pain in excess of the accompanying physical basis for the pain, or even in the absence of a physical basis for the perceived pain. In such cases, and in cases similar to the one presented, in which pain behaviors serve the patient's immediate needs while hindering long-term rehabilitation, a behavioral approach is a significant component of a total management program for chronic-pain-producing conditions.

It is important to note that the managing personnel were successfully enlisted in this program as a result of demonstrating changes in pain and well behaviors with changes in the social environment and also as a result of the proposed rationale for the program—that reinforcing immediate requests for comfort and avoidance of procedures were producing long-term physical and psychological risks. While many parents and professionals who manage patients with chronic-pain disorders will respond to the proposed rationale, we have found the objective demonstration of environ-

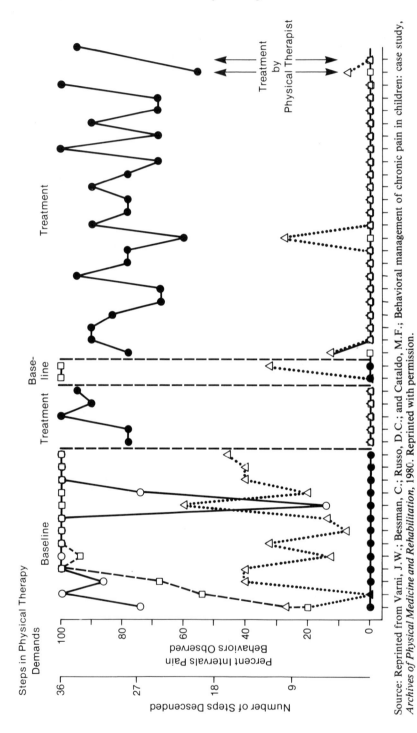

Source: Reprinted from Varni, J.W.; Bessman, C.; Russo, D.C.; and Cataldo, M.F.; Behavioral management of chronic pain in children: case study, *Archives of Physical Medicine and Rehabilitation*, 1980. Reprinted with permission.

Note: The vertical broken line indicates when treatment or a return to baseline was initiated. The date abscissa indicates the distribution of sessions across days.

Figure 12–3. Number of Steps Descended and Percent of Intervals in which Pain Behaviors Were Noted When Either Demands or No Demands Were Being Made on the Child to Participate in Physical Therapy.

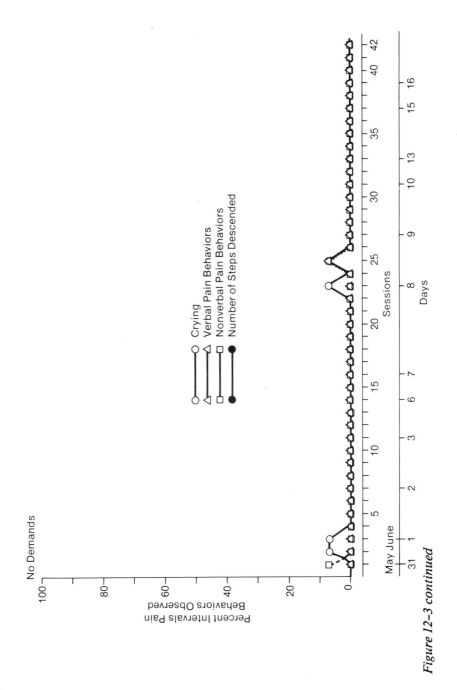

Figure 12-3 continued

mental influences on pain to be invaluable in convincing other parents or staff who have difficulty accepting the rationale.

Emotional Stress. The emotional stresses often associated with a chronic disorder such as hemophilia may greatly impede interpersonal development and physical-activities exploration (Agle and Mattsson, 1976), as well as lead to secondary dysfunction such as chronic insomnia (Varni, 1980*b*). The most frequently used behavioral technique for stress and anxiety management is relaxation training, in one or another of its popular variants, including the relaxation response (Benson, 1975), progressive muscle relaxation training (Jacobson, 1938), hypnosis (Kroger, 1977), autogenic training (Schultz and Luthe, 1969), and stress inoculation training (Meichenbaum and Turk, 1976). The common denominators of all these techniques consist of imagery conditioning and muscle relaxation in an attempt to reduce sympathetic nervous system dominance or the "fight-or-flight" response (Benson, 1975). The essential components involve the concentration on a single word or pleasant scene; self-statements suggesting relaxation, heaviness, warmth, and coping; and regulated breathing (Varni, 1979*a*). Combining relaxation training with desensitization techniques (Wolpe, 1973), that is, the gradual exposure of the patient to the feared object or situation, has allowed management of a number of fear or phobic responses, including needle phobias or fear of injections (Katz, 1974), an important consideration given the number of transfusions a hemophiliac must endure. Such relaxation-desensitization training also has been found useful for anxiety and fear associated with interpersonal interactions, as described in the next subsection.

Unassertiveness/Social-Skills Deficits. With repeated incidents of pain, bleeding, and immobilization, the hemophilic individual often finds himself or herself removed from the normal flow of everyday social contact (Agle, 1977). These episodes which interrupt interpersonal interactions may ultimately impede the normal development of assertiveness and social skills, potentially resulting in passivity and mood depression, leading to even further isolation. This deteriorating interpersonal skills cycle requires vigorous intervention to prevent further psychological adjustment difficulties. Most often, unassertiveness is not a pervasive personality trait, but rather is situationally specific (Eisler et al., 1975); that is, certain interpersonal encounters are anxiety provoking, whereas others do not represent any difficulties (for example, parents versus peer interactions). Behavioral-assessment inventories exist to aid in delineating specific areas of unassertiveness or social skills deficit (Gambrill and Richey, 1975). A number of assertion training manuals are available, both for children (Palmer, 1977) and adolescents and adults (Bower and Bower, 1976).

Teaching the differentiation between passivity, assertion, and aggression involves distinguishing assertion as the expression of one's feelings and rights, without impinging on the rights of others (aggression). Assertiveness focuses on negotiating reasonable changes in social interactions, without the use of manipulation or guilt (passive aggression). Assertiveness includes such components as duration of eye contact, body posture, speech volume, appropriate affect, and number of speech disturbances (Eisler et al., 1975). Once the unassertiveness situations have been identified, training consists of practice interactions set up by the therapist, whereby the patient emits his or her typical response to the problem and the therapist then models a more appropriate response. Through behavioral rehearsal, the patient practices the more adaptive behavior in front of the therapist, receiving constant feedback to refine style. Once the behavior has been mastered during the sessions, the patient then employs the new skills in real-life situations that had originally been problem areas. The usefulness of assertion training cannot be overemphasized, not only in reducing interpersonal anxiety and skills deficits, but also in decreasing generalized mood depression (Lewinsohn et al., 1976) as the patient moves toward exercising more control over his or her life situation.

Weight. Excessive weight and obesity place a greater burden on the musculoskeletal structure, potentially leading to an increased number of hemorrhages into the joints, increased pain, and decreased mobility (Boone, 1976). A behavioral approach to weight control emphasizes modification of eating patterns rather than pound reduction per se (Stuart and Davis, 1972). The most frequently employed techniques involve self-monitoring of food and calorie intake, analysis of the time and situations associated with food intake, stimulus modification, cognitive restructuring of self-statements regarding food and weight, and the designing of an activity or exercise program (Mahoney and Mahoney, 1976). Figure 12–4 contains an example of an eating-patterns data sheet. Specific techniques such as separating eating from other activities, making high-calorie foods unavailable, eating slowly, and reinforcing eating changes have been reported to be successful components of an overall behavioral weight-control program (Stunkard and Mahoney, 1976).

Substance Abuse. In an attempt to reduce the chronic pain associated with arthritic joints and the acute pain indicative of hemorrhage, many hemophiliacs rely on a number of analgesic or narcotic substances (Varni, 1979). Unfortunately, over time, a problem of substance abuse may develop, whether it be analgesic medication overuse, narcotic dependency, or alcohol abuse. Behavioral management of substance abuse is a relatively recent development and consists of an intense and multifaceted program combin-

Food and Beverage Intake Record

Day	Time	How Much	Food Eaten (What Kind)	Where	With Whom	Doing What	Calorie Count
First meal							
Snack(s)							
Second meal							
Snack(s)							
Third meal							
Snack(s)							
Activities							

Comments

Figure 12–4. Self-Report Eating Patterns, Calorie Consumption, and Activity Data Sheet Utilized in Weight Management

ing analysis of stimulus–consequent environmental events, problem-solving skills training, behavioral contracting, and self-monitoring (Sobell and Sobell, 1977).

Behavioral Disorders. Epidemiological research has suggested that children with chronic illness and disabilities are at high risk for developing behavioral and emotional disorders secondary to their chronic condition (Rutter et al., 1970). A behavioral approach to the modification of behavior disorders consists of training the child's parents and teachers, when indicated, in behavioral-management techniques (Patterson, 1975; Varni, 1980*b*) and teaching the child self-control skills. Behavioral self-regulation skills training has been applied to a diversity of child behavior problems in both the school and home (Glynn and Thomas, 1974; Lovitt and Curtiss, 1969; Rekers and Varni, 1977*a* and *b*; Varni et al., 1978). In addition, self-instructional training, utilizing observations that children's motor behaviors are often accompanied by related verbal statements (Lovaas et al., 1977; Meichenbaum and Goodman, 1969), relies mainly on verbally mediated self-regulation of behavior and has been successfully employed with children described as impulsive and hyperactive (Bornstein and Quevillon, 1976; Meichenbaum and Goodman, 1971; Varni and Henker, 1979).

As previously mentioned, patients with chronic medical disorders often evidence depression as a result of a general feeling of not being in control. Through the training of such coping skills as behavioral self-control strategies and assertiveness, patients can develop a sense of internal control and a sense that they can affect their environment and the events affecting them. Such skills acquisition not only may provide a sense of internal control, but also may significantly contribute to the patient's successful psychological development. The learning of coping skills may prevent the chronically disabled patient from developing further behavioral and personality disorders secondary to the disability (Yule, 1977). To take this concept one step further, we may in fact be able to help chronically disabled patients *overcompensate* in other areas from their disorder through the use of assertion, social skills, and self-management training (Cataldo et al., 1980*b*). Thus through coping skills, patients can be taught not only to remedy behavioral deficits, but also to excel.

Health-Care Delivery

Adherence to treatment regimens for chronic disorders represents a continuing problem, with estimates of noncompliance ranging from 4 to 92 percent (Marston, 1970) and averaging from 30 to 35 percent (Davis, 1966). In a review on medical-regimen compliance, Kasl (1975) suggests that noncompliance may very well be a function of social-environmental events, as well as the lack of immediate change in symptomatology. Zifferblatt (1975) also suggests that antecedent stimuli and consequent events are the major functional variables influencing medical-regimen compliance. In hemophilia, examples of compliance would be administering concentrate as soon as a hemorrhage has been identified; reasonably restricting "risk-taking" behaviors, such as football; and performing physical-therapy exercises necessary to rehabilitate affected musculoskeletal structures. Gentry (1977) proposes behavioral self-control training as a potential method for improving medical-regimen compliance. While the investigations reporting the successful use of behavioral procedures in medical compliance (for example, Bigelow et al., 1976) are promising, further research must be conducted over extended follow-up periods to determine the ultimate utility of the procedures. In terms of drug-effectiveness evaluation, behavioral-medicine methodologies provide the empirical designs necessary to assess outcome on an individual-by-individual basis (Varni et al., 1978). Single-subject, multiple-baseline, and reversal designs (see figures 12–2 and 12–3) have proved to be effective devices for demonstrating experimental control and treatment effectiveness over a wide range of behaviors (Hersen and Barlow, 1976). In terms of assessment, the data sheet shown in figure 12–1 illustrates a behavioral-assessment technique for pain associated with hemophilia. Through the use of the pain-assessment data sheet and multiple-baseline and reversal designs, the effectiveness of analgesic medications, coagulation-factor concentrates, and/or behavioral strategies may be evaluated with regard to pain reduction. Often hemophiliacs rely on analgesic medication to control the pain associated with hemorrhage. The empirical demonstration of pain relief with concentrate administration and/or behavioral strategies may serve an essential educational function for the reluctant patient. Thus, through the delineation of effective and efficacious interventions, behavioral methodologies may aid in optimizing the delivery of health-care services.

Conclusion

In the foreword to *Behavior Therapy and Health Care* (Katz and Zlutnick, 1975), Stewart Agras of the Stanford University School of Medicine pointed out that behavioral influences on disease and health maintenance have been both long known and long minimized or overlooked by medical researchers and clinicians. Agras suggests that this state of affairs has resulted primarily from a lack of empirically demonstrated clinical procedures designed to change health-related behaviors. It is hoped that the field of behavioral medicine can significantly change this state of affairs.

Unquestionably, the field is emerging, with a new journal (*Journal of Behavioral Medicine,* Plenum Press) and the formation of an Academy of Behavioral Medicine Research (Institute of Medicine, National Academy of Sciences, 1978). Indicative of a field in its formative stages, the Academy's definition of the term *behavioral medicine* represents some significant changes from the Yale conference definition quoted earlier in this chapter. The Academy of Behavioral Medicine definition reads as follows:

> Behavioral medicine is the interdisciplinary field concerned with the development and integration of behavioral and biomedical science knowledge and techniques relevant to the understanding of health and illness and the application of this knowledge and these techniques to prevention, diagnosis, treatment and rehabilitation.

Thus the emphasis has moved from "behavioral science contribution to biomedicine" to "integration of biomedical and behavioral science"—in essence, a combining of perspectives, strengths, and talents in a truly comprehensive research effort (Weiss et al., 1978). With further communication between the medical and behavioral sciences and their resulting collaborative empirical investigations, significant advances in health care can be anticipated.

References

Agle, D.P. (Ed.). *Mental Health Services in the Comprehensive Care of the Hemophiliac.* New York: National Hemophilia Foundation, 1977.

Agle, D.P., and Mattsson, A. Psychological complications of hemophilia. In *Hemophilia in Children*, ed. M.W. Hilgartner, Littleton, Mass.: Publishing Sciences Group, 1976.

Agras, W.S., Barlow, D.H., Chapin, H.N., Abel, G.G., and Leitenberg, H. Behavior modification of anorexia nervosa. *Archives of General Psychiatry* 30: 279–286, 1974.

Barlow, D., Reynolds, E., and Agras, W.S. Gender identity changes in a transsexual. *Archives of General Psychiatry* 28: 569–576, 1973.

Barnes, M.R. Token economy control of fluid overload in a patient receiving hemodialysis. *Journal of Behavior Therapy and Experimental Psychiatry* 7: 305–306, 1976.

Benson, H. *The Relaxation Response.* New York: Avon Books, 1975.

Bigelow, G., Strickler, D., Liebson, I., and Griffiths, R. Maintaining disulfiram ingestion among outpatient alcoholics: A security-deposit contingency contracting procedure. *Behavior Research and Therapy* 14: 378–381, 1976.

Bird, B.L., and Cataldo, M.F. Experimental analysis of EMG feedback in treating dystonia. *Annuals of Neurology* 3: 310–315, 1978.

Birk, L., ed. *Biofeedback: Behavioral Medicine.* New York: Grune and Stratton, 1973.

Black, R.G. Management of pain with nerve blocks. *Minnesota Medicine* 57: 189–194, 1974.

Black, R.G. The chronic pain syndrome. *Surgical Clinics of North America* 55: 999–1011, 1975.

Blanchard, E.B. Behavioral medicine: A perspective. In *Behavioral Approaches to Medical Treatment.* ed. R.B. Williams and W.D. Gentry Cambridge, Mass.: Ballinger, 1977.

Boone, D.C., ed. *Hemophilia: A Total Approach to Treatment and Rehabilitation.* Los Angeles: Orthopaedic Hospital, 1968.

Boone, D.C., ed. *Comprehensive Management of Hemophilia.* Philadelphia: Davis, 1976.

Bornstein, P., and Quevillon, R. The effects of a self-instructional package on overactive preschool boys. *Journal of Applied Behavior Analysis* 9: 179–188, 1976.

Bower, S.A., and Bower, G.H. *Asserting Yourself.* Reading, Mass.: Addison-Wesley, 1976.

Boyer, J. Coronary heart disease as a pediatric problem: Prevention through behavior modification. *American Journal of Cardiology* 33: 784–786, 1974.

Breslow, L. Risk factor intervention for health maintenance. *Science* 200: 908–912, 1978.

Cataldo, M.F., and Risley, T.R. Infant day care. In *Control of Human Behavior,* Vol. 3., ed. R. Ulrich, T. Stachnik, and J. Mabry Glenview, Ill.: Scott, Foresman, 1974.

Cataldo, M.F., Russo, D.C., and Freeman, J.M. Behavior modification treatment of a 4½ year old girl with myoclonic and grand mal seizures. *Journal of Autism and Development Disorders,* 1980a.

Cataldo, M.F., Russo, D.C., Bird, B.L., and Varni, J.W. Assessment and management of chronic disorders. In *Comprehensive Handbook of Behavioral Medicine,* ed. J. Ferguson and C.B. Taylor. Holliswood, N.Y.: Spectrum Publications, 1980b.

Cataldo, M.F., Russo, D.C., Ciulla, R., and Bessman, C.A. Procedural aspects of a monitoring system for professional staff. Unpublished manuscript, 1978.

Cataldo, M.F., Varni, J.W., Russo, D.C., and Estes, S. Behavior therapy techniques in the treatment of exfoliative dermatitis. *Archives of Dermatology,* 1980c.

Childs, B. Approaches to genetic counseling. *Annuals of New York Academy of Science* 240: 132, 1975.

Davis, M.S. Variations in patient's compliance with doctor's orders: Analysis of congruence between survey responses and results of empirical investigations. *Journal of Medical Education* 41: 1037-1048, 1966.

Dietrich, S.L. Musculoskeletal problems. In *Hemophilia in Children,* ed. M.W. Hilgartner Littleton, Mass.: Publishing Sciences Group, 1976.

Ebersold, M.J., Laws, E.R., Stonnington, H.H., and Stillwell, G.K. Transcutaneous electrical stimulation for treatment of chronic pain: A preliminary report. *Surgery and Neurology* 4: 96-99, 1975.

Eisler, R.M., Hersen, M., Miller, P.M., and Blanchard, E.B. Situational determinants of assertive behavior. *Journal of Consulting and Clinical Psychology* 43: 330-340, 1975.

Engel, B.T., Nikoomanesh, P., and Schuster, M.M. Operant conditioning of rectosphincteric responses in the treatment of fecal incontinence. *New England Journal of Medicine* 290: 646-649, 1974.

Epstein, L.H., and Masek, B.J. Behavioral control of medicine compliance. *Journal of Applied Behavior Analysis* 11: 1-9, 1978.

Epstein, M.H., and Harris, J. Children with chronic pain: Can they be helped? *Pediatric Nursing* 4: 42-44, 1978.

Fabrega, H., and Tyma, S. Language and cultural influences in the description of pain. *British Journal of Medical Psychology* 49: 349-371, 1976.

Fink, R., Shapiro, S., and Lewison, J. The reluctant participant in a breast cancer screening program. *Public Health Reports* 83: 479-484, 1968.

Fordyce, W.E. *Behavioral Methods for Chronic Pain and Illness.* St. Louis: Mosby, 1976.

Fordyce, W.E., Fowler, R., Lehmann, J., and Delateur, B. Some implications of learning in problems of chronic pain. *Journal of Chronic Diseases* 21: 179-190, 1968.

Friar, L.R., and Beatty, J. Migraine: Management by trained control of vasoconstriction. *Journal of Consulting and Clinical Psychology* 44: 46-53, 1976.

Fuller, G.D. Current status of biofeedback in clinical practice. *American Psychologist* 33: 39-48, 1978.

Gaarder, K.R., and Montgomery, P.S. *Clinical Biofeedback: A Procedural Manual.* Baltimore: Williams & Wilkins, 1977.

Gambrill, E.D., and Richey, C.A. An assertion inventory for use in assessment and research. *Behavior Therapy* 6: 550-561, 1975.

Gentry, W.D., and Bernal, G.A. Chronic pain. In *Behavioral Approaches to Medical Treatment,* ed. R.B. Williams and W.D. Gentry. Cambridge, Mass.: Ballinger, 1977.

Glynn, E.L., and Thomas, J.D. Effect of cueing on self-control of classroom behavior. *Journal of Applied Behavior Analysis* 7: 299-306, 1974.

Goldstein, M.K., Stein, G.H., Smolen, D.M., and Perlina, W.S. Bio-behavioral monitoring: A method for remote health measurement. *Archives of Physical Medicine and Rehabilitation* 57: 253–258, 1978.

Halpern, L.M. Treating pain with drugs. *Minnesota Medicine* 57: 176–184, 1974.

Hamburg, D.A., and Brown, S.S. The science base and social context of health maintenance: An overview. *Science* 200: 847–849, 1978.

Hersen, M., and Barlow, D.H. *Single Case Experimental Designs.* New York: Pergamon, 1976.

Hersen, M., and Bellach, A.S. A multiple-baseline analysis of social skills training in chronic schizophrenics. *Journal of Applied Behavior Analysis* 9: 239–245, 1976.

Hilgartner, M.W. (ed.). *Hemophilia in Children.* Littleton, Mass.: Publishing Sciences Group, 1976.

Ince, L.P. *Behavior Modification in Rehabilitative Medicine.* Springfield, Ill.: Thomas, 1976.

Jacob, R.G., Kraemer, H.C., and Agras, W.S. Relaxation therapy in the treatment of hypertension. *Archives of General Psychiatry* 34: 1417–1427, 1977.

Jacobson, E. *Progressive Relaxation.* Chicago: Univ. of Chicago Press, 1938.

Kamiya, J., Barber, T.X., Miller, N.E., Shapiro, D., and Stoyva, J. *Biofeedback and Self-control: 1976/77.* Chicago: Aldine, 1977.

Kasl, S.V. Issues in patient adherence to health care regimens. *Journal of Human Stress* 1: 5–17, 1975.

Kasper, C.K. Hematologic care. In *Comprehensive Management of Hemophilia,* ed. D.C. Boone, Philadelphia: Davis, 1976.

Katz, C.R. Single session recovery from a hemodialysis phobia: A case study. *Journal of Behavior Therapy and Experimental Psychiatry* 5: 205–206, 1974.

Katz, R.C., and Zlutnick, S. *Behavior Therapy and Health Care.* New York: Pergamon, 1975.

Kohlenberg, R.J. Operant conditioning of human anal sphincter pressure. *Journal of Applied Behavior Analysis* 6: 201–208, 1973.

Kroger, W.S. *Clinical and Experimental Hypnosis.* Philadelphia: Lippincott, 1977.

Lalonde, M. *A New Perspective on the Health of Canadians: A Working Document.* Ottawa: Government of Canada, 1975.

Lewinsohn, P.M., Biglan, A., and Zeiss, A.M. Behavioral treatment of depression. In *The Behavioral Management of Anxiety, Depression, and Pain,* ed. P.O. Davidson. New York: Brunner/Mazel, 1976.

Liberman, R.P., Teigen, J., Patterson, R., and Baker, V. Reducing delusional speech in chronic, paranoid schizophrenics. *Journal of Applied Behavior Analysis* 6: 57–64, 1973.

Lovaas, O.I., Varni, J.W., Koegel, R.L., and Lorsch, N. Some observations on the nonextinguishability of children's speech. *Child Development* 48: 1121-1127, 1977.

Lovitt, T.C., and Curtiss, K.A. Academic response rate as a function of teacher and self-imposed contingencies. *Journal of Applied Behavior Analysis* 2: 49-53, 1969.

Magrab, P.R., and Papadopoulou, Z.L. The effect of a token economy on dietary compliance for children on hemodialysis. *Journal of Applied Behavior Analysis* 10: 573-578, 1977.

Mahoney, M.J., and Mahoney, K. *Permanent Weight Control.* New York: Norton, 1976.

Margolis, S. Physician strategies for the prevention of coronary heart disease. *Johns Hopkins Medical Journal* 141: 170-176, 1977.

Marks, I.M. New approaches to the treatment of obsessive-compulsive disorders. *Journal of Nervous and Mental Disease* 156: 420-426, 1973.

Marston, M.V. Compliance with medical regimens: A review of the literature. *Nursing Research* 19: 312-323, 1970.

Masek, B.J., Epstein, L.H., and Russo, D.C. Behavioral perspectives in preventive medicine. In *Handbook of Clinical Behavior Therapy,* ed. S.M. Turner, K.S. Calhoun, and H.E. Adams. New York: Wiley, 1980.

Meichenbaum, D., and Goodman, J. Reflection-impulsivity and verbal control of motor behavior. *Child Development* 40: 785-797, 1969.

Meichenbaum, D., and Goodman, J. Training impulsive children to talk to themselves: a means of developing self-control. *Journal of Abnormal Psychology* 77: 115-126, 1971.

Meichenbaum, D., and Turk, D. The cognitive-behavioral management of anxiety, anger, and pain. In *The Behavioral Management of Anxiety, Depression, and Pain,* ed. P.O. Davidson New York: Brunner/Mazel, 1976.

Merritt, A.D., and Conneally, P.M. Hemophilia: Genetics and counseling. In *Hemophilia in Children,* ed. M.W. Hilgartner Littleton, Mass.: Publishing Sciences Group, 1976.

Merskey, H. On the development of pain. *Headache* 10: 116-123, 1970.

Meyer, A.J., and Henderson, J.B. Multiple risk factor reduction in the prevention of cardiovascular disease. *Preventive Medicine* 3: 225-236, 1974.

Palmer, P. *The Mouse, the Monster, and Me: Assertiveness for Young People.* San Luis Obispo: Impact Publishers, 1977.

Patterson, G.R. *Families: Applications of Social Learning to Family Life.* Champaign, Ill.: Research Press, 1975.

Rekers, G.A., and Varni, J.W. Self-monitoring and self-reinforcement processes in a pre-transsexual boy. *Behavior Research and Therapy* 15: 177-180, 1977a.

Rekers, G.A., and Varni, J.W. Self-regulation of gender-role behaviors.

Journal of Behavior Therapy and Experimental Psychiatry 8: 427–432, 1977*b*.

Renne, C.M., and Creer, T.L. Training children with asthma to use inhalation equipment. *Journal of Applied Behavior Analysis* 9: 1–11, 1976.

Rutter, M., Tizard, J., and Whitmore, K. eds. *Education, Health, and Behavior.* London: Longmens, 1970.

Schultz, J.H., and Luthe, W. *Autogenic Therapy.* New York: Grune and Stratton, 1969.

Schwartz, G.E., and Weiss, S.M. Yale conference on behavioral medicine: A proposed definition and statement of goals. *Journal of Behavioral Medicine* 1: 3–12, 1978.

Scott, R.W., Blanchard, E.B., Edmunson, E.D., and Young, L.D. A shaping procedure for heart-rate control in chronic tachycardia. *Perceptual and Motor Skills* 37: 327–338, 1973.

Seligman, M.E.P. *Helplessness.* San Francisco: Freeman, 1975.

Sobell, L.C., and Sobell, M.B. Alcohol problems. In *Behavioral Approaches to Medical Treatment,* ed. R.B. Williams and W.D. Gentry. Cambridge, Mass.: Ballinger, 1977.

Stravino, V.D. The nature of pain. *Archives of Physical Medicine and Rehabilitation* 51: 37–44, 1970.

Stuart, R.B., and Davis, B. *Slim Chance in a Fat World: Behavioral Control of Obesity.* Champaign, Ill.: Research Press, 1972.

Stunkard, A.J., and Mahoney, M.J. Behavioral treatment of the eating disorders. In *Handbook of Behavior Modification and Behavior Therapy,* ed. H. Leitenberg. Englewood Cliffs, N.J.: Prentice-Hall, 1976.

Surwit, R.S. Biofeedback: A possible treatment for Raynaud's disease. *Seminars in Psychiatry* 5: 483–490, 1973.

Swanson, D.W., Swenson, W.M., Manuta, T., and McPhee, M.C. Program for managing chronic pain: 1. Program description and characteristics of patients. *Mayo Clinic Proceedings* 51: 401–408, 1976.

Varni, J.W. Behavioral medicine in hemophilia arthritic pain management. *Archives of Physical Medicine and Rehabilitation,* in press. a.

Varni, J.W. Behavioral treatment of disease-related chronic insomnia in a hemophiliac. *Journal of Behavior Therapy and Experimental Psychiatry,* 1980, *11,* in press b.

Varni, J.W. Behavioral medicine approach to chronic arthritic pain and analgesia abuse in hemophilia. *Blood, 54,* (Abstract), 1979.

Varni, J.W. Behavior therapy in the management of home and school behavior problems with a 4½-year-old hemophilic child. *Journal of Pediatric Psychology, 5,* 17–23, 1980.

Varni, J.W., and Henker, B. A self-regulation approach to the treatment of three hyperactive boys. *Child Behavior Therapy,* 1: 171–192, 1979.

Varni, J.W., Boyd, E., and Cataldo, M.F. Self-monitoring, external reinforcement, and timeout procedures in the control of high rate tic behaviors in a hyperactive child. *Journal of Behavior Therapy and Experimental Psychiatry* 9: 353–358, 1978.

Varni, J.W., Russo, D.C., and Cataldo, M.F. Assessment and modification of delusional speech in an 11-year old child: A comparative analysis of behavior therapy and stimulant drug effects. *Journal of Behavior Therapy and Experimental Psychiatry* 9: 377–380, 1978.

Varni, J.W., Lovaas, O.I., Koegel, R.L., and Everett, N.L. An analysis of observational learning in autistic and normal children. *Journal of Abnormal Child Psychology* 7: 31–43, 1979.

Varni, J.W., Bessman, C.A., Russo, D.C., and Cataldo, M.F. Behavioral management of pediatric chronic pain. *Archives of Physical Medicine and Rehabilitiation, 61,* 375–379, 1980.

Weiss, S.M., Clayman, D.A., and Cataldo, M.F. Developments in behavioral medicine. *Behavior Therapist* 1: 3–4, 1978.

Weiss, T., and Engel, B.T. Operant conditioning of heart rate in patients with premature ventricular contractions. *Psychosomatic Medicine* 33: 301–321, 1971.

Weissenberg, M. Pain and pain control. *Psychological Bulletin* 84: 1008–1044, 1977.

Williams, C.L., Arnold, C.B., and Wynder, E.L. Primary prevention of chronic disease beginning in childhood. The "Know Your Body" program. *Preventive Medicine* 6: 344–357, 1977.

Wolpe, J. *The Practice of Behavior Therapy.* New York: Pergamon, 1973.

Wolpe, J., and Lazarus, A.A. *Behavior Therapy Techniques.* New York: Pergamon, 1966.

Yule, W. The potential of behavioral treatment in preventing later childhood difficulties. *Behavioral Analysis and Modification* 2: 19–31, 1977.

Zifferblatt, S.M. Increasing patient compliance through the applied analysis of behavior. *Preventive Medicine* 4: 173–182, 1975.

Zlutnick, S., Mayville, W., and Moffat S. Modification of seizures disorders: The interruption of behavioral chains. *Journal of Applied Behavior Analysis* 8: 1–12, 1975.

13 Pain and Its Management: A Behavioral-Medicine Perspective

Jo Ann Brockway

Pain has long been one of the primary concerns of human beings, and the alleviation of pain has long been one of the major concerns of the health-care professionals. Chronic pain may be one of the most common disabling conditions of humanity. It is a complex phenomenon, affecting millions of people each year. Weisenberg (1977) states that "pain is a reason for seeking health care and a reason for avoiding it. It is the basis of a multimillion dollar drug industry that promises relief to the thousands who are guided by the societal norm in which ills are dealt with by popping the right pill." Pain is also the reason for innumerable medical evaluations, surgeries, and a myriad of other therapies. The cost of pain in economic terms has been estimated to be between $10 billion and $25 billion each year (Bonica, 1973); its cost in human suffering is immeasurable. In spite of this expenditure of money and professional effort, for many persons pain continues, seemingly without end.

Perhaps for this reason, pain has been the focal point of a burgeoning interest from many disciplines, research and clinical alike, in recent years. yet pain remains a puzzling and multidimensional problem. While pain has been approached from many points of view, a unified and comprehensive perspective on pain remains elusive. The biochemist may view pain as metabolic changes across cell membranes, while the neurophysiologist may see it as the transmission of nerve impulses in specific spatial patterns. To the experimental psychologist, pain may be a particular level of sensation; to the psychotherapist, it may represent suffering and guilt. The medical practitioner may view it as an indication of tissue damage or perhaps as a nagging and insoluble problem, while the patient in pain may view it as an unpleasant physical sensation, a reason for alarm, or a cause for despair.

What is this many-faceted disorder called pain? Most definitions of pain include some reference to the physiological aspects of pain, yet pain is more than a physiological stimulus. Melzack (1973) states that "pain has

This chapter was supported in part by Research and Training Center Grant 16–P–56818/0 from the Rehabilitation Services Administration. The author wishes to acknowledge the major contribution made by Wilbert E. Fordyce, Ph.D., to the behavioral approach to pain management. Most of the conceptual framework, evaluation techniques, and treatment strategies presented in this chapter are based on his work.

obvious sensory qualities, but it also has emotional and motivational properties. It is usually caused by intense, noxious stimulation, yet it sometimes occurs spontaneously without apparent cause. It normally signals physical injury, but it sometimes fails to occur even when extensive areas of the body have been seriously injured; at other times it persists after all the injured tissues have been healed and becomes a crippling problem that requires urgent, radical treatment." Sternbach (1974) calls pain "an abstraction that we use to refer to different feelings which have little in common except the quality of physical hurt, . . . the injured or affected locus, i.e., the apparent source of the pain, . . . a class of behaviors which operate to protect the organism from harm or to enlist aid in effecting relief." Although the preceding definitions include physiological, sensory, emotional, motivational, and behavioral aspects of pain, as well as some reference to some of the complexities of pain, they do not manage to adequately define pain, nor to convey the difficulties in successfully treating problems of chronic pain.

Perhaps more relevant to a discussion of clinical pain and its management than a definition of pain is a discussion of some of the variables that influence the experience of pain. Pain in its acute phase generally serves as a warning of impending or actual tissue damage; it means that something is wrong somewhere in the body. For example, severe acute abdominal pain may indicate appendicitis, and an acute pain in the ankle may mean a sprain. However, most authors indicate that the relationship between the experience of pain and the extent of physical injury is not dependable. Beecher's (1956) study is illustrative of this point. Beecher compared requests for narcotics for pain relief in two populations: a group of soldiers wounded on the battlefield and a group of civilian patients with comparable surgical wounds. On the battlefield, only 25 percent of the men requested narcotics, while over 80 percent of the hospitalized surgical patients requested such medication. Beecher ascribes the difference to the meaning of the pain experience. The soldier's wounds incurred on the battlefield meant a ticket to safety, while the civilian's surgical wounds meant a threat to safety.

Emotional state influences pain perception. For example, it has been noted that pain increases with increased anxiety (Sternbach, 1968). The experience of pain also appears to be related to cognitive variables. Surgical patients who receive preoperative instruction and preparation for surgery request fewer postoperative narcotics (Egbert et al., 1964). Expectancy also influences pain. Beecher (1972) reported that administering a placebo resulted in significant decreases in clinical pain in 35 percent of the patients studied. The variables listed here are but a few of the many factors that have been reported to influence the perception of pain. The reader who is interested in a review of the relevant literature might begin with Weisenberg's (1977) review.

Given that pain is more than a physiological phenomenon, it makes sense that the successful treatment of pain often necessitates more than purely physical or medical techniques. In fact, in recent years, many psychology-based techniques have been developed for use in the treatment of pain. These strategies have included stress-management and anxiety-reduction techniques, such as biofeedback, autogenic training, and hypnosis, as well as special inpatient and outpatient pain programs that use behavioral techniques such as operant conditioning to decrease pain.

This chapter will not attempt to review all such techniques. Rather, the chapter will focus on pain management from a primarily behavioral or operant point of view. A brief review of the behavioral rationale will be included to provide a framework within which behaviorally based treatment strategies can be discussed. The process by which operant pain is acquired will be discussed, with particular reference to the role of the health-care system in the development and maintenance of operant pain. Guidelines for identifying operant pain will be presented, along with techniques for treating problems of chronic operant pain.

The Learning Approach to Pain

Traditionally, pain has been approached via the medical or disease model, as shown in figure 13-1. From the disease-model perspective, pain is seen as

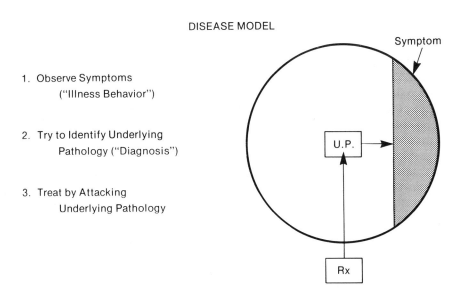

Source: Wilbert E. Fordyce, *Behavioral Methods for Chronic Pain and Illness* (St. Louis, Mo.: Mosby, 1976). Used by permission of the publisher.

Figure 13-1. Disease Model of Chronic Pain

the symptom of an underlying organic pathological condition. The treatment of pain is not aimed at the symptom per se; rather it is directed toward eradicating the underlying etiologic factor. The elimination or correction of the underlying pathology will, presumably, result in the alleviation of the symptoms of pain.

The learning-approach model of pain was first described by Fordyce and his colleagues (1968). From the learning-model perspective, shown in figure 13-2, pain symptoms are viewed as behaviors that are in themselves problems that can be treated directly. The treatment of pain, using a learning approach, is aimed directly at eliminating the symptoms or problem pain behaviors and substituting more adaptive behaviors.

A critical aspect of the learning-model approach to pain is the conceptualization of pain as behavior. In order for the patient to have a clinical pain problem he or she must behave in some way that communicates to the health-care professional (or family or friends) that he or she is experiencing pain. Tissue damage may be visible, but damaged tissue may or may not be accompanied by pain (for example, the patient with spinal cord injury may have severe tissue damage below the level of sensation and experience no pain). The biochemical or neurophysiological aspects of the pain problem are not visible. It is only the behavior of the person in pain that signals to the environment, purposefully or not, that pain exists.

Pain behaviors may be verbal messages, such as a description of the locus or intensity of the pain, a moan or sigh, or a request for medication, or nonverbal messages, such as a limp, a grimace, or a particular body position. If there are no observable pain behaviors, there is no clinical pain problem. Instead there is only a private experience unknown to others.

The pain behaviors not only signal the environment that the patient is experiencing pain, but also simultaneously elicit a response from the environment. The response may be a prescription for medication, a directive to "take it easy," a family member taking over a household chore, or an angry outburst. These responses play a major role in determining the future of the patient's pain problem. This is so because the principles of learning and conditioning apply to pain as behavior as they do to other behaviors. A brief and certainly oversimplified review of some relevant points related to learning will be included here. The reader who wishes a more thorough discussion of these principles should consult Skinner (1953), Miller (1969), or Krasner and Ullman (1966).

It is important to distinguish operant from respondent behavior. *Respondent behavior* occurs automatically when an adequate stimulus is present; that is, the behavior is a reflexive response to a specific stimulus condition. *Operant behaviors* also may be elicited by specific stimulus conditions. In addition, however, operant behaviors are influenced by their outcomes. When a given behavior is systematically followed by a positive

LEARNING MODEL

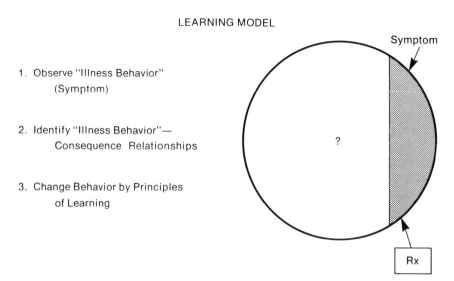

1. Observe "Illness Behavior"
   (Symptom)

2. Identify "Illness Behavior"—
   Consequence Relationships

3. Change Behavior by Principles
   of Learning

Source: Wilbert E. Fordyce, *Behavioral Methods of Chronic Pain and Illness* (St. Louis, Mo.: Mosby, 1976). Used by permission of the publisher.

Figure 13–2. Learning Model of Chronic Pain

consequence, it is likely to increase in frequency; when a behavior is systematically followed by a neutral or negative consequence, it is likely to extinguish or decrease in frequency. Thus, when systematic behavior-consequences occur, learning occurs. It is important to note that the learning or conditioning process occurs automatically when there are systematic and contingent behavior-outcome relationships.

With regard to pain as behavior, respondent pain behavior occurs in response to specific antecedent conditions or nociceptive stimuli. Operant pain behavior may occur in response to an antecedent nociceptive stimulus, but in addition has come under the control of environmental contingencies. Thus, when pain behaviors consistently elicit a positive response from the environment, they tend to occur more frequently. An example may help to clarify these points. A small child drops a heavy toy on his or her foot, the foot hurts and the child begins to cry. Crying in this case may be an example of respondent pain behavior. If the child consistently receives a positive response from his or her parents (environment) for crying when he or she drops toys on his or her foot, the crying may occur even when the child drops a toy only near the foot instead of on it, or when he or she drops a light object on the foot. The crying here has become an operant pain behavior; it continues to occur even when the original painful stimulus condition does not occur.

The Problem of Chronicity

The preceding discussion notwithstanding, the medical or disease model for pain is a useful model that is quite appropriate for acute pain. In the acute-pain situation, very often pain is indeed a symptom of an underlying pathological condition, for example, a broken leg. The treatment is quite properly aimed at healing the broken leg (that is, eradicating the underlying pathology), which should eliminate the pain symptoms.

The problem arises when treatment of the acute-pain problem is not successful in alleviating the pain. When the patient thus fails in the health-care system, the pain problem becomes chronic. With chronicity comes the opportunity for learning to occur. Inevitably, chronicity brings repeated occurrences of pain-behavior positive-reinforcement sequences that lead to systematic changes in behavior. In the acute situation, pain may cause modifications of the daily activities and lifestyle of the patient and his or her family. If the patient's problem is correctly diagnosed and successfully treated, then these modifications are temporary. If, however, the problem is not properly diagnosed, or if treatment continues for several months, chronicity occurs, and these disruptions become changes in behavior patterns. Similarly, with chronicity, learning occurs with respect to what the patient says and does around his or her pain; that is, his or her pain behaviors are modified to an undetermined extent by reinforcement from the environment. Thus the pain behaviors may or may not reflect any particular organic pathology.

Another difficulty often arises once the pain problem has become chronic, frequently after a series of health-care practitioners has been consulted for diagnostic evaluations and treatment recommendations without much success. The patient is referred into another treatment system, which also traditionally has been based on the disease model. In this system, the pathological condition underlying the pain problem is considered to be psychogenic, rather than organic, and may be labeled a personality problem or an emotional disturbance. Treatment, for example, psychotherapy, is aimed at eradicating the underlying emotional disorder in order to eliminate the pain. This diagnosis is often made by exclusion; that is, since no underlying organic cause can be found to explain the pain, the problem must be an underlying psychogenic cause. This is often interpreted by the health-care professional, the patient, and the patient's family to mean that no "real" cause can be found for the pain, so it must not be "real." Instead the pain is often thought to be "all in the head" or "imagined."

Labeling a patient's pain as psychogenic is unfortunate in several respects and is rarely, if ever, beneficial to the patient. First, the authenticity of the patient's pain problem is challenged. The patient knows that he or she hurts and that the hurt is "real." The patient seeks to prove the pain is "real"—often by becoming involved in yet more evaluations and treatments, which may result in the patient's becoming even more disabled. Second, few patients with chronic pain will follow through with a referral for psychotherapy. Of those who do, many do not continue or may continue with little investment in it. Even for those who invest themselves in it, psychotherapy by itself is most often not sufficient to bring about a reduction in the pain problems. Third, the patient becomes angry and embittered at the health-care system, making it more difficult to successfully treat his or her pain problem. This is not to say that patients with chronic pain do not have emotional problems; some do. It is simply to say that labeling pain as psychogenic and treating the patient as having an emotional disorder is not likely to be a successful approach to managing chronic pain.

Once the pain problem has become chronic, the issue is not "What is causing the pain?" or "Is the pain real?" The pain problem that has become chronic is most likely some combination of residual nociceptive stimulus plus learned behaviors. The important issues at this point are "what factors are maintaining the pain problem?" and "What can be done to help the patient?"

The Acquisition of Operant Pain

The acquisition of chronic pain is a simple process that requires only that pain behaviors be systematically followed by positive reinforcement. Under these circumstances, learning occurs automatically, and pain comes under the control of environmental contingencies. Then the pain problem continues without any effort on the part of the patient to prolong it.

Pain behavior may be reinforced directly; that is, direct positive consequences such as rest or attention may systematically follow the occurrence of the pain behavior, thereby increasing its strength. For example, a spouse who is generally minimally attentive may massage the patient's area of pain or be solicitous to the needs of the patient when he or she exhibits pain behaviors. Rest often results in decreased pain and thus is a positive reinforcer. Patient displays of pain behavior may be followed by resting and by decreased discomfort and thus are reinforced.

Pain behavior also may be reinforced by indirect means, such as the avoidance of some unpleasant or stressful situation. One frequent example is the person who, prior to injury, experienced a change in vocational situation, such as a promotion or a move to another work area, which resulted in increased responsibility or stress. The occurrence of pain may be succeeded by "time out" from work and thus the avoidance of stress. In the older person with somewhat vague pain complaints, pain behavior is often reinforced by providing an avoidance of situations that might reveal declining intellectual abilities. The development of certain pain behaviors such as a limp may be reinforced by avoidance of pain. Although the patient originally developed the limp as a means of avoiding or decreasing pain, the limp may become a habit pattern and may continue long after the original problem has been resolved.

Pain behavior may be maintained not only because it is followed by positive consequences, but also because competing well behaviors are punished by the environment. Frequently, it occurs that a patient who has engaged in little acitivity in an attempt to alleviate pain now begins to feel better and so undertakes an activity previously put off because of the pain. Quite often, this sudden increase in activity is followed by pain, which effectively punishes the patient's well behavior. Family and friends may punish well behavior by instructing the patient not to do too much and by reacting with displeasure when the patient engages in activity. At the least, family members may simply ignore well behavior and thus extinguish it.

The very nature of the health-care delivery system aids in the development and maintenance of operant-pain problems. To begin with, traditional medical management is largely illness-contingent. Except for periodic (such as yearly) examinations and the occurrence of medical problems, one generally has little contact with the health-care system. Under this arrangement, the correct circumstances may provide series of pain-behavior positive-reinforcement sequences.

The attention of the physician or other health-care professional is often a potent reinforcer. The health-care professional's attention and concern may fill a void for the patient who gets little attention or understanding from family and friends. Such attention is usually contingent on patient illness or exhibition of pain behavior. In order to interact with the health-care professional, the patient must have a problem. Additionally, the practitioner's attention is focused on the patient's description of the various aspects (for example, locus, intensity) of the pain problem. The health-care professional's attention may serve as a reinforcer of pain behavior in yet another way. Continued contact with a health-care professional may provide witness to the authenticity of the pain problem for the patient to whom it has been suggested that his or her pain problem is "psychogenic."

The health-care system may reinforce pain behavior via medications. Many patients with chronic-pain problems are addicted to or reliant on pain medications or other medications prescribed for "sleep" or "relaxation." Such medications are often prescribed *prn* (on an "as needed" basis). The positive effects of the medication, whether anxiety reduction, pain alleviation, or "it still hurts, I just don't care anymore," are then contingent upon the patient's continuing to display pain behaviors. The patient must hurt in order to receive medication. Thus pain is maintained, even though the original painful stimulus condition may have been resolved.

General directions to the patient to "take it easy" or "do as much as you can and stop when it hurts" may contribute to the development and maintenance of pain behavior. The directive to "take it easy" may, in effect, become a physician-prescribed avoidance of unpleasant activity or time out from stress and thus a reinforcer of pain behavior. The "do what you can" prescription may result in the patient engaging in activity until pain occurs, resulting in the systematic punishment of well behavior (activity ⟶ pain) coupled with the systematic reinforcement of pain behavior (pain ⟶ rest ⟶ decreased pain).

Identifying Operant Pain

The presence of a chronic-pain problem does not, by itself, necessarily indicate operant pain. Chronic pain may be essentially respondent in nature, as in some cases of rheumatoid arthritis or cancer. In order to effectiely treat chronic pain using an operant approach, there must be evidence for a significant operant component to the pain problem. Operant pain should not be identified by exclusion; that is, a pain problem should not be considered operant simply because no "organic" pathology can be found to account for the pain. In order for there to be a significant operant component to the chronic-pain problem, all of the following must be true:

1. There must be insufficient organic pathology to account for the extent of the expressed pain, or there must be only questionable or speculative pathology.
2. Medical evaluation does not indicate a medically based treatment of choice.
3. There must be systematic relationships between pain behavior and well behavior and reinforcement.

A thorough medical evaluation, or sometimes an evaluation by each of several specialists, should address the issues in points 1 and 2. A discussion of these issues would be outside of the scope of this chapter and outside of my area; they will therefore not be pursued here. The reader interested in such a discussion might begin with Bonica (1975).

A determination of whether there are systematic relationships between pain and well behavior and reinforcement is best made via a behavioral analysis, that is, a detailed examination of the pain- and well-behavior reinforcement contingencies and the factors that influence pain. The behavioral analysis may include interviews with both the patient and family members, psychological test results, and patient diaries of activities. It should be conducted by a health-care professional trained in interviewing skills, knowledgeable in the behavioral approach, and experienced with problems of chronic pain.

The behavioral-analysis interview should provide specific information about the patient's pain problem, such as the time pattern of the pain (for example, decreased pain in the morning, increasing at midafternoon, and remaining at a high level until evening), what pain behavior the patient exhibits, how those around him or her respond to the pain behavior, what activities lead to increased or decreased pain, what the patient no longer does or does less frequently because of pain, and what significant others now do (or no longer do) because of the patient's pain. It is important to obtain information from both the patient and a significant family member since, not infrequently, each will have a differenct perspective on the pain problem.

The Minnesota Multiphasic Personality Inventory (MMPI) has been found to be useful in identifying patients who appear to readily display somatic symptoms and yet are less concerned about their physical complaints than might be expected (Fordyce, 1976). Additionally, the MMPI appears to be helpful in identifying some people for whom pain is not the primary problem, but rather is a part of a major psychiatric disorder, for example, schizophrenia.

Patient-activity diaries, where patients record activities, pain level, and medication usage over several 24-hour periods, have proven useful in evaluating patient-activity patterns and the relationship between activity and pain and medication use. There is often a discrepancy between what the patient does and what he or she says he or she does. Activity diaries, if completed appropriately, help elucidate these relationships.

Information from the behavioral analysis is compiled to determine whether there is a significant operant component to the patient's pain problem. Where it appears that the patient is deriving some positive outcome from the pain (that is, something good happens because of the pain and/or something bad does not happen because of the pain), there is frequently a significant operant component to the pain problem. It should be cautioned here that the existence of a significant operant component to the pain problem does not preclude the existence of respondent pain. The results of the behavioral analysis must be combined with the results of the medical evaluations to determine whether an operant approach to treatment is indicated. For a more complete discussion of the components and interpretation of the behavioral analysis of chronic pain, see Fordyce (1976).

Behavioral Management of Chronic Operant Pain

There are many problems the health-care professional faces in treating the patient with a chronic-operant pain problem. Chronic-operant-pain patients are often difficult to deal with. They are frequently suspicious and angry—suspicious of the health-care professional's view of the validity of their pain problem and angry that other health-care professionals have not accepted the authenticity of their pain and/or have not solved their pain problem. Additionally, the health-care professional is often faced with the patient's demand that something be *done* about his or her problem; that some treatment, be it medication, surgery, transcutaneous stimulation, or something else, be prescribed for the pain. Third, the health-care professional is faced with the knowledge that if he or she does not respond in some way to the patient's pain, the patient may seek help elsewhere, perhaps going for treatment to someone less conservative in prescribing medication or more willing to perform risky procedures.

In order to effectively manage the chronic-operant-pain problem, the health-care professional must show considerable clinical sensitivity and skill in early contacts with the patient to enable him or her to understand that the professional is not challenging the authenticity of the patient's pain problem, but is intent on finding out how he or she may help the patient.

Once it has been determined that the patient does have an operant-pain problem, the health-care practitioner must decide on the course of action most likely to be of benefit to the patient. The question of inpatient versus outpatient treatment often arises. A highly structured, intensive inpatient operant-pain treatment program is indicated for (1) those patients for whom medication addiction or abuse is in evidence or for whom there are other chemical-dependency problems; (2) those patients whose significant others either strongly and directly reinforce pain behavior, actively punish well behavior, or make excessive demands on the patient such that engaging in activity is aversive; and (3) those patients who will not, in your judgment, maintain a regular exercise program at prescribed times in prescribed amounts without supervision. For these patients, an inpatient treatment is necessary. Such inpatient operant programs have been described in detail elsewhere (Fordyce, 1976; Roberts, 1978); space does not permit a detailed description of such programs here. Instead, general guidelines for the operant-based management of chronic pain will be discussed.

The first step is to provide the patient and significant family members with an orientation or explanation of the evaluation results and proposed treatment plan. This is particularly important since the operant-based treatment approach is likely to be unfamiliar to the patient and somewhat different than what was expected. This provides both a basis for informed consent for treatment and an opportunity for patient and family members to receive equal information.

The orientation should include a brief explanation of the concept of pain as behavior and the means by which behavior, including pain behavior, can be modified. It is particularly important to help the patient and family understand that the notion that pain is learned is quite different from the notion that pain is psychogenic or "all in your head." It should be emphasized that learning occurs automatically when conditions are right and is not suggestive of emotional problems.

The objectives of treatment should be made clear. That is, the patient and family should be told what treatment is expected to accomplish in terms of patient function, that is, what the patient is likely to be able to do when treatment is complete and what limitations on activity might remain. The methods by which treatment will proceed should be fully explained: what is expected of the patient and family, what the patient and family can expect from the personnel involved in treatment, what will be done about medications, and so forth.

The health-care professional-patient interactions must often be modified in order to effectively treat the patient with chronic operant pain. The health-care professional, whether he or she is a nurse, a physician, a physical therapist, a physician's assistant, or other, should learn to neutrally respond to complaints and descriptions of pain. It should be reemphasized here that this is to be done after the pain problem has been thoroughly evaluated with the resulting conclusion that the pain is operant in nature. To say that the pain behaviors should receive a neutral response is *not* to say that they should be ignored or punished. The health-care professional should note the occurrence of pain behavior to himself or herself, but should respond to it neutrally.

It is not enough, however, to neutrally respond to pain behaviors. The patient will need some interim reinforcement to replace the reinforcement previously occurring in response to pain behaviors until he or she begins to increase his or her activity enough to derive reinforcement from increased functioning. The health-care practitioner, then, must provide positive reinforcement for appropriate nonpain behaviors, such as appropriate social conversation or performance of prescribed activity.

Patients with chronic operant pain often have restricted levels of activity and high levels of rest and reclining. As was discussed before, it often occurs that activity results in pain, which is followed by rest, which results in decreased pain. Thus activity is punished and so tends to decrease in frequency, while rest is reinforced and so tends to increase in frequency. In order to increase activity and decrease rest, the activity-pain and pain-rest sequences must be broken.

In order to accomplish this, exercises must be prescribed in a systematic way. Exercises appropriate to the patient's general medical status should be prescribed. This informs the patient and family that activity is okay. The second step is to obtain "baselines" for each exercise. That is, the patient is told to "do as many of this exercise as you can before fatigue, weakness, or pain causes you to want to stop" over several exercise sessions. The amount of each exercise done is recorded, and exercise quotas are set for each exercise. Quotas should begin at a level that is less than what the patient could do during baselines and should increase by a set amount each day to a level reasonable for the patient based on age and general medical status. In this way, activity is not punished by pain, and rest occurs after (reinforces) activity. Exercises should be done to quota, no more and no less.

It is often quite helpful to have patients keep records of their exercises in the form of graphs. This provides visual feedback of the patient's progress to both the patient and the health-care professional. Additionally, the health practitioner can use the graphs as a basis for focusing attention and positive reinforcement on patient activity.

Learning-model methods have been developed for managing medications (Fordyce, 1976; Halpern, 1973). Except where there is clear evidence of currently ongoing bodily damage factor, as, for example, in an ongoing cancer, there is no justification for, and many objections to, the use of injectable medications, which have more potent conditioning effects, both physiologically and psychologically, than orally administered medication.

Medications should be prescribed on a time-contingent rather than pain-contingent basis. This breaks up the pain-behavior positive-reinforcement (hurting-taking medications) sequence. Pain no longer needs to occur in order for medication to be given/taken, which allows for the extinction of medication-related pain behaviors. Narcotic medication, if used, should be prescribed for a preset limited time, which usually includes the length of time that pain requiring narcotics is reasonably expected to occur plus two to three "buffer" days to allow for a margin of safety. The medications are best administered via the "pain cocktail," in which medications are combined with a masking agent (for example, cherry syrup) to total 10 cc per dose. The amount of active ingredient can then be modified over time. (The patient should be told clearly beforehand that medication in the "pain cocktail" will be modified and decreased over the course of treatment, and that the patient will not be told when medication modifications are made but will be informed when there are no active ingredients in the cocktail.)

Some patients with operant pain indicate that tension and stress result in increased pain. Here it is often the case that a stressful situation leads to pain, which punishes engaging in the stressful activity; the pain is followed by leaving the situation, which results in decreased pain. Thus the avoidance of stress is reinforced. Biofeedback and general relaxation-training procedures may be employed in these cases as a method of more effectively dealing with stress such that stress is followed by relaxation rather than by pain and avoidance behavior.

Earlier, the problem of well behaviors was discussed. Well behavior is often punished by family and friends. Often the well-behavior repertoire, in terms of social, recreational, and vocational skills, may have diminished significantly over the course of the pain problem. Merely reducing the frequency of pain behaviors will not necessarily result in an automatic increase in well behavior. Management of the pain problem must address the issue of what the patient will do in place of exhibiting pain behaviors. Treatment must provide for some generalization of increased activity via exercises to increased functional "real-life" activity. The target functional well behaviors should be in the patient's repertoire, or if not, treatment should be directed toward remedying these gaps, perhaps by referral.

Pain and Depression

One further issue that should be addressed is that of pain and depression. Pain and depression frequently occur together (Merskey and Spea, 1967). Depressed patients not infrequently complain of pain problems; in fact, depression is often mislabeled as pain by the patient and health-care professionals alike. Patients with chronic-pain problems are often depressed. Determining which is the major problem may not be an easy task.

When the question of pain versus depression arises, a psychological or psychiatric evaluation is appropriate to help resolve the issue. Where the major problem is depression, appropriate treatment, perhaps including chemotherapy, should be instituted.

Depression in patients with chronic-pain problems may often be a result of a lowered level of reinforcers. Patients with chronic-pain problems tend to limit their activities and thereby limit the reinforcers available to them. When this is the case, depression may be a self-liquidating problem; it may resolve as the patient becomes more active and receives more reinforcement from others and from the widened range of activities in which he or she is engaged. Increasing patient activity levels acts to treat both the chronic-pain problem and the depression. Where necessary, antidepressant medication can be included along with the rest of treatment.

References

Beecher, H.K. The placebo effect as a non-specific force surrounding disease and the treatment of disease. In *Pain: Basic Principles—Pharmacology—Therapy,* ed. R. Janzen, W. Keidel, A. Herz, C. Steichele, J.P. Payne, and R.A.P. Burt Baltimore: Williams and Wilkins, 1972.

Beecher, H.K. Relationship of significance of wound to the pain experienced. *Journal of the American Medical Association* 161:1609–1613, 1956.

Bonica, J.J. The management of pain. *Postgraduate Medicine* 53:56–57, 1973.

Bonica, J.J., ed. *The Management of Pain*. Philadelphia: Lea and Febeger, 1975.

Egbert, L.D., Battit, G.E., Welch, C.E., and Bartlett, M.K. Reduction of postoperative pain by encouragement and instruction of patients. *New England Journal of Medicine* 270:825–827, 1964.

Fordyce, W.E., *Behavioral Methods for Chronic Pain and Illness*. St. Louis: Mosby, 1976.

Fordyce, W.E., Fowler, R.S., Lehmann, J.F., and deLateur, B.J. Some implications of learning in problems of chronic pain. *Journal of Chronic Diseases* 21:179–190, 1968.

Fordyce, W.E., Fowler, R.S., Lehmann, J.F., deLateur, B.J., Sand, P.L., and Trieschmann, R.B. Operant conditioning in the treatment of chronic clinical pain. *Archives of Physical Medicine and Rehabilitation* 54:399–408, 1973.

Halpern, L.M. Analgesics and other drugs for relief of pain. *Postgraduate Medicine* 53:91–100, 1973.

Krasner, L., and Ullman, L.P. *Research in Behavior Modification*. New York: Holt, Rinehart and Winston, 1966.

Melzack, R. *The Puzzle of Pain*. New York: Basic Books, 1973.

Merskey, H., and Spear, F.G. *Pain: Psychological and Psychiatric Aspects*. Baltimore: Williams & Wilkins, 1967.

Miller, N. Learning of visceral and glandular responses. *Science* 163:434–445, 1969.

Skinner, B.F. *Science and Human Behavior*. New York: Macmillan, 1953.

Sternbach, R.A. *Pain: A Psychophysiological Analysis*. New York: Academic, 1968.

Sternbach, R.A. *Pain Patients: Traits and Treatment*. New York: Academic, 1974.

Weisenberg, M. Pain and pain control. *Psychological Bulletin* 84: 1008–1044, 1977.

14 Obstetrics and Gynecology: The Well-Being of the Total Woman

Cathie-Ann Lippman

Introduction

The woman seeking medical care most often does so in the context of female problems, and thus this experience, often her first medical contact, carries with it the potential for setting the tone of her total future health care. The goal of this chapter is to delineate the psychologic aspects involved in the health care of women. It is not meant to teach doctors and nurses to become psychiatrists, but to help them provide total care to their patients as they apply the psychological aspects to obstetrics and gynecology. While obstetricians and gynecologists specialize in women's medicine, it is the responsibility of all health-care practitioners to recognize the special aspects of women's health care.

What is it a woman wants from her doctor? A woman wants to be treated like a human being, not like an object or an organ. In this wish she is, or course, not unique, but what is important is an appreciation and understanding of her special psychological, sexual, and physical characteristics. She wants to be treated with respect, not in a condescending fashion. Although women often assume women doctors are more understanding because the woman physician personally undergoes the same experiences when she needs medical care, being a woman is no guarantee of empathy. Whether male or female, the physician is expected to be empathetic, sensitive, competent, self-assured, knowledgeable, conscientious, able to take care of anxiety-provoking aspects of medical practice, honest, flexible, able to listen, and able to communicate in simple, understandable terms (Haar et al., 1975).

While the preceding list of qualities is somewhat awesome in scope, certainly many benefits may accrue from an effort to employ some degree of sensitivity, perspective, and empathy. The resulting rapport creates an atmosphere in which the patient is more inclined to comply with suggestions and prescriptions of the practitioner. In addition, in this time when patients

The author is grateful to Cedars-Sinai Medical Center, in particular Carole Hurvitz, M.D. and Marilyn Plasek, and to Helen Lippman for their technical assistance, to Jules H. Kamin, Ph.D. and Terry Anne Preston, Ph.D. for their ideas and criticism, and to the many women who generously contributed their opinions and suggestions for this chapter.

are generally more intelligently informed about doctoring and better able to evaluate their medical care, the rapport can serve as a constructive foundation for personal discussion rather than litigation should some medical mishap occur. "If the physician meets the expectations of his/her patients with respect to hearing their problems, demonstrating a sincere effort to solve the problems, and supplying emotional support as needed, it is much less likely that the patient will become an adversary even should some medical misadventure occur" (Hinshaw, 1977).

Patients and other physicians do not, however, expect any practitioner to know absolutely everything. Any woman respects a physician who is willing to seek consultation, just as she wants a physician who helps her to seek a second opinion instead of becoming defensive or making derogatory comments to her for not trusting his or her opinion. "The request by one physician of another for a medical opinion and judgment in a particular case in no way implies that the physician requesting the consultation feels inferior in knowledge, skill, or ability to the one of whom the consultation is asked. Even a physician who is a recognized authority in a given specialty may advisably seek consultation of another expert. The chosen consultant should be a physician whose opinion is respected and who can be trusted to stand by that opinion" (Hinshaw, 1977). This will increase, not detract from, the respect the woman has for her physician.

At times, the act of coming to a physician per se has been taken as consent for care. Increasingly though, it is recognized that this is only one step in that direction. Physicians are advised to inform their patients about differential diagnoses and findings; educate them about the need for procedures and how they are carried out, which can include how a physician goes about evaluating a complaint; and obtain informed consent verbally for routine procedures, such as pelvic examinations, and written consent for more extensive procedures. The assumption behind this advice is that every woman has the right of self-determination, and in order to exercise that right, she must be informed and knowledgeable enough to refuse her doctor's recommendations should she choose (Hinshaw, 1977). The person who ultimately decides what will be done to the woman's body is not the physician, but the woman patient herself. The fact that she seeks care makes it likely that she will comply with the physician's suggestions; the physician can increase that likelihood by attending to these issues.

Gynecology

The Interview with the Patient

The interview is the practitioner's major tool for developing a working relationship with his or her patient. Busy practices do not seem to provide opportunity for extensive discussions with patients. However, the time taken, especially in the first interview, is a worthwhile investment compared with what may later be a series of nonproductive office visits, laboratory tests, or operating procedures that are not of observable significant benefit from the patient's point of view (Donovan and Benson, 1976).

The first interview should take place preferably in a room other than an examining room. Any woman feels more secure to meet the doctor for the first time when she is fully dressed. When a woman is seen for gynecological reasons, she frequently has intimate and embarrassing (to her) complaints or confessions to make. It is most important for the physician and the nurse to be sensitive to this. Even if she is accompanied by her husband, a significant other, or another relative or friend, it is wise to talk with the patient alone at first (Greenhill, 1959). This demonstrates the physician's respect for the patient's private concerns and helps him or her assess the patient's maturity without the support of the other person. Then a few moments may be spent with the husband or significant other, if available. This allows the physician to evaluate the status of the relationship. Conflicts there may impair or at least complicate the care he or she wishes to give. In addition, physicians commonly find themselves called upon to act as advisor on issues other than strictly medical ones (Greenhill, 1959). The physician will need to decide for himself or herself how comfortable he or she feels with this role and to evaluate how much he or she can do for any individual.

How is rapport established? Listen to the patient. Leave her with the impression that her doctor is interested in her and willing to hear what she has to say. Note the degree of embarrassment or anxiety associated with topics. This can be determined by listening for ambiguous terminology, for example, saying "down there" instead of referring specifically to the genitals, watching for fidgety posture, hesitancy to look directly at the interviewer, or the expression of embarrassment or nervousness when she talks about something. This commonly arises with questions about sexual activity. The straightforward yet sensitive manner of the practitioner can alleviate much anxiety. Mention that many people find it difficult to talk about such a personal issue as sexual activity, but that it is a vital part of the gynecological history. If she is still too hesitant, tell her the topic can be put off till later (Long, 1976).

Rapport is also aided by attending to the kind of language used by the patient and using the same phrases as she in order to clarify that you understand what she means and to ensure that she understands your terminology. Summarizing her complaint as you understand it, and asking her to repeat her understanding of your explanations, helps ensure that you are taking the information accurately and that she will be able to more accurately follow through with your suggestions. Most patients are willing to be informed and educated. Answer questions. There are several "Don'ts," however.

Do not say: "Don't worry about that, you don't need to know all the complexities" or "Don't worry about the test results; I'll let you know if there are any problems."

Do not offer to answer questions and then evade them.

Do not pretend to know an answer if you do not.

Do not offer to answer questions unless you are willing to ensure your patient understands the answer.

Do not say you are available at all hours and then not be reachable.

Do not assume the patient understands all your terms.

Do not assume a woman is comfortable in the setting of her doctor's office.

Rather, assume the patient wants to know and understand what you are talking about, the terms you are using, and the steps and indications for procedures. Some women are not assertive enough to ask for explanations, but they still want to know. It is natural to worry about the results of diagnostic procedures until the answers are available. If you do not know the answer to a question—which probably happens very rarely—say, "I don't know, but I can find out for you," or refer her to someone who might know, or just leave if at "I don't know." If a question seems unrelated to what you have been discussing, ask her why she asks. This can reveal a lot of information about her, how she thinks, her expectations, and so forth. Clarify your hours. Some practitioners find it very helpful to establish certain hours of the day or certain days when they may be called for questions. If you are not immediately available, say you will call back—and then be sure to do so. To not follow through on a phone call conveys the message "I am not dependable." The physician who ensures coverage when he or she is away is seen as dependable and responsible. The physician who is seen as uncaring to his or her patients will be spoken of by them as haughty and inconsiderate and will lose patients.

As much as a woman respects her doctor and feels comfortable with him or her, one can never assume that she feels fully comfortable in the office or hospital. She might feel quite vulnerable and hopeful that her physician will respect her and treat her with courtesy.

The Physical Examination

The manner in which the practitioner manages the first complete physical examination demonstrates to the women patient the sort of concern, thoroughness, and helpfulness she will receive thereafter (Long, 1976). Women like the examination to be conducted in an aesthetically pleasing atmosphere, that is, colorful, cheerful and warm, yet one that also reflects the professionalism and dignity of the physician. The patient wants a clean gown and drape, and one that is large enough to prevent embarrassment. The physician or his or her assistant should escort the woman to the dressing area and give explicit instructions about what to take off, what she may leave on, and how to put on the gown. The assistant should then leave her to accomplish this. The assistant or physician should ensure that the woman is draped prior to beginning any discussion or examination.

It is generally held that a chaperone is no longer required on a routine basis. The physician should be alert and selective as to which patients may require the presence of his or her assistant. Instruct the assistant to be alert and available for the overly fearful or potentially seductive patient. Often a woman wants her husband, relative, or friend to be present. The decision rests with the physician as to how comfortable he or she feels with this other person present. Unless some impropriety might result, or if the physician fears the examination will be interfered with, allowing this other person to be present will relax your patient and aid the examination. If you do have an assistant in the room, introduce the patient to him or her before she is up in stirrups.

The Pelvic Examination

The gynecological examination shares similar problems and requirements with any other medical examination, but the psychological issues are more prominent because the site of the procedure is a woman's genitals (Emerson, 1970). Many women find the pelvic examination not only unpleasant, but dehumanizing, degrading, and insensitive (Green, 1975). Very few patients accept the examination calmly. Most women find this the most distasteful aspect of any general physical. The most important contributors to this seem to be the exposure and manipulation of the woman's genitals, the fear of discovery of pathology in a location that is not readily visible to herself, the violation of her body privacy by a person who is at most an awesome, friendly stranger, confusion about the covert and overt sexual overtones of the examination regardless of the sex of the examiner, the expectation of physical discomfort from the procedure, memories of prior examinations, horror stories other women have related about their own examinations, and the inaccessibility and hidden nature of a woman's genitals because of their anatomic location.

The physician can alleviate some anxiety and improve rapport with the patient by saying to her: "Most patients are a little nervous about pelvic examinations (or other procedures as it applies), so let me tell you what I'll be doing'' (Settlage, 1975). The rapport is established before the patient lies down on the table in the lithotomy position. (The standard position for pelvic examination, the lithotomy position, has a woman lying on her back with her legs flexed and spread apart—either supported by stirrups or flexed on her belly.) After the first meeting, for future examinations, the patient may already have disrobed, gowned and been covered on the examining table when the physician enters. Rapport is established during the time before the patient lies down in the lithotomy position. For the patient you have seen before, this can be the time to explore current medical problems or to update the routine history. Then explain the purpose of the examination, especially any change in procedure should one have been established since you previously saw the patient. Do not assume she knows step by step and understands the need for each step. Repetition is acceptable, even if the woman has heard the explanation before.

After discussion, the patient is told to lie down (Settlage, 1975). She can then be helped in putting her feet in the stirrups while her perineum is still covered. This respects her modesty appropriately and avoids unnecessary exposure. For example, she can be told, ''Next, move to the head of the table'' and helped by holding the drape in position over her abdomen as she moves down to the end of the table with your instructions. These attentions convey concern for her comfort and feelings, especially if they are done while the physician is standing in a location where she knows he or she is looking at her and not at her genitals. The physician also conveys this by not leaving her alone at this delicate moment, only to return to the room after she is all ready. Some physicians prefer to leave the room while the nurse positions the patient. This is acceptable, but it loses some continuity, as well as psychological advantages of the doctor in charge being there. Some doctors prefer to have the patient lie down for a standard examination, reserving the move to the lithotomy position for the pelvic examination alone. Many women prefer this also.

Starting the examination with a less threatening area, for example, the abdomen, again conveys, ''I understand the common thoughts and concerns and respect them.'' Breasts are also anxiety-provoking in a physical (Settlage, 1975). The tremendous public awareness of breast cancer exacerbates the conflict between sexual fantasies and the need for careful examination.

Women like to know the doctor is interested in looking at more than her genitals. Maintain eye contact whenever possible; for example, once the patient is in the lithotomy position, flattening the drape or providing the patient with a pillow for her head permits her to watch the doctor and the doctor to watch her.

Talk to the patient in a natural manner as you explain step by step what you are going to do, what she is likely to feel, for example, pressure sensations, possible types of discomfort, and answer any questions or comments she has about discomforts or concerns.

Allow the patient adequate time to carry through your requests. For example, if you tell her to relax before you put in the speculum, give her several seconds to do so. If she says "ouch," do not insist that it does not hurt. Some women have a harder time relaxing.

Most women find speculum insertion to be the most crucial part of the examination (Magee, 1975). Just telling her to relax may not explain how or what to relax. Some suggestions include instructing the woman that "she has a muscle she squeezes closed when she has to urinate and cannot get to a bathroom, and she should do the opposite of that," or contract it first, and then relax.

The speculum itself is frightening. Many patients call them clamps and are afraid of what the "clamp" will do inside (Magee, 1975). Tell the patient what the speculum actually does; that is, it is not a clamp, but it holds the skin apart so you can see. The metal ones are very cold unless warmed up. Fingers should be inserted slowly, just as a speculum should. Avoid compressing the urethra—it is very painful (Magee, 1975). Inform the patient that the feel of the speculum inside as it opens might produce in her the urge to urinate and defecate (Magee, 1975). The click of the lock on the plastic speculum is also frightening; warn the patient in advance that she will hear it and what it is.

"It is particularly important during the bimanual examination that the patient be aware of your movements and the sensations she will have. Her anxieties will be maximal because you have in effect invaded her vagina and pelvis with a portion of your body" (Settlage, 1975). The doctor can allay much of this anxiety with the earlier educative and empathetic approach to the patient, "but unless care is taken during this last portion of the exam, you will not gain potentially important information and she will remember the entire process as unpleasant. Be extremely cautious in considering the woman's reactions as a painful response. Elicit information which differentiates pressure, sensation of movement, urge to defecate, and urge to urinate, which are always normally present in the bimanual examination" (Settlage, 1975).

Education is an essential part of the gynecological examination (Settlage, 1975). Familiarity with her own body is a woman's right and helps her to become a more knowledgeable patient and aide to the doctor who cares for her. The doctor has the authority to give the woman permission to explore and learn more about her own body; for example, during the examination, give her the choice of using a mirror so she can see what she looks like as you explain her anatomy. An attitude that says a woman does not need to know is self-defeating and deprives the doctor and the patient of a convenient avenue for establishing the working relationship needed to maximize health care.

Specific Gynecological Issues

Menstruation and Contraception

Menstruation is called the "curse" for more reasons than the Biblical attribution. For most women, the "period" at some time is a source of pain, disability, unpleasant mood change, shift in body sensation and image, nuisance, and embarrassment. Many women often find it a convenient excuse from full effort, while others minimize the physiologic changes. Women bleed 1/6 to 1/4 of their lives during child-bearing years. While a few women may seem to exaggerate the disabling features of the period, most take it in stride. It would be crass, however, for any physician to assume that the menses have no meaning for any woman patient.

Control of contraception lies within any individual's domain. The various methods are not without their psychological side effects. Birth control pills provide the greatest security according to statistical data. Their physiological side effects, however, may be discomforting and dangerous. A woman who prefers other forms of contraceptive devices is not perforce an unreliable gambler nor disrespectful of her male partner's needs. The unrelenting fact of life remains that only females become pregnant. While this capability provides for joy-filled and exciting dreams and experiences, the vulnerability carries an ever-present burden. As long as women are considered second-class, less competent citizens, theirs will be the disproportionately greater responsibility for mature family planning.

The Emergency

Like other medical emergencies, the gynecological variety demands the most of those qualities of the doctor-patient relationship, with the doctor as the authority-expert and the patient as submissive to the speedy efforts at diagnosis and treatment (Donovan and Benson, 1976).

It is important that during the emergency, and as soon as possible afterward, the patient gradually be given back decision-making function in order to resume responsibility for her own physical and emotional welfare. Keeping the patient totally dependent increases the burden on the doctor rather than gradually removing it and leaving him or her room and energy to devote to other crises that arise. At the extreme, the patient who must remain dependent to receive the doctor's attentions can develop new or extended symptoms in an unconscious attempt to sustain the relationship with the doctor. The patient recovering from surgery or serious ill health must not suddenly be abandoned to care for herself. She needs her doctor's help and support and the opportunity to "hasten her return to full health and vigor and a life without continued dependence on her doctor."

Dilatation and Curettage

By encompassing features of anatomic anonymity, invasion of body parts, and removal of some unseen toxic material, the "D and C" procedure possesses significant psychological impact. It may leave a woman with a fearful fantasy of what has remained behind and what was removed. While most women cope very well, the physician is advised not to minimize the potential effect of this procedure and to schedule a follow-up session in order to monitor the patient's well-being.

Hysterectomy

Even for the postmenopausal woman or for the woman who has decided not to use her childbearing capacity any longer, the uterus is psychologically essential to the image she has of her whole body. Except for dire emergency, talk of its removal should not be done in haste. Hysterectomy is not necessary for sterilization. However, loss of it does not mean a woman will go "crazy."

The uterus is a symbol of strength, health, and general effectiveness. Loss of the uterus means loss of childbearing ability and loss of menstruation. The fantasy of many women and men is that the removal of the uterus is associated with obesity, masculinization, premature aging, loss of sex drive, and loss of coital pleasure. This is true for heterosexual or homosexual women. In general, hysterectomy is associated with fears, as well as with positive and negative feelings about the effect the loss may have on marital and sexual relationships and on the woman's feminine role functions (Raphael, 1972). Some women see it as retribution for sins they have committed during their lives.

When appropriate indications for hysterectomy are present (that is, retaining the uterus would be more harmful than losing it), a discussion between the patient and the physician should occur about the physical implications and the meaning this has for her life and for her continued sexual fulfillment. A minimum of two interviews is required to allow the woman to evaluate the data the physician presents her and how she thinks and feels about it. In evaluating the patient's response, the physician can ask such questions as: "What is your attitude about losing a part of your body through surgery?" "What results do you expect from the operation?" "How have you experienced surgery in the past, and what was your reaction?" "What is your present life situation?" Also include questions concerning emotional supports and marital and sexual compatibility: "How have you responded to stressful situations in the past?" "Do you have any previous psychiatric history?" Some anxiety by the patient is appropriate. Beware of the patient who lacks anxiety altogether or who is overly agitaged about the surgery, since these are prognostic indicators of postoperative difficulties (Polivy, 1974). Educate the patient and her mate to dispel myths and convey support and understanding; this will help minimize psychiatric sequelae. Grieving after hysterectory is normal. The physician should be prepared to give support for longer than just a few weeks. However, within a couple of months, the woman should have returned to normal functioning (Roeske, 1978).

There is no scientific evidence for increased incidence of mental illness after hysterectomy over any other kind of surgery. The woman who grieves for a long time and who is disabled in her everyday life because of prolonged mourning should be referred for psychiatric evaluation.

Sterilization

Sequelae from voluntary sterilization are generally fewer and less damaging than when sterilization is required by medical necessity. It is important to determine whether or not the woman feels under pressure to submit to the procedure (Donovan and Benson, 1976). Most women, especially with increasing public awareness, know all that is involved in making this decision, but it is important for the physician to evaluate the patient's knowledge about the procedure and its consequences (for example, never having more children) and the variety of ways it is performed (with the pros and cons and success rates for each) and to educate her to arrive at a mutually satisfactory conclusion. The woman needs the opportunity to ask questions and to express her feelings. Again, a minimum of two meetings is usually necessary to allow for this. Postoperatively as well, most women would like the opportunity to discuss the issues further. This helps the patient adjust better and comply better with the practitioner's medical advice.

For any surgery or procedure that requires regional or general anesthesia, the woman who is well-informed and has a good rapport with her doctor generally is more calm and cooperative and therefore a better surgical risk (McDonald, 1976).

Adolescence

Adolescence is a period of growth and change, of adjustment to change in one's physical size and shape, and of increased intellectual comprehension of abstract concepts. It is also a period of increasing independence and desire for separation, while still being dependent on one's family for emotional and financial support. Peers become one's social focus.

Most adolescent girls reach menarche while still under the care of a pediatrician or family practitioner. This is the time for introduction to information about physical development and the responsibilities of womanhood. The concept of pelvic examinations can be introduced by examinations of the genitals. Adolescents are naturally very shy and modest about their bodies, in particular about exposing them or, worse, being touched by an adult male. This is one reason why many teenage girls would prefer to be seen by a female physician.

The changes in a young girl's body can be frightening, a focus of curiosity, and symbolize a new role—becoming a woman—and all that it encompasses. Breast development draws attention from boys and girls. Few girls are prepared for or feel comfortable with this attention. The development of breasts is the first publicly noticeable sign of change for the girl, her parents, and her peers. Thus it is important for the health practitioner in caring for adolescents to be sensitive to their modesty and their uncertainty about self vis-à-vis confusing societal expectations. The health practitioner must also appreciate their lack of knowledge or experience in managing situations related to their newly developed reproductive capacities. It will help the practitioner to determine the level of knowledge and sophistication of the girl and her mother. For example, is she a young pubescent new to her body changes and the attention of others—especially males—or is she almost an adult, taking upon herself responsibility for her sexual activity. The practitioner also needs to determine for himself or herself how willing and able he or she is to be a resource for the teenager—someone who can speak to her in her language, gives her accurate information not platitudes, and does not think that her questions are trivial or that she is too young to be asking them. By ensuring proper care and attention, the practitioner can help the teenage girl to become an aware woman and a good patient for the rest of her life (Senarclens, 1972).

Menopause

The *menopausal woman* is a commonly used term in Western countries, yet the simplicity in the concept has come increasingly into question. There is a general concensus that the symptoms of vasomotor instability, hot flashes, flushes, and episodes of perspiration are among the consistent symptoms accompanying menopause and presumably result from hormonal imbalance (Flint, 1975; Notman, 1978; Wentz, 1976). Specifically, *menopause* refers to the cessation of menstruation, while the "change of life" stage is called the *climacterium*. Most confusion arises around this difference, that is, the biological changes versus the larger implications this period has in a woman's life.

There is a general tendency, albeit incorrect, to assume the variety of complaints of the 40 to 60-year-old woman are a result of the menopause. The complaints are varied—they can include cold, moist, and numb extremities; chills; palpitations; headaches; dizziness; fatigue; joint pain; nervousness; irritability; insomnia; depression; self-depreciation; jealousies; and a number of gastrointestinal complaints (Flint, 1975). Women have been told that these are a normal part of the menopause. Rather, there is increasing appreciation for the diversity of responses both in our culture and cross-culturally.

Factors that place a woman at higher risk for adjustment include dependence on her role as wife and/or mother and/or homemaker, her self-esteem and personal identity, limited financial resources, marital instability, and the impression that she has few alternatives for herself (VanKeep and Kellerhals, 1976). Societal expectations for women in this age group also influence the outcome. And for the married woman, the husband's response to the midlife event as it affects both himself and his wife is also significant. Our society views the menopausal and postmenopausal women as occupying lowered status. She is less "feminine," is getting old, and according to some myths, has "outlived her reason for being," namely, child bearing (Parlee, 1978). In other cultures, where the older woman has been viewed with higher esteem for centuries, adjustment to the climacterium is easier (Flint, 1975; Notman, 1978; Parlee, 1978).

Taking these issues into consideration, then, the physician who works with a woman during the perimenopausal years must be aware of the psychosocial changes the woman has to cope with. It would be inappropriate to assume that all her complaints can be treated via "pharmaceutical juggling" (Notman, 1978; VanKeep and Kellerhals, 1976; Wentz, 1975). The physician must evaluate the woman's perception of herself and her self-esteem as it is affected by the menopause, the alternatives she sees for herself in the years to come, her responses to stresses in the past (for example, pregnancy, a child's leaving home, a change in her or her husband's or significant other's career), and the financial and intellectual resources available to her. With this information available, the physician can better decide the etiology of the complaints and thus the appropriate recommendations as to medication, verbal support, and/or referral for other counseling.

The Aging Patient

One might think that the older women has been through it all, so there is no need to explain anything to her (Gray, 1977). Really, she too is looking for a competent professional who will provide opportunities for counseling and education in a warm and supportive environment. Cessation of reproductive capabilities may make it harder for the older woman to maintain regular checkups, pelvic examinations, and Pap smears.

Increasing physical limitations present new demands for an older woman. The normal height of the examining table may be harder to maneuver onto. Fragility and shrinkage of tissues make normal-sized instruments more threatening. Older women often require more time dressing and undressing and may need physical support.

Sexual feelings do not diminish with old age, however. The good physician reassures the patient about the normality of her feelings and helps her maintain her body properly. Additionally, the physician can make suggestions and give advice about sexual questions. The older woman does not want someone to tell her that she is too old, or that it is time to set aside sex, or that if she is a widow or divorcee that she "shouldn't do it."

For the older woman who has lost many emotional supports, the gynecologist or physician provides important support. She looks to him or her for encouragement to maintain personal care and nutritional and dietary requirements. It is hard enough facing old age. Such a woman does not want to be reminded by others and, worse, told by the treatment she receives from professionals that she is as good as gone. Any patient wants to be, and should be, evaluated as an individual.

All too often in aging, depression presents covertly as physical symptoms or as senility. In some women, after menopause, autonomic nervous system instability can cause or aggravate emotional disturbances (Overstreet, 1976). Many times older women need aid in the form of social services. The physician is advised to know of resources in the community to whom such a woman may be referred, for example, the Visiting Nurse Association, the Department of Public Health, the Department of Social Services at state and local levels, and community centers.

Changes in the Doctor-Woman Relationship

Expertise about organs and functions that are so intimate and personal has a tendency to carry with it a sense of power to dominate the patient. Many women are increasingly less inclined to look for qualities of power in a doctor or nurse.

The summary "What to Expect from Your Doctor" describes the background, education, and expectations women are bringing with them to their doctors:

1. An accurate diagnosis of your condition, healthy or otherwise, at your request.
2. Results and meaning of any tests or examinations performed by him or by others at his discretion as soon as they are available.
3. Indications for treatment, varieties and alternatives, pros and cons of particular treatments in the opinion of other experts, as well as the doctor's own preference and the reasons for it.
4. Answers to your questions about any examination or procedure he may perform, in advance of or at any time during the performance of it. Stopping any examination or procedure at any moment, at your request.
5. Complete information about purpose, content, and known effects of all drugs prescribed or administered, including possible risks, side-effects and contraindications, especially of any combination of drugs.
6. Willingness to accept and wait for a second medical opinion before performing any elective surgery which involves alteration or removal of any organ or body part.
7. Answers to your questions about your body or your general physical health functioning, in addition to any particular condition. Or, encouragement to seek these answers from another source [Boston Women's Health Collective, 1973].

These items may sound pedantic or trivial, but they arise because women have felt subjugated and mistreated by their physicians for centuries. A woman who complains of gynecological problems dislikes being told she is childish or "hysterical," particularly by a man who has never endured the same treatment or by the man's nurse who seems an extension of his ego. Women's desires for increasing participation in their own treatment extends, too, to their needing to ask questions about their sexuality. In answering such questions, physicians need to be as sensitive as they are in other matters mentioned in this chapter. Women are developing the courage to stand up for their own rights. They want to work with nurses, receptionists, and doctors who will treat them as respectable human beings rather than as mindless second-class citizens.

Obstetrics

Pregnancy is a special time for a woman and her family. Normal emotions and expectations range from joy, fulfillment, and a sense of creation to stress, fear, and anxiety. Conflicts arise over sexual relations, physical attractiveness and change in one's own body image, and implications for family life, such as the father's feelings, the mother's attention, work schedule, and meanings for the couple as a pair (Nadelson, 1973).

Many complex and varied motivations may contribute to the act of becoming pregnant. Pregnancy may serve as a means of holding a relationship together, as an expression of sexual identity, as a means of establishing a separate identity for an adolescent, as a means of caring for oneself by taking care of a product of oneself, and, for a healthy mature couple, as an expression of the wish to procreate.

Controversy surrounds the degree of interaction between physiological and psychological concomitants of pregnancy and how they feed into each other (Nadelson, 1973). For example, moderate nausea, fatigue, vomiting, and some emotional lability are common changes early in pregnancy. Physiological etiologies can explain these, yet psychological factors such as guilt or ambivalence also may predominate. Disappointment may be experienced because of the lack of well-being or at the first noticeable sign of life. With quickening and noticeable changes in body shape, disappointment may disappear along with the other unpleasant first-trimester symptoms. Feelings of dependency commonly increase in the second trimester. By the third, anxieties over labor, delivery, and the baby's health and well-being abound.

The Normal Pregnancy

A pregnancy does not occur in a vacuum. The couple constitutes a family, and there may be children as well. Grandparents are usually close emotionally, if not geographically. Everyone is influenced by a pregnancy. The expectant mother becomes the center of attention. How a woman copes with this attention will in turn influence the course of her pregnancy and the dedegree to which she will cooperate with medical instructions. In addition, a family's attitude toward the pregnancy, childbirth, children, and doctors will be influenced by each person's own family experience, religious beliefs, and cultural expectations. The physician will need to take all these into account when working with the pregnant woman and her husband. Occasionally, nowadays, single women bear children. The same issues apply. In addition, the physician may serve a larger role for this woman because she does not have a spouse or partner with whom to share the experience.

In general, families wish to be involved with and have the right to affect decisions concerning pregnancy, labor, and delivery (Nielsen, 1975). The physician and his or her nurse should educate the couple in order that they may give truly informed consent for procedures or make decisions affecting their care. The practitioner should respect the attitudes of the family and how they are reflected in the woman's or couple's decisions. It is important for the physician and nurse to know their own beliefs in order to keep them separate from their patient's beliefs. If the practitioner cannot offer good care because his or her beliefs are so different from the patient's, he or she must inform the patient and help her find care that will be more acceptable.

Once the practitioner has decided to care for the patient, he or she is responsible for evaluating the family's level of knowledge and ensuring that they have the opportunities to learn facts and helpful aids for pregnancy, childbirth, and care of the newborn. Various educational arrangements include didactic discussions with the patient and her spouse, an educational corner in the office with audio and/or visual tapes and illustrated books, filmstrips, self-evaluation questions, and public classes, preferably those which the practitioner has evaluated for the comprehensiveness of the material and quality of teaching.

The primipara woman, that is, the woman who is pregnant for the first time, in particular wants to know about the normal physiological and psychological changes associated with pregnancy; they are new to her. For example, changes in the pelvic floor and turgescence may change the time durations in intercourse so that, especially during the second trimester, orgasm may be reached sooner. A woman normally becomes more inwardly preoccupied with herself. One possible result of this is a mild decline in sexual interest. Couples should be advised that this is temporary for the pregnancy and that they can expect return to their usual sexual experience after. It is common during the third trimester for the woman to find herself being treated as a delicate object. Many men have an aversion to sexual relations with a pregnant woman. Thus the couple should be advised that comfort, warmth, and supportive needs are as great as ever and that physical attention and affection are needed even if sexual intercourse is avoided, (Donovan, 1976).

Women involved in sports will want advice from their physicians about what activities are safe to continue during pregnancy. Women no longer consider themselves unfeminine for being athletically oriented. Those who are athletically inclined will look with disfavor on a physician who tries to tell them that athletics are unfeminine or unhealthy. Popular literature is spreading the "word" about physical fitness, and the up-to-date physician will become informed about the "do's and don'ts" in this area.

With the approach of the delivery date, the pregnant woman and her husband or partner commonly have fantasies or dreams about the new baby. Themes include the sex and health of the infant, what changes will occur in the family, and the possibilities of injury, ill-health, or even death to the child or the mother (Nadelson, 1973). Other thoughts include the change in the mother's relationship to the fetus when, at delivery, it becomes a separate individual, as well as concern about the ability to properly care for and love the infant. Clues as to how the new baby will affect the marital relationship arise during pregnancy in the form of how much the wife is distracted from the husband by pre-occupation with the infant.

Labor

Each process of labor and delivery is unique, even for the women with several previous experiences (Nadelson, 1973). Women wish for the presence of someone who is supportive and warm, someone who provides a sense of sharing and familiarity. This person can be a woman or a man. The point is that this person helps alleviate some of the anxiety inherent in the experience.

Many couples and single women today are choosing natural childbirth, or at least part of the instruction to relieve tension and fear. It is important for the physician to understand each couple, that is, how they have responded to stress previously, and how they have prepared to respond to the stress of the present labor and delivery. The single woman who has no partner may have family who will help her. Some women with husbands and many family members still find that their relatives are unable to provide enough support. The demands on the physician will increase inversely with the support available to the mother. In one instance the physician may find a stable, mature woman able to make appropriate use of hospital systems for adequate support, and in another instance he or she will find a woman who needs both the nursing staff and physician to help her.

Human being are complex, and each is different. No cookbook recipes can adequately prepare the medical staff to work with each individual family. Thus the staff will need to evaluate each situation anew, be flexible, and work to make the hospital environment as flexible as possible within the rules of the institution.

Labor is a painful experience, and the amount of pain felt and suffered will vary with each mother. While heavy medication may at times be necessary, it may leave the woman with a sense of unreality. The medication may make her less conscious, less aware of labor and delivery, and less able to appropriately perform mothering care at and after delivery.

Companionship is one of the best means of support during labor (Nielsen, 1975). Fears increase if a woman is left alone at this time, and common ones include fear that the baby may be born suddenly or that if problems arise, someone will not respond quickly enough. Those attending the woman should be empathetic, reassuring, and encouraging, as well as knowledgeable of the labor process. The physician models for the nursing staff the atmosphere and behavior he or she feels are important. Each staff member has the responsibility to be warm and supportive. Conflicts and inconsistencies among the professionals diminish the care to the patient.

Fathers do not want to be forgotten. The father can give his support to the mother whether he stays in the labor room or waits elsewhere. A father's absence places more demand for support on the labor room staff.

During labor and delivery, the woman or the pair (that is, the mother and father) wish to be treated as in a working relationship with the obstetrician. High on the list of qualities desired for the practitioner, aside from technical competence, ranks the ability to establish and maintain a warm, respectful relationship. The birth of a child is a uniqe moment in a couple's life, and a cool, business-as-usual attitude from the practitioner or staff detracts from their experience and leaves resentment.

Delivery

Delivery is similar to a pelvic examination in that a woman wishes respect for her body and modesty as much as possible. Most women never become comfortable baring their bodies to hospital personnel. It is understood that some disrobing is required for delivery, but as with surgery, minimal exposure is desired.

Part of the preparation for labor and delivery should be to inform the couple of the standard operating procedure for each phase. If this is done, the couple will not be taken by surprise when handed the infant or if the infant is taken away. Also, they can help the staff rather than create obstacles.

After Delivery

The obstetric staff has the responsibility of ensuring that all mothers are educated in techniques about self-care and baby care. The education process must be flexible and acknowledge differences according to culture and tradition as long as nothing is harmful to the infant or mother. The staff also must be flexible according to the amount of knowledge the mother and father already have. Many hospital staffs and public health instructors find that fathers are eager to take part when classes are held in the evenings. After delivery, physicians may need to encourage the mother to resume her intellectual, social, and other activities at a normal pace. There are some myths still circulating that set restrictions on the recovery process. Unnecessarily restrictive instructions can be limiting not only to physical activity, but to mental activity as well; this simply adds stress rather than relief to an already stressful period.

Formal instructions also should vary with the individual. Women who have difficulty making decisions may do better with very specific instructions. However, more independent and self-confident parents may prefer basic knowledge. Providing written instructions in clear, simple language extends the hospital staff's influence and effect to the home after discharge.

A complete educational program includes the topic of feelings normally experienced by women as mothers and as wives and by men as husbands and fathers. Knowing that others tend to feel as they do helps people experience the normal range of feelings, not feel alone, and not expend energy inappropriately feeling guilty. These feelings can include ecstacy, joy, a sense of adventure, and a sense of being drawn closer to the spouse. Women may experience a sense of loss (that is, having grown accustomed to the special relationship with the being within her). There may be anger and resentment at the baby for the change in the woman's body shape and image, for the demands on her for nurturance, attention, love, and care. These are magnified by fatigue (Donovan, 1976). Many women worry about wanting to get away from the baby for awhile. The woman who has delivered for the first time may be concerned about her own mothering abilities and about her husband's skills as a father. If either parent had an unhappy childhood, their doubts can increase as they try not to repeat the mistakes of their own parents.

Husbands as new fathers commonly wonder how much time the new infant will demand and may see child care as an exclusively feminine activity that detracts from their masculinity. This deprives the father of the chance to partake in his own growth and the growth of his child, as well as the intimate relationship he can develop with the child. It also may produce disagreements with the wife over responsibilities.

A new infant demands more time, energy, and money than most parents ever expect. They should not feel stupid or misled at not realizing this in advance. The physician and his or her staff can alleviate many of these concerns by educating both parents in advance and by carefully monitoring them during follow-up visits.

Infant Feeding

Some women have decided in advance of talking with the doctor which form of infant feeding will be used, that is, breast or bottle. Many wish educated advice of the physician who may honestly have his or her own opinions, but who also can attempt to objectively integrate the pros and cons for each method. The woman who chooses the bottle or who is unable to breast feed wants to know that she is no less of a mother, even though many feel that way. It is the quality of the interaction between the mother and her child that is important for child development and maternal-infant bond development, not whether the breast or bottle is used specifically (Donovan, 1975).

Special Obstetrical Problems

Teenage Pregnancy

Pregnancy creates a crisis for teenage girls (La Barre, 1972). Teen years normally require adjustment to body changes—size, shape, and inner impulses. These arise in the context of increasing capacity for understanding abstract concepts and changes in social relationships. The adolescent girl struggles with her independence from her family, while still needing them for emotional and financial support. There is increasing reliance on friends to replace the family, and sexual maturity predates the emotional maturity needed to manage it. Teenage pregnancy taxes an incomplete adjustment to the developmental changes of adolescence and requires adjustments to unfamiliar roles as new wives or unwed mothers-to-be.

Teenage pregnancies are rarely planned and are rarely approved of by the families. The girl is faced with the decision of keeping or giving up the baby and whether to tell her family. If she keeps it, most schools will not allow her to remain; she will be forced to attend a special program away from her friends and classmates. Most teenagers and their families require professional help during this process.

The physician is in a special position to provide education, and to monitor how well the girl and her family are coping, or whether they may need professional counseling to weigh decisions and return to normal life afterward (La Barre, 1972). One parameter by which to monitor coping is to inquire about the following:

1. The quality and stability of the relationship with the boy involved.
2. Strength of peer relationships; any evidence of increasing isolation or downward drift in the choice of peers.
3. Marked conflict with the family.
4. Increasing inadequacy and failure in school performance.
5. Severe or unusual mood or affect shifts with evidence of depression or withdrawal.
6. Increasing frustration and inadequacy in the care of the child after delivery.

Evidence of problems in any of these areas is indication for referral for psychiatric evaluation and input before the situation worsens (Bernstein, 1972).

In general, families will respond to this crisis as they have to others in the past. Healthy families maintain family stability, survive the crises, and commonly become closer through the experience. The decision to keep the child raises issues of financial and emotional support for the girl and the child. The teenager is faced with adjusting to the maternal role while still developing her own identity through adolescence.

Complicated Pregnancies

Note: These descriptions are brief. Whether a women's medical course proceeds simply or with complications, it is important for the physician and staff to treat her emotions and her body with the respect referred to throughout this chapter.

Hyperemesis Gravidarum. Excessive vomiting during pregnancy is generally viewed as a treatable disorder with which psychiatric intervention is the therapy of choice. Various psychiatric etiologies are extant. Biologic contributions to the problem remain controversial.

Spontaneous Abortion. "There is no convincing evidence that emotional factors can cause abortion " (Donovan, 1976). The couple should be assured that the "miscarriage" is not a reflection of something physically or emotionally wrong with them. Women often feel guilty that they have thought or done something wrong, and it is not uncommon for husbands or parents to blame her. Rather, this is nature's way of getting rid of a nonviable fetus.

Habitual Spontaneous Abortions. The contribution of emotional factors is controversial and hard to assess. For the couple who has tried repeatedly to maintain a pregnancy, each loss is especially discouraging and may be a source of conflict between husband and wife as each searches for blame in an attempt to understand what they cannot comprehend.

Therapeutic Abortion. Previously, psychiatric opinion was that therapeutic abortions were fraught with psychological complications. Since 1960, several good scientific studies have shown that this threat of serious sequelae is a myth (Pasnau, 1972; Barnes et al., 1971; Niswander and Patterson, 1967; Patt et al., 1969). Most normal women respond to abortions with a sense of relief, often with a mild feeling of depression. Even women with psychiatric illness respond with improved mental attitudes or with no change in their psychiatric problems. One sequela of therapeutic abortions is a significant increase in effective birth control techniques used by these women.

Recommendations for obstetricians include

1. No routine psychiatric consultation. Rather the decision should rest

with the patient and her physician. She is not crazy or malicious to make the request.

2. Psychiatric evaluation is recommended for the following cases:
   a. If the patient exhibits signs and symptoms of a major psychiatric illness including psychosis, suicidal ideation, significant depression, or severe personality or behavior disorder.
   b. If the patient has a history of a previous postpartum psychosis.
   c. If the patient exhibits ambivalence over her decision and/or requests psychiatric assistance in discussing motivational issues.
   d. If the patient is massively compliant with the wishes of parents or spouse, but does not herself wish to have an abortion.
3. Followup the patients for several visits in order to adequately monitor physical and emotional status (Pasnau, 1972).

Caesarian Section. This operation differs from regular delivery in three main ways. First, the woman is usually unconscious for the delivery of her infant, although some anesthesiologists keep her awake and anesthetize her below the trunk. If she is not awake, she loses her sense of boundaries and does not experience closure on the pregnancy. Second, surgery leaves a scar and thus a permanently visible change in the woman's body. Most women adjust to this well, but for the woman who frantically needs an intact body image, this is a tremendous threat. Third, major surgery prolongs recuperation time and postpones full opportunity for development of the mother-infant bond. This may not be a problem of great significance in the long run, but diminishes the experience in the short run.

Problem Births

Instead of the happy experience in giving birth, tragedy strikes those families where there is delivery of a stillborn, malformed, or distressed infant, or where there is injury to the mother.

The parents suffer from loss of the expectation of a normal child. They grieve, as with any mourning. The staff helps them by being supportive and by giving them permission to feel the wide range of feelings they are likely to experience. They blame in attempt to understand. At times, this is directed at the hospital staff, at other times at each other. The staff aids resolution by advising against a quick and simple solution—like a tubal ligation or vasectomy to prevent recurrence. No matter how many children in a family, the loss of one child or birth of an abnormal child is unique and nonreplaceable. Parents need to be advised of the special requirements of the malformed child. Here the practitioner works closely with the pediatrician to help the parents learn about the care of the child and to find other parents with similar problems. Staff encouragement can help them overcome obstacles to parenting. All too often the mother is blamed because the baby comes from her body. Genetic education and counseling can alleviate this. Should the physician find continued marital conflict over this on following visits, marital counseling is advised (Lippman and Carlson, 1977).

Postpartum Illness

Significant physical illness in a mother or infant will impede development of mother-infant attachment or at least make it more difficult. The long-term outcome probably depends on the quality of life and relationships over years. In the beginning, though, there can be a serious assault on the mother's sense of herself as a mother and on her self-esteem. One example is placental complications, infection, and prolonged hospitalization. These parents need the encouragement and support of the physician and staff during the illness and during follow-up afterward.

Psychiatric Illness

The risk of a severe disturbance increases when a greater-than-usual physical stress has occurred and commonly repeats with future pregnancies. Biological and psychological factors are recognized. The practitioner must watch for bizarre behavior, delirium, restlessness, and confusion, particularly in the first month postpartum. Depression commonly presents later, and with the first signs of potentially destructive attitudes or acts, psychiatric consultation should be sought. In general, the earlier the problems are recognized and treatment sought, the better chance for recovery.

Amniocentesis

Like any other invasive procedure, amniocentesis is felt as an intrusion into a woman's body and into the special relationship she has with the fetus. These feelings are not excessive for most women, but should be recognized.

Motherhood

Pregnancy, labor, and delivery are a time of maturation and growth; most women cope well with these major stresses. Motherhood is learned from experience with one's own mother, watching friends and relatives, movies, and television shows, and is also a product of the experience. The bond between a mother and her child develops over months and as each interacts with the other through smiles, looks, talking, and moving.

Fathers are an important factor in motherhood. The relationship between a mother and father can enhance motherhood or make it a refuge or a burden. The physician working with the pediatrician can assess the progress of these relationships over several visits.

For the unmarried woman, the physician may serve a special means of support. Single status does not imply poor coping or mothering skills.

In general, the history of the patient will give clues to the physician, regarding possible maladaptive responses to pregnancy, labor, and delivery. Important areas of concern include

1. Previous history of psychiatric treatment or hospitalization.
2. Past history of difficult response to pregnancy and delivery and post-partum.
3. Marital or family discord.
4. Familial or congenital diseases in previous deliveries, birth of a defective child.
5. Major individual or family medical problems or deaths.
6. Conflicts about the role as a mother and the capabilities to care for a child.
7. History of pseudocyesis, infertility, habitual abortion, premature births, still births, hyperemesis, prolonged or difficult labor.
8. Extremes in age range, that is, under 17 or over 40.
9. Previous poor relationships with physicians (may guide the present approach to this patient).
10. Past difficulties at other critical maturational stages, for instance, puberty.
11. History of early maternal deprivation.
12. Conflicts with sexual identity.
13. Unmarried status (Nadelson, 1973).

Summary

In the final analysis, women are not identical copies of each other, but distinct individuals. Because of these personal differences, women will seek various qualities in their physicians. Some seek a person who is firm in his or her opinions and is quick to inform the patient. Others prefer someone who is more flexible. No one physician can meet the personal needs of every patient. Any one woman will continue to select the physician who most satisfies her medical needs and addresses her psychological and intellectual expectations.

References

Barnes, A.B., Cohen, E., Stoeckle, J.D., and McGuire, M.T. Therapeutic abortion: Medical and social sequelae. *Annals of Internal Medicine* 75:881–886, 1971.

Bernstein, D.M. The distressed adolescent—pregnancy vs. suicide. In *Psychosomatic Medicine in Obstetrics and Gynecology,* ed. B. Karger. London: Karger, 1972, pp. 372–374.

Donovan, J. Emotional aspects of pregnancy. In *Obstetric and Gynecologic Diagnosis and Treatment,* ed. Ralph C. Benson. Los Altos, Calif.: Lange Medical Publications, 1976, pp. 850–856.

Donovan, J.C., and Benson, R.C. Psychologic aspects of gynecologic practice, In *Obstetrics and Gynecologic Diagnosis and Treatment,* ed. Ralph C. Benson. Los Altos, Calif., Lange, 1976, pp. 398–402.

Emerson, J. Behavior in private places: Sustaining definitions of reality in gynecological examinations. In *Patterns of Communicative Behavior,* ed. Hans Peter Dreitzel. New York: Macmillan, 1970, pp. 73–94.

Flint, M. The menopause: Reward or punishment. *Psychosomatics* 16:161–163, 1975.

Gray, M.J. Ambulatory gynecologic services: Special needs and perspectives of the aging patient. *Clinical Obstetrics and Gynecology* 20:183–189, 1977.

Green, R., ed. *Human Sexuality.* Baltimore: Williams & Wilkins, 1975, p. 123.

Greenhill, J.P. *Office Gynecology.* Chicago: Yearbook Publishers, 1959, p.21.

Haar, E., Halitsky, V., and Stricker, G. Factors related to the preference for a female gynecologist. *Medical Care* 13:782–790, 1975.

Hinshaw, A.L. Preventive aspects of liability in obstetrics and gynecology. *Clinical Obstetrics and Gynecology* 20:19–24, 1977.

Kroger, W.S. Hysterectomy: Psychosomatic factors of the preoperative and postoperative aspects and management. *Western Journal of Surgery, Obstetrics, and Gynecology* 65:317–323, 1957.

LaBarre, M. Emotional crisis of school-age girls during pregnancy and early motherhood. *Journal of the American Academy of Child Psychiatry* 11:537–557, 1972.

Lippman, C., and Carlson, K. A model liaison program for the obstetrics staff: Workshop on the tragic birth. In *The Family in Mourning,* ed. Charles E. Hollingsworth and Robert O. Pasnau. New York: Grune and Stratton, 1977. pp. 167–179.

Long, A.E. Gynecologic history, examination, and diagnostic procedures. In *Current Obstetric and Gynecologic Diagnosis and Treatment.* ed. Ralph C. Benson. Los Altos, Calif.: Lange, 1976, pp. 78–95.

Magee, J. The pelvic examination: A view from the other end of the table. *Annals of Internal Medicine* 83:563–564, 1975.

McDonald, J.S. Obstetric analgesia and anesthesia. In *Obstetric and Gynecologic Diagnosis and Treatment,* ed. Ralph C. Benson. Los Altos, Calif.: Lange, 1976, pp. 544–564.

Nadelson, D. "Normal" and "special" aspects of pregnancy. *Obstetrics and Gynecology* 41:611–620, 1973.

Nielsen, I. A midwife-physician team in private practice. *American Journal of Nursing* 75:1692–1695, 1975.

Niswander, K.R., and Patterson, R.T. Psychologic reaction to therapeutic abortion. *Obstetrics and Gynecology* 29:702–706, 1967.

Notman, M. Women and mid-life: A different perspective. *Psychiatric Opinion* 15:15–25, 1978.

Our Bodies, Our Selves, Boston Women's Health Collective. New York: Simon and Schuster, 1973, p. 255.

Overstreet, E. Menopause and postmenopausal syndrome. In *Obstetric and Gynecologic Diagnosis and Treatment.* ed. Ralph C. Benson, Los Altos, Calif.: Lange, 1976, pp. 456–468.

Parlee, M.B. Psychological aspects of the climacteric in women. *Psychiatric Opinion* 15:36–39, 1978.

Pasnau, R.O. Psychiatric complications of therapeutic abortion. *Obstetrics and Gynecology* 40:252–256, 1972.

Patt, S.L., Rappaport, R.G., and Barglow, P. Follow-up of therapeutic abortion. *Archives of General Psychiatry* 20:408–414, 1969.

Polivy, J. Psychological reactions to hysterectomy: A critical review. *American Journal of Obstetrics and Gynecology* 118:417–426, 1974.

Raphael, B. The crisis of hysterectomy. *Australia and New Zealand Journal of Psychiatry* 6:106–115, 1972.

Roeske, N. The emotional response to hysterectomy. *Psychiatric Opinion* (February 1978), pp. 11–20.

Senarclens, M.D. The adolescent's approach in gynecology. In *Psychosomatic Medicine in Obstetrics and Gynecology.* Basel: Karger,: pp. 375–378.

Settlage, D.S. Fordney. Pelvic examination of women. In *Human Sexuality.* ed. Richard Green, Williams & Wilkins, 1975, pp. 124–131.

VanKeep, P.A., and Kellerhals, J.M. The ageing woman. About the influence of some social and cultural factors on the changes in attitude and behavior that occur during and after the menopause. *Acta Obstetricia Et Gynecologica Scandinavica* [Supplement 51]:18–27, 1976.

Wentz, A.C. Psychiatric morbidity and the menopause. *Annals of Internal Medicine* 84:331–333, 1976.

15 Health Psychology and Older People: Toward Eradicating Agism from Attitudes and Practices

Richard Steinman

Initiated in earnest shortly before World War II, *gerontology,* the scientific study of aging, has snowballed during the intervening decades, together with professional applications of scientific findings. The rapid and eclectic generation of knowledge and clinical insights has accompanied an escalation in the proportion of the population that is older and of health policy, politics, and dollars concerned with older Americans.[1] This escalation is expected to continue—in something resembling a geometric progression. Whereas today's percentage of Americans aged 65 and older amounts to 11 percent of the nation's population, this proportion is expected to reach 20 percent by the year 2030. These developments must inevitably have a profound impact on the practice of health psychology, whether sooner or later.[2] A number of telling reasons support this prediction.

The physical or social well-being of older people is profoundly interlaced with psychological (both mental and emotional) dynamics. In recent years, a new appreciation has emerged of human development as lifespan development, together with the recognition that in later life the capacity for social/psychological development continues, even if physical development has been curtailed, terminated, or reversed.

Living in a complex industrial society has profound implications for health and illness, and these implications are replete with psychological meaning—especially for today's old people, who have been among the first in history to live through such rapid social change. There is increasingly widespread recognition among social gerontologists that, to be effective, efforts to restore the health of the aged must involve multidisciplinary teamwork.

Old age rehabilitation has implications that are not only profoundly physical, but psychological as well. Currently, there is a pressing need to evaluate both the fiscal and psychic benefits and costs—for older people, their families, and the larger society—of vast interventive programs based on certain public policies, as well as proposed alternatives.

Research psychology's contribution continues to be needed in the form of both new knowledge and a reconsideration of stale assumptions about

211

the personalities and cognition of the aged. Now that a breakthrough has recently been made in the form of tools for periodic assessments that (re)evaluate the impairments and latent potentialities of the elderly, psychology's critical contribution is needed for the utilization and refinement of such tools.

Finally, there is the striking contrast in the occurrence of new cases of psychopathology of all types: 236.1 cases per 100,000 for the population over age 65, in contrast with 76.3 cases per 100,000 for those between 25 and 34 years of age and 93 cases per 100,000 for those between 35 and 54 years.[3] This incidence, alone, should place the mental health of the elderly high among psychology's priorities.

The following postulates concerning stereotypes about older people, and the consequences of those stereotypes, are the underpinnings of this chapter:

Stereotypes about older people are limited neither to American culture nor to industrial societies. Rather, they have been prevalent in all but a handful of the societies about which evidence is available to scholars.[4] (However, among industrial societies there are some distinctions in the nature and degree of the stereotyping.)

During their formative years, most people, including most of those who will become professionals, are acculturated to incorporate primarily negative views of aging.

Unless curricular innovations occur, academic and professional education frees neither scientists nor clinicians from the burden of largely unconscious and negative assumptions about the aged.[5]

It is feasible to educate professionals to become aware of and to reexamine—both cognitively and empathically—previously unquestioned stereotypes about older people and about professional roles assumed in relation to them.

It is the purpose of this chapter to contribute in some small way to this latter process: by identifying key assumptions concerning older people, in general, and the well and the frail elderly, in particular; by highlighting the impact of these assumptions on the behaviors of society and many professionals (which, in turn, strongly influence practices affecting older patients); by illustrating alternative perceptions and practices on the part of those professionals who have become relatively free of traditional stereotypic views; and be delineating seven principles basic to such practice.

Impact of Acculturation on Many Health-Care Professionals

Attitudes and assumptions about aging and the aged are so pervasive that it must be concluded that psychology and health psychologists have been affected by them to an extent comparable with other professions. Robert N. Butler, a geropsychiatrist and first director of the National Institute on Aging, has coined the term *agism* to sum up these attitudes:

Agism: The Prejudice Against the Elderly

The stereotyping and myths surrounding old age can be explained in part by lack of knowledge and by insufficient contact with a wide variety of older people. But there is another powerful factor operating—a deep and profound prejudice against the elderly that is found to some degree in all of us. "Agism [is] a process of systematic stereotyping of and discrimination against people because they are old, just as racism and sexism accomplish this with skin color and gender. Old people are categorized as senile, rigid in thought and manner, old-fashioned in morality and skills. . . . Agism allows the younger generations to see older people as different from themselves; thus they subtly cease to identify with their elders as human beings."

At times agism becomes an expedient method by which society promotes viewpoints about the aged in order to relieve itself of responsibility toward them. At other times, agism serves a highly personal objective, protecting middle-aged individuals—often at high emotional cost—from thinking about things they fear (aging, illness, death).[6]

Butler details six of the most pervasive myths—out of "the multitude . . . surrounding old age"—with which older people are confronted in addition to "the difficulties of physical and economic survival":

The Myth of "Aging": The idea of chronological aging is a kind of myth. There are great differences in the rates of physiological, chronological, psychological and social aging within the person and from person to person. In fact, physiological indicators show a greater range from the mean in old age than in any other age group, and this is true of personality as well. Older people actually become more diverse rather than more similar. Organic brain damage can create extensive intellectual impairment, but most older people do not suffer impairment of this magnitude.

The Myth of Unproductivity: Many believe the old to be unproductive. But in the absence of diseases and social adversities, old people tend to remain productive and actively involved in life. Substantial numbers of people become unusually creative for the first time in old age. In 1971,

1,780,000 people over 65 were working full time and 1,257,000 part time. Many more would work if jobs were available. When productive incapacity develops, it can be traced more directly to a variety of losses, diseases or circumstances than to that mysterious process called aging. Even then, in spite of the presence of severe handicaps, activity and involvement are often maintained.

The Myth of Disengagement: This is related to the previous myth and holds that older people prefer to disengage from life, to withdraw into themselves. There is no evidence to support the generalization that mutual separation of the aged person from his society is a natural part of the aging experience. Disengagement is only one of many patterns of reaction to old age.

The Myth of Inflexibility: The ability to change and adapt has little to do with one's age and more to do with one's lifelong character—though one is not necessarily destined to maintain one's character in earlier life permanently. True, the endurance, the strength and the stability in human character structure are remarkable and protective. But most people change and remain open to change throughout the course of life. The old notion that character is laid down in final form by the fifth year of life can be confidently refuted. Change is the hallmark of living. Scientific studies of healthy older people living in the community do not support the notion that older people become less responsive to innovation and change.

The Myth of "Senility": "Senility" is a popularized layman's term used by doctors and the public alike. Some of what is called senile is the result of brain damage. But anxiety and depression are also frequently lumped within the same category even though they are treatable and often reversible. Old people, like young people, experience a full range of emotions, including anxiety, grief, depression and paranoid states. Drug tranquilization is another frequent, misdiagnosed and potentially reversible cause of so-called senility. Malnutrition and unrecognized physical illnesses may produce "senile behaviors." Alcoholism, often associated with bereavement, is another cause. Because it has been so convenient to dismiss all these manifestations by lumping them together under an improper and inaccurate diagnostic label, the elderly often do not receive the benefits of decent diagnosis and treatment. Actual irreversible brain damage, of course, is not a myth . . . [but] similar symptoms can be found in a number of other conditions which *are* reversible through proper treatment.

The Myth of Serenity: In contrast to the previous myths, which view the elderly in a negative light, the myth of serenity portrays old age as a kind of adult fairyland. But, in fact, older persons experience more stresses than any other age group, and these are often devastating. The strength of the aged to endure crisis is remarkable, and tranquillity is an unlikely as well as inappropriate response. Depression, anxiety, psychosomatic illnesses, paranoia, garrulousness and irritability are some of the internal reactions to external stresses. Depressive reactions are particularly widespread in late life. To the more blatant psychotic depressions and the depressions associated with organic brain diseases must be added the everyday depressions that stem from long physical illness or chronic discomfort from grief, despair and loneliness. Physical disease and social isolation can follow bereavement. Anxiety is another common feature. There is much to be anxious about. Anxiety may manifest itself in many forms: rigidity, help-lessness, manipulativeness, restlessness and suspiciousness, sometimes to the point of paranoid states.[7]

With this compendium of stereotypes, Butler contributes to our under-standing of the impact of lay tradition on professional (mis)perceptions. All six of the myths delineated are relevant to the health-care professional's work with older patients. However, with few exceptions, professionals tend to be largely unappreciative of the true nature of the elderly because the professions have been very slow to educate their future practitioners as to the dynamics of aging, the multiple dimensions of diagnosis and treatment, and the capacity of even fragile older people to exploit their hidden poten-tialities if encouraged to do so. Unless academic and professional school curricula are revised to provide the (future) professional with systematic alternatives to lay myths, professional attitudes toward the aged are likely to remain similar to, rather than dissimilar from, traditional assumptions.

Psychology, itself, is a case in point. There is reason to believe that psy-chology has sometimes been influenced by perceptions of the aged that do not stand up to the rigors of inquiry conducted by scientists immune to pre-vailing assumptions. Eisdorfer, for example, offers "findings, coupled with the works of others, [which] suggest the need for reappraisal of our concept of a 'normal' age-related loss of intellectual function."[8] "Serious doubt has been cast on the idea that older persons cannot profit from experi-ence."[9]

Moreover, the British gerontologist Malcolm Johnson reports that there is a

general belief that the old are rigid and dogmatic and unable to learn. This . . . has been reinforced by the findings of most psychologists working in this area. However, a . . . piece of new research by Dr. A. Angleitner of the Psychological Institute at the University of Bonn casts considerable doubt on the conclusions of these earlier studies.

Angleiter claims that previous researchers into rigidity in old age reached false conclusions. . . . the elderly are no more rigid than younger people of the same level of intelligence and schooling. Angleitner's own study of 70 and 80 year olds in West Germany replicated the 13 established psychologi-cal tests of rigidity and flexibility. But he controlled for the two variables of intelligence and schooling and found no real evidence of increase on the rigidity or dogmatism scales. From this analysis he asserts psychological measures of rigidity are based on the flexibility of thought which is encour-aged by our education systems. What is measured is attainment in these skills.

If Angleitner's hypothesis holds, we can expect an increasing "flexibility" among the older population as educational change "works its way through," and society will have an even richer field of talent to draw on. It will topple the belief that people inevitably grow too old to learn.[10]

Dichotomizing the Elderly

To better understand the impact of societal, including professional, responses to older Americans, it is useful to distinguish those who have several significant "strikes against them" from the well aged. In the United Kingdom, and increasingly in the United States, the former have come to be referred to as "the frail elderly."[11] Webster states that to be frail is the equivalent of being fragile, easily broken, not firm or durable, destructible, or liable to fail or perish.[12] The Federal Council on Aging and the Aged states that frail older people have experienced "a reduction of physical and emotional capacities and loss of a social support system, to the extent that the individual is immobilized and unable to maintain a household or social contacts without continuing assistance from others."[13] Let us consider, from the standpoint of prevailing societal and professional attitudes and behaviors, the nature of the dichotomy that is perceived to exist between the well and the frail.

Reactions to the Well Elderly

The community at large seldom doubts the validity of independent living for the "well aged"—those who are self-sufficient—in their day-by-day functioning, living out their lives privately and autonomously. Among such elders, some even receive positive reinforcement, especially if their physical or intellectual capacities fly in the face of societal age stereotypes. For example, admiration for the continued virtuosity of the nonagenarian, Artur Rubinstein, is widespread, and some families appear to afford similar recognition to well-functioning elders in their midst. However, the overwhelming remainder—more ordinary senior mortals—are usually taken for granted or ignored most of the time. Being ignored may not be an entirely negative experience, for from it may be inferred a "live and let live" expectation of the well aged, even, perhaps, a kind of unspoken affirmation that the totally self-caring are just doing what they ought to be doing, like the rest of the community.[14] Such acceptance of the "rugged individualism" of some elderly people is consistent with the puritan ethic, which has profoundly affected the development of American culture.

It is perhaps paradoxical that the well elderly are more likely to receive a range of support than the frail. According to folk wisdom, "nothing succeeds like success," or "the rich get richer and the poor get poorer." Reality appears to be consistent with these sayings. In a nation such as ours, without a national health service, superior purchasing power equates with better access to medical care. Furthermore, according to Representative William S. Cohen (R-Me.) of the House Select Committee on Aging, the Older Americans Act has catered mainly to the needs of those who are in good health. The health and social needs of the more than 8.5 million elderly who have chronic impairments have not received adequate attention under the Act.[15]

Recent research findings reveal a positive correlation between the degree of an aged parent's well-being and the degree of contact and support—emotional, social, financial, or in the form of services—furnished by adult offspring: the greater the older person's independence, the more likely it is that adult offspring are attentive.[16]

Reactions to the Frail Elderly

What, then, of those aged persons with multiple "strikes against them?" Perhaps most insidious for them is one of the stereotypes that leaves the well elderly relatively unscathed, namely, the view that it is a novelty for older persons to be vigorously healthy and independent. As already indicated, when there is public approval of healthy aging, it stems, in part, from a prevailing contrary expectation, to wit: older people are ordinarily decrepit, malfunctioning, unchanging (except to deteriorate still further)—in short, "ready for the scrap heap," "all washed up." When a frail older person gives evidence of vulnerability—socioeconomic, emotional, mental, and/or physical—all too often this evidence serves as a self-fulfilling prophecy on the part of those who, owing to stereotypes, expect to find older people in this state anyway. Truly the "book" is prejudged by its wrinkled, gray, or faded "cover." In consequence, inordinate attention is usually paid to the person's limitations, without comparable emphasis on her (or his) remaining strengths or capacities for restoration and development.

Psychological assaults on the older person are exacerbated when illness or disability strikes. Often a dramatic shift occurs from society's benign neglect of many of the well aged to a heavy dose of overprotection in the case of the frail elderly. This is often coupled with expectations of helplessness, which further induce dependency and further undermine the older person's sense of self-worth.

Alternative Perceptions and Practices of Some Professionals

Many Americans, including many professionals, assume there is little or no alternative to institutionalizing older people when they become frail. A small but growing cadre of professionals, however, in concert with some politicians and administrators, has been developing alternative findings, perceptions, and practices.

The Psychological Benefits of a Home of One's Own

A familiar and stable residence is implicated not only in the physical, but also in the psychological well-being of many of the elderly. Butler and Lewis provide the following insights:

> Home is extraordinarily significant to many older persons. It is part of their identity, a place where things are familiar and relatively unchanging, and a place to maintain a sense of autonomy and control. Some insist on remaining at home "at all costs" to their emotional and physical health and personal security. Such tenaciousness can be laid to a desire for freedom and independence; a fear of loss of contact with family and loved people, places and things; a fear of dying because of the reputation of hospitals and nursing homes as "houses of death" from which there is no return; and a trepidation about change and the unknown, which frightens people of all ages. In this nation of homeowners where 67 percent of older people own their homes, the idea of a personal house is deeply ingrained; and communal living is viewed as a loss of personal liberty and dignity. The notion of home can refer primarily to the four walls surrounding one, to the neighborhood in which one is located, or to the possessions that make one feel at home. Home may mean certain other individuals living with one or it may mean neighbors, pets, and plants. It can either be a place where one has lived a good part of one's life or be a new place, as when older people move into a retirement community or leave the farm for a home in town. Thus home is whatever the "concept of home" means to each person.[17]

The current generations of the elderly have been particularly imbued from their formative years onward with the value of independence and autonomy. Butler and Lewis tellingly convey the high degree of association, for today's aged, between remaining in one's own home and maintaining a sense of autonomy and security.

In addition, Butler's and Lewis's statement demonstrates that living arrangements have implications for the health of older people. This is corroborated by a nurse who reports on the functional dependency on their familiar home environment that many aged persons gradually develop over the course of years, often without being aware of it:

> They prefer to remain in familiar surroundings, and do things the way they have always done them, because as one grows older, one requires more reminders and signposts along the way to avoid becoming confused and disoriented. So sudden changes are something to be avoided. . . . They need to stay in that old and inconvenient house on the hill. They need the sound of the old boards under their feet more than they need electricity or plumbing. . . . They have to make so many adjustments to new things (losses of physical ability or the sudden death of an old friend, for example) that they begin to hoard whatever it is within us that allows us to face change without seeing it as chaos.[18]

No wonder older people have such a strong preference to remain at home rather than enter homes for the aged, hospitals, or nursing homes. Whether it is the long-term contact with a friendly neighborhood shopkeeper or the accustomed position of the arms of a chair that enable one to rise, independently, even in the face of gradually declining strength in one's leg muscles, the familiar environment provides a network of subtle supports and affirms one's continuing ability to function on one's own.

Most of the relevant knowledge that has been generated by Americans since World War II has found its way across the Atlantic, where, coupled with European findings, it has been put into practice to good effect. In several European nations, health and social services do far better at actualizing such principles as those of Butler and Lewis and Curtin than do their American counterparts. For example, in Sweden, the proximity of familiar places and people has been considered so fundamental to the well-being of the aged that, as a matter of national policy, hundreds of small homes for the aged have been built throughout the country in local villages and towns. It was considered unthinkable that an aged Swede should have to leave her or his familiar environs in order to enter a retirement home.[19]

In Scotland, consultant physicians in geriatric medicine visit the homes of frail aged persons referred for possible hospitalization in order to assess each patient's debility *in the context of the environment* that exists (or fails) to support that patient in the community. Each geriatrician makes an informal assessment of the mental-emotional-relational-social-architectural-neighborhood supports, while at the same time performing the more traditional roles of the physician, effecting an assessment of current physical health and ills, chronic or acute. The geriatrician depends heavily on this total assessment in adjudging what it will require to restore the patient to competence in his or her setting. This may result in the avoidance of hospitalization altogether or until some future date (when further deterioration has occurred in relationships, environmental supports, or the patient). If and when the patient is hospitalized, the geriatrician, for the duration of his or her professional service, retains an image of each patient's "baseline" back in the community, adjusting that perception continually in the light of new evidence furnished by others (district nurse, social worker, psychologist, general practitioner, hospital intern, or resident) who are in touch with changes in the patient's home situation during the course of hospitalization. The physician interrelates two issues continually: What is the level of restoration this debilitated patient must be enabled to achieve in order to be able to negotiate his or her environment, upon his or her return, better than he or she was able to do at the time of admission? and How can that environment be adapted to support the patient better upon his or her return than it was able to at the time of hospitalization? Each of these variables affects the other.

During this decade, Britain has created a whole new profession, the health visitor, whose functions have now been extended to provide a useful link facilitating and enhancing the general practitioner's cognizance of how the older patient's social-psychological needs and functions influence his or her state of health.

In recent years, Americans have begun to improve community-based supports to older Americans under the leadership of the new National Institute on Aging, the Administration on Aging of the Department of Health, Education and Welfare, and the Federal Council on Aging. (The latter two have counterparts in each state government, importantly supplemented by approximately 650 area agencies on aging dispersed throughout the United States.)

Yet the American surface has only just been scratched. On this side of the Atlantic there has recently been talk of redefining the "long-term care" continuum to include health services in the patient's home, but policies and funding are still very much skewed in favor of underwriting institutional programs for older people. For example, of the $4.826 billion that Medicaid expended on the health care of eligible older people during fiscal year 1976, 97.4 percent (all but $126 billion) was used to provide institutional care. Serious as is this imbalance in the expenditure of such vast sums, the psychological cost to older people is also a matter of great concern—particularly when it is kept in mind that it has been variously estimated that from 30 to 80 percent of nursing home admissions are inappropriate or unnecessary.[20]

Upgrading Institutions

The realization is fairly widespread that institutions must be upgraded in order to avoid unnecessary psychological and physical deterioration among older patients.

Older people in general are opposed to the use of institutions; this . . . is most obvious in the clearly mentally ill, the subtly mentally disturbed, and in the oldest and the most impaired. Thus those who need protective care the most want it the least . . . whereas those who may need it the least are less resistant to accepting the change in residence. . . . One reason aged persons who need protective institutions also need psychiatric assistance is the intensity of their feelings that institutional use constitutes rejection by family and friends and a loss of independence.

Unfortunately, the low quality of institutional care in the past, however attractive the physical plant, has tended to reinforce such beliefs and attitudes. Institutions are for the most part so poorly equipped, staffed, and organized that the resistance of families of aged persons to making use of them is more frequently related to realistic appraisal . . . than to guilt based on giving the care of the parent over to others; or, as is so often asserted, on unconscious hostility.

Institutional care is usually regarded as a prelude to death by applicants and their families rather than as a new, useful experience in community living. It can be such an experience in the best old-age homes and could be in many state hospitals that attempt to become communities in themselves as well as to remain related to the outside world. Unfortunately, most institutions are not self-contained communities and are by no means a part of the larger community. Therefore, they become places in which old persons with little or nothing to do and with their senses, minds, and emotions blunted by drugs simply wait for death.

Entrance into residences of such poor quality tends to downgrade the person's image of himself. His disability may become greater, and there may be development or exaggeration of psychological and emotional disorder. Institutional deterioration can be counteracted by the provision of community-type activities: sheltered workshops in hospitals or homes, recreational therapy, hotel-type accommodations, and the contagion of high morale in a well-motivated staff. These improve self-concepts and behavior and help decrease objections to entrance into homes as well as to continued residence in them.[21]

Challenging Misguided Policies

If few citizens—lay or professional—seem concerned about the horrendous cost ($10 billion annually) of maintaining 1 million older Americans in nursing homes, it is no wonder. Neither our educational institutions nor our popular culture provide much of a vision of the alternatives that do, in fact, exist—even for the frail. Too many shrug helplessly, assuming that long-term institutional care is the only resource for older people who no longer appear vigorous and self-caring. These cultural factors both influence and are complicated by policy decisions made at the national level that affect vast millions of people—both the aged and those concerned with their welfare. These policies operate to inhibit the delivery of in-home health and social services, even by enlightened practitioners who would wish to do so. Ricker-Smith and Trager have documented that in 1967 an artificial emphasis was imposed

> on in-home health services by Medicare and Medicaid; that is, they defined organized home health care as essentially a supplement to medical and acute care and, consequently, short-term clients were favored. While in-home health services [are appropriate for the latter] . . . , they are also appropriate for long-term conditions. Failure to provide them frequently hastens need for more expensive care and for inappropriate institutionalization. . . . As a result of legislative and regulatory emphasis on post- or sub-acute care, . . . [services] are skewed in the direction of short-term clients.[22]

The grim harvest reaped by such short-sighted policies is illustrated by the findings of a recent study conducted in Cleveland, Ohio by the U.S. General Accounting Office (GAO). The GAO discerned that except for the severely impaired, frail older people—ranging from mild to serious degrees of impairment—could be maintained with the benefit of home-health services at a cost less than that of institutional care.[23]

Developing Continuums (or Clusters) of Care

Even good-quality institutionalization must be weighed against alternative resources made available along the total continuum of care. Many such resources (see table 15–1) are summed up by the term *in-home health services*. Considerable knowledge exists about how to enable older people— even those who are distinctly frail—to maintain themselves in their own homes or in other community-based facilities such as housing projects or the homes of relatives. (A fraction of older people have even begun to live in collectives or communes.) Not only does this methodology conserve older people, physically and psychologically, but, as we saw earlier, it conserves health-care dollars as well.

The Federal Council on the Aging, an advisory body to the legislative and executive branches of the federal government, has concluded that to a significant extent, the limitations that exacerbate the frailty of the aged are not primarily physical in nature.[24] Granted, serious chronic physical impairment does contribute to placing older people seriously at risk, but key social-psychological factors consistently discriminate between aged persons with comparable physical impairments who are and are not at risk. Paramount among these factors are

Bereavement (usually loss of spouse; correlates with widowhood as a risk factor).

Lack of proximity to significant others.

Being single (nonexistence of offspring and grandchildren as sources of emotional and concrete support; correlates with lowered access, over the course of a lifetime, to higher education and higher incomes).

Lowered income; lifelong poverty (the latter correlates with other risk-precipitating factors such as more limited problem-solving skills).

Involuntary or precipitous disruption of familiar, secure living arrangements.

Advanced old age.

Social isolation (correlates with a number of the preceding as well as with residency in the midst of urban density or rural seclusion).

Several resources on the continuum are designed to relieve such risk factors. Once community planners and budget managers begin to make such continuums truly available to America's elderly, it becomes feasible for competent professionals to cluster a combination of services, selected from the continuum according to the individual needs of a given older person at a given stage of her or his development and debilitation.

Table 15-1
A Comprehensive Compilation of Services and Supports Enabling the Elderly to Remain in the Community

Adult education	Geropsychiatry	Prescription service (cut-rate, mail order)
After-care	Group experiences	Protective services
Bank loans and other banking services	Health screening	Psychiatry (outpatient)
Chore services	Home-health services	Recreation
Clergy	Home renovation and home repairs	Retired Senior Volunteer Program
Clinical psychology	Homemaker service	Revolving door policies in nursing homes
Communal living arrangements	Hospice services (including death and dying counseling)	Sales of services or arts and crafts
Community health nursing	Housing relocation	Self-help organizing
Congregate meals	Income maintenance (including Social Security and SSI)	Senior centers or clubs
Consumer services		SCORE (Senior Corps of Retired Executives)
Cooperative buying	Information, advocacy, referral, and follow-up services	Shopping services
Counseling, family (or marital)	Legal services	Social action and lobbying
Day health centers	Meals, home-delivered	Speech pathology and audiology
Driver refresher courses	Medicaid and Medicare	Surplus foods
Employment and employment assistance	Multidimentional, functional assessment (including multiphasic screening)	Talking books
Environmental modification		Tax counseling
Flexible retirement policies	Nutrition education	Telephone reassurance
Food stamps	Occupational therapy (outpatient or in the home)	Therapeutic recreation
Foster care	Psychiatry	Transportation, feasibly priced
Foster grandparents (and other opportunities to perform meaningful roles)	Physical therapy (outpatient or in the home)	Vocation (re)training
Friendly visiting	Preparation for retirement	Well-aged clinic
General practice		

Multidimensional Functional Assessment

Only quite recently has a methodology for matching resources to the individual vulnerability and strengths of older persons begun to emerge.[25] This is a particularly crucial skill in serving older people because their social, psychological, and physical needs tend to be so intermeshed and therefore complex to diagnose and prescribe for:

> A crucial aspect of the functional assessment of elderly individuals is that they are likely to have a conglomerate of social, physical, and psychological problems. Their status is influenced by many factors and it is sometimes all but impossible to determine which factors are most influential. A clear distinction between the effects of aging and the effects of disease processes is often very difficult to establish. The functional status of various systems is typically interdependent; physical and psychological functions are often intricately interrelated . . . and are frequently complicated by social factors and cultural attitudes. In general, the likelihood that a patient will have both physical and psychiatric illnesses, usually in combination with social problems, increases with age. Consequently, when functional assessment of elderly persons is undertaken, social, psychological, and physical dimensions all demand attention. . . . [In contrast to the typical younger patient], a thorough investigation of aged persons usually reveals multiple impairments, an observation which constitutes a strong argument for a multifunctional diagnostic appraisal as the foundation for a treatment plan.[26]

Thus we see that skillful functional assessment, individualizing the needs of one older person and differentiating them from the needs of others, leads logically to a distinct treatment plan, on the basis of which the continuum of care is tapped for a cluster of services that may or may not include institutionalization.

Seven Principles Basic to Serving Older People

The preceding catalog of alternative perceptions and practices is illustrative rather then comprehensive. Nevertheless, it demonstrates that substantial progress is being made toward the development of enlightened practices and enlightened critiques of retrograde policies. The following principles are put forth as guides in differentiating such professional perceptions and behaviors from those of practitioners who have not yet freed themselves from the burden of traditional assumptions, myths, and stereotypes about older people. These principles also can assist helping professionals in progressing toward more enlightened work with and on behalf of the aged.

1. In all societies, persons excluded from social exchanges or interchanges are devalued and stigmatized. Such exclusion deprives them of

being a part of the basic social fabric. Nations, social institutions, communities, organizations, professionals, and relatives can all help to enhance the state of well-being of the aged by encouraging and expecting them to participate in the performance of numerous reciprocal roles, in every sphere of life, irrespective of the limitations of their individual conditions.[27]

2. When life is present, the capacity for development is also present. This in no way implies that in order for development to be taking place, no deterioration or losses may be in evidence. It does imply that the two processes are not mutually exclusive and that from evidence of deterioration—whether normative or pathogenic—the absence of developmental potentiality may not be inferred.

3. To a great extent, the way for humans to preserve competence, to slow down the deterioration of competence, or to restore competence is to utilize the widest possible range of their psychological and physical faculties, with as much autonomy as they are capable of. To sum up, "use or lose."[28]

4. When there is a suspension or debilitation of functional ability, it is crucial that any and all supportive therapy or services be prescribed and administered in such a way as to supplement, rather than supplant, the remaining capacities of the older person.[29]

5. An older person's achievements with regard to restoration or development, no matter how modest, should be measured not only against standardized norms, but also relative to a baseline derived from her or his own individual potentialities and limitations.

6. Therapy or social services that contribute to the restoration of function, or to the deterrence of deterioration, not only constitute competent remedial services, but may open up to some older persons avenues of development that would otherwise have remained closed to them.

7. Therapy or services are most likely to be proffered developmentally by those who are capable of perceiving, relating to, and serving older people: as adults rather than children, as individuals rather than stereotypes, as persons in a dynamic rather than a static state. Professionals and others who are characterized by the former of these attributes are assumed to be capable of respecting and challenging the potentialities of the living for as long as they are alive; those characterized by the latter are assumed to be unwitting repositories of agism.

Some will ask themselves: "But are not these principles basic to good professional service to people of *all* ages?" The answer is an emphatic "Yes"—what's good for older people tends very strongly to be good for all people because older people are, first and foremost, fully alive and fully human. However, because so many of their fellow citizens have lost or never had such a perception, these humane-service principles must be reenunciated specifically on behalf of the aged.

Notes

1. Psychology's contribution is illustrated by James E. Birren ed., *Handbook of Aging and the Individual: Psychological and Biological Aspects* (Chicago: Univ. of Chicago, 1959); James H. Barrett, *Gerontological Psychology* (Springfield, Ill.: Thomas, 1972); Jack Botwinick, *Aging and Behavior* (New York: Springer, 1973); Joseph H. Britton and Jean O. Britton, *Personality Changes in Aging* (New York: Springer, 1972); Dennis B. Bromley, *The Psychology of Human Ageing,* 2d. ed. (Baltimore: Penguin Books, 1966); and Robert Kastenbaum, ed., *New Thoughts on Old Age* (New York: Springer, 1964).

2. Along with the other mental-health professions, clinical psychology does not have a good track record of service to older people, whether measured quantitatively or qualitatively. Extremely little therapy has been made available to older people, and diagnostic services are seldom comprehensive. See Robert N. Butler and Myrna I. Lewis, *Aging and Mental Health,* 2d. ed., (St. Louis: Mosby, 1977), pp. 141–151. Despite at least a decade of criticism from the field of aging, "only 3 percent of the budget of . . . NIMH [The National Institute of Mental Health of the U.S. Health Service] is devoted to the study of mental problems of old age. NIMH's program in aging has always been limited. . . . NIMH directors have not taken major leadership in pressing for higher budgets within the Department of Health, Education and Welfare or with Congress in proportion to the incidence, prevalence and costs of mental illnesses among the elderly. In 1972, under pressure from organizations interested in the elderly [which did include the American Psychological Association and the American Psychiatric Association], NIMH created the office of special assistant on aging, which has given the impression of activity and the illusion of change. . . . But no substantial increase in funds has appeared. The . . . anticipated priorities for the 1970s proposed by NIMH do not include aging. They do include crime and law enforcement, drug use and abuse, all more important politically as far as legislative support and funding are concerned."

"NIMH is currently having difficulties maintaining the programs it now has [which] affords an understandable reason why NIMH may be reluctant to get involved with the elderly at this time. It does not, however, explain NIMH's neglect of the old when it was in its well-financed heyday in the late 1950s and 1960s, nor does it explain the unwillingness of the NIMH leadership to re-examine its priorities and reallocate its present budget more in keeping with the prevalence of psychiatric problems. As matters stand, any hopes for expansion in the field of aging and mental health will probably have to come from congressional pressure" [Robert N. Butler, *Why Survive? Being Old in America* (New York: Harper & Row, 1975), pp. 254–256].

Given this recent history at NIMH, it is no surprise that in the 507 community mental-health centers operating across the United States (in February 1976), older people made up only 4 to 5 percent of the clientele (Butler and Lewis, *Aging and Mental Health,* pp. 228–229).

Clinical psychologists may point to the preceding indictment as an explanation for their relative inability to attend to the psychological needs of the elderly. However "scant attention to the mental-health needs of older people," for which Butler indicts "*all* the various professional groups that work in mental-health settings," cannot be explained solely on the basis of federal recalcitrance. Since mental-health neglect "mirrors what we have seen in every area of late life" (Butler, *Why Survive?* p. 231), it seems reasonable to suggest that psychology and its colleagues in community mental health have not extricated themselves from the more general pattern of societal neglect of the aged.

3. Butler, *Why Survive?* p. 227.

4. Leo William Simmons, *The Role of the Aged in Primitive Society* (New Haven, Conn.: Yale Univ. Press, 1945); Simone de Beauvoir, *The Coming of Age* (New York: Putnam, 1972), pp. 38–215.

5. Butler, *Why Survive?* pp. 4–5, 178–183, 229–234 (*passim*).

6. Ibid., pp. 11–12; includes a quotation from Butler and Lewis, *Aging and Mental Health.*

7. Ibid., pp. 7–10.

8. Carl Eisdorfer, "Intelligence and Cognition in the Aged," in *Behavior and Adaptation in Later Life,* ed. E.W. Busse and E. Pfeiffer, (Boston: Little, Brown, 1977), p. 217.

9. Ibid., p. 221.

10. Malcom Johnson, "Old Age and the Gift Relationship," *New Society* (3 March 1975): 640.

11. See, for example, "National Policy for the Frail Elderly," *Annual Report to the President, 1977* (Washington: Federal Council on the Aging, 1978), pp. 35–42.

12. *Websters New International Dictionary of the English Language,* 2d ed. Unabridged (Springfield, Mass.: 1960).

13. Cleonice Tavani, et al., *Report on National Policy for the Frail Elderly,* Federal Council on the Aging, Washington, September 1976.

14. There are at least two important ways in which even the well aged are subject to threats to their self-caring ability. Major phenomena beyond their control are the plummeting of income upon retirement (representing a 53.1 percent average loss exacerbated by present-day, never-ceasing inflation) and the lack of a well-rationalized system to affirm and maintain the ongoing health of America's aged. The latter has recently been referred to by a bipartisan congressional group as the "overlapping, fragmented, slipshod organization of Federal social and health programs affecting the

elderly'' (News release, Subcommittee on Health and Long-Term Care, U.S. House of Representatives Select Committee on Aging, January 16, 1978).

15. Ibid.

16. Personal communication at 30th Annual Scientific Meeting, Gerontological Society, Inc., San Francisco, November 22, 1977.

17. Butler and Lewis, *Aging and Mental Health,* p. 211.

18. Sharon R. Curtin, *Nobody Ever Died of Old Age* (Boston: Little, Brown, 1972), pp. 72–73.

19. Reports have recently reached the United States of a cutback in this program owing to the high cost of building so many widely dispersed facilities with a maximum occupancy of forty residents.

20. *Home Health—The Need for a National Policy to Better Provide for the Elderly,* Comptroller General's Report to the Congress, U.S. General Accounting Office, Washington, undated.

21. Alvin I. Goldfarb, "Institutional Care of the Aged," in *Behavior and Adaptation,* ed. E.W. Busse and E. Pfeiffer, *Behavior and Adaptation in Later Life,* pp. 288–289; see also, Robert N. Butler, "Houses of Death Are a Lively Business," *Why Survive?* pp. 260–299.

22. Katherine Ricker-Smith and Brahna Trager, "In-Home Health Services in California: Some Lessons for National Health Insurance," *Medical Care* 16 (3): 188, 1978.

23. *Home Health—The Need for a National Policy to Better Provide for the Elderly.*

24. Tavani et al., *Report on National Policy for the Frail Elderly.*

25. See, for example, H. Grauer and F. Birnbom, "Geriatric Functional Rating Scale to Determine the Need for Institutional Care," *Journal of the American Geriatric Society* 23 (10): 472–476; Butler and Lewis, *Aging and Mental Health,* Chapter 9, "Diagnostic Evaluation: How to Do a Work-Up," pp. 158–210; and *Older Americans Resource and Service Program Manual,* Duke University Center for the Study of Aging and Human Development, 1975.

26. Charles M. Gaitz and Paul E. Baer, "Diagnostic Assessment of the Elderly: A Multi-functional Model," *Gerontologist* (Spring 1970): 47.

27. This principle was derived with the help of Johnson, "Old Age and the Gift Relationship," pp. 639–641.

28. Grace deCarlton Ross, personal communication, May 1972.

29. If a slight error is to be made as to the exact dosage of supplemental treatment or service to be appropriately prescribed, it should be on the side of a bit too little rather than a bit too much. The very act of bridging from the deteriorated state to the supplement may constitute, for the older person, a significant episode of restoration, even, in some few instances, of development.

16 Work Stress: Effects on Physical and Mental Health of Patients and Treatment Personnel

Barbara L. Smith

Work Stress: General Comments

Some occupations seem to have an affinity for certain kinds of illnesses. Indeed, the job one chooses could determine the sickness one gets. Nurses develop blood clots in their legs and chronic back pain. Nurses also have more spontaneous abortions and defective babies if working when pregnant around anesthetic gases and infectious diseases. Beauticians and stewardesses complain of chronic fatigue.[1] Executives and attorneys seem to suffer from cardiovascular diseases; accountants and middle managers are ulcer-prone.[2] Stress-related illnesses are gaining more attention, as is the whole area of the effects of stress at work on the physical and mental well-being of the worker.

Working in a counseling center (Los Angeles County Occupational Health Service) serving 80,000 employees from many different fields, I have had many opportunities to observe occupational stress, particularly its emotional components in the human-service fields. Workers' Compensation claims for "stress and strain" have certainly become fashionable in the last few years. The numbers of people dissatisfied with their jobs have increased as has the incidence of "burnout" among helping professions.[3] These trends suggest to me that there have probably been some changes in our general relationship to work, as well as in the work systems themselves, that have produced this phenomenon of occupational stress.

Occupational stress, or *work stress,* can be very simply defined as the response of workers to stressors in the work environment. As with any stress response, the individual responds automatically if a situation is perceived as stressful.[4] Stress can be a response to physical stimuli, such as heat or cold, but usually the stressor is in the interpersonal environment.

All stress is not negative, although the term has been most generally used in the negative sense. The usage of occupational stress in Workers' Compensation jargon is most definitely negative and refers to chronic stress states more often than an acute reaction. The innate stress response is highly adaptive; too much or too little stress can reduce productivity. It is not

229

stress, but chronic stress, that is maladaptive.[5] Stress, chronic stress, and burnout, a particular variant becoming quite common among helping professions, will be discussed in more detail in subsequent paragraphs.

Symptoms of Chronic Work Stress and the Medical-Leave Escape

The work environment can be the source of many stressors. Attendance, morale, productivity, intragroup conflict, and industrial injuries are symptoms known to employers as manifestations of the stress reactions of their employees. Much work on occupational stress has resulted in the following simplistic assumptions: (1) that certain occupations are stressful, (2) that the inherent stressors are the cause and should be modified, (3) that some employees are basically poorly equipped to handle ordinary stressors, and/or (4) that personal problems, not work problems, are the cause of stress symptoms at work.[6] Examining highly competent employees or the executives capable of "handling stress" reveals that they too can be and often are the victims of chronic stress.[7] A commonly used term, *burnout,* clearly describes what can happen to highly dedicated, hardworking individuals.[8]

The work of Holmes and Rahe on life changes and illness can be applied to the interaction between stressors at work and home and the onset of a significant illness.[9] Any life changes 6 months to 1 year before the illness require adaptation, that is, trigger the stress response. Positive events, such as promotions and vacations, require adaptation and as such are stressful. In some instances, our own interpretation of a success can be negative, and the automatic stress response that follows may surprise ourselves and others. A discussion of any changes and any personal losses should be part of the medical history taken. What the patient has to say about work or the spouse about the other's work pressures is likely to reveal both acute and chronic stress.

Prior to becoming seriously ill, people commonly experience a number of symptoms that can be related to work stress. These are all side effects of being in a state of chronic stress as opposed to a short-term crisis, where it is possible to return to a less stressed level of functioning. Chronic fatigue is perhaps the most common complaint where work stress is occurring. This symptom often goes along with mild depression, multiple somatic complaints, nervousness, and more than usual irritability.

When these symptoms are reported to the family doctor, the treatment recommended is often time off from work in order to "rest," with some tranquilizing medication. Medical leaves, sometimes following an industrial injury, usually are needed, in my experience, when the individual has depleted all coping resources or other forms of perceived escape (leave, absenteeism). Job modifications, transfers, or disabilities are often part of such an extreme chronic occupational stress syndrome.

Time off alone is not sufficient for full recovery or future stress management. In order for an employed person to cope with stressful work pressures and to manage that stress while working, it is necessary for the person to understand the nature of the stressors and the coping mechanisms involved, both adaptive and maladaptive. During the time off work, the individual will need to make some changes in managing stress or the cycle is likely to repeat itself. Selye calls such chronic stress reactions "distress."[10]

A person in a human-service field who has "burned out" can recover and prevent future burnout by applying knowledge about the phenomenon to changing how the emotional demands of working with people are managed. Education about burnout and coping with stress should reach employees while still at work. Once a medical leave is necessary, the burned out worker may need professional counseling.

Definitions of Stress and Burnout: Physiology and Emotions

The terms *stress* and *burnout* need some further definition. Our normal way of coping with demands to change, to threats that are real or imagined, is a set of reflexive physiological reactions known as the *stress response.*[11] Our bodies, like those of our cave-dweller ancestors, do everything necessary for survival in a crisis; we are literally prepared for fight or flight. Once the crisis is over, these same physiological systems go through a period of recovery and then return to their normal levels of functioning. We are physically well equipped for dealing with short-term stressors, particularly if additional energy, strength, and speed are needed.

There are few stressful situations in which this automatic stress response is useful, particularly in the work setting. Punching out your boss when enraged at his or her ridiculous demands is not a very wise solution to a problem. Most sources of frustration seem repetitive or never-ending. Our bodies cannot maintain a state of physiological alarm for such long periods of time; however, continuing to sense a situation as stressful can prevent the recovery spoken of earlier. We may even become used to functioning at a constant level of tenseness, relaxing fully again only when far removed from the work situation.

Elevated blood pressure, muscle tension, headaches, and hyperventilation may all be indicators of a chronic state of stress, or distress, where the body is still responding to a perceived threat, but not at the maximal level possible. This continued exertion of the muscle, respiratory, gastrointestinal, and particularly cardiovascular systems can and does result in damage and serious illness.

A sudden demand for coping with a crisis can precipitate serious physical damage, for example, a heart attack, in the person who is constantly drawing on the body's stress-response mechanisms. By preventing the normal recovery from stress, we enter a chronic state of distress and are at risk for a major illness.

Chronic stress can be maintained by a hard-driving lifestyle. A lifestyle known as "hurry sickness" or the type A personality is characterized by trying to accomplish an increasing number of things under time pressures, usually self-imposed. This lifestyle is correlated with heart attacks.[12] High achievement orientation and extreme time consciousness are quite common. "Hurry sickness" probably compounds the difficulties caregivers, in particular, have in taking time to recuperate when they could be helping more people.

Burnout: The Emotional Drain and Its Physical Consequences

I consider burnout a chronic-stress phenomenon. However, for the purpose of this chapter, I wish to restrict the usage of this term to the human-service fields. The reason for this is to underline the tremendous significance of the emotional drain experienced in the giving, helping relationship.[13] Burnout seems to be most severe and reached most rapidly when the client problems are severe, traumatic, overwhelming, and not quickly or more than superficially dealt with by the human-service system.

The crisis of our clients and their extreme emotions are experienced by us as caregivers. Although we learn objectivity in our training, as we become more drained we find ourselves seeing clients in a stereotyped manner and becoming quite uninvolved emotionally. Reacting to their feelings or taking unhealthy responsibility for their problems also can occur; we can lose objectivity when our internal resources are depleted. We carry problems home and may even take our clients with us.

We may rationalize going beyond our professional role by saying that the agency or "system" is inadequate. Typically we overextend ourselves. We become involved in another client's crisis before recovering from helping the preceding client, who may not have been the first crisis that day. I feel that caregivers must do something about their own crises, which follow clients' crises. We need to discuss our involvement in the clients' crises with coworkers, or else carry with us the burden of unexpressed feelings, built up tensions, and so forth, which will lead to burnout. Pacing, which is discussed later, definitely applies to emotionally draining client contacts.

Carrying work problems home proves to be mentally and physically fatiguing. The attention given to work problems detracts from enjoying a personal life and family relationships. Someone who is burning out on the job is very likely to develop personal problems in addition because of this withdrawal of involvement. Worrying about work, talking about it without solving any problems, seeking momentary escapes through drugs and alcohol, and the neglect of diet and sleep that is correlated with this burnout phenomenon alter the person's physical health. Often muscle tensions and worrying prevent restful sleep, and the person always feels tired, fatigued, and drained.

This chronic fatigue leaves the individual feeling less and less able to cope. Each new demand or reminder of unresolved problems increases frustration, hopelessness, feelings of inadequacy, confusion, and a sense of being overwhelmed. While the automatic stress response may be triggered, the individual in a state of chronic stress has not felt fully recoverd from the last crisis. Indeed his or her physiological systems have not returned to baseline, and the constant low level of tension is a physical reality. Any susceptibility to colds, muscle aches, headaches, and other minor nonspecific physical distress leaves the person neither seriously ill nor ever well. It is not at all surprising that after a series of crises that have elicited a stress response, the individual does become seriously ill. How the person has been handling stress prior to a new problem determines what kind of physical and mental resources are available.

Advantages of Managing Stress at Work

The whole point of managing stress is to achieve a state of mental and physical wellness, not just to avoid serious illness. Persons in a state of distress do not feel well, lack energy, lack motivation and interest in living fully, and have a host of minor physical problems to lower their overall resistance and ability to cope with additional demands. Prevention and healthful living require that our lifestyles promote our well-being.

In working with executives, sheriffs, firefighters, judges, attorneys, nurses, social workers, therapists, librarians, and welfare workers with special education or training programs on stress management, I have integrated diet, exercise, interests, and personal and spiritual relationships. For example, the program aimed at heart attack prevention involves habit changes in the area of eating behaviors, not just weight loss through a standard diet. Along with changing eating habits, drinking, exercising, and relaxing are targets for habit change. I have consistently observed the interaction between excesses in eating and drinking with elevated stress levels, particularly at the end of the work day. Changing what one does after work by introducing a period of exercise or relaxation helps a person to decompress from work pressures.

Stress management usually requires lifestyle changes. With a daily awareness of fluctuating stress or discomfort levels, individuals are able to pace themselves at work, taking time out for minirecovery breaks when needed. Longer periods of exercise and relaxation after work are a means of recovering from the accumulation of stress. This "decompression" period allows the worker to leave work pressures at the job. In his book, *Stress without Distress,* Selye (1974) indicates how the constructive energizing qualities of stress are maximized for a fuller, more satisfying and productive life. In a recent survey of job satisfaction in *Psychology Today,* Renwick and Lawler indicate that most people use exercise as a means of coping with job stress, which would certainly produce physiological recovery from stress responses.[14]

Other means of coping with and reducing the effects of work stressors will be discussed from the perspective of what the individual can do alone and with coworkers to survive work stress and burnout. Health professionals can apply these principles to themselves as well as to their patients in counseling regarding work stress. Total stress management in the work environment will require more than individuals making lifestyle changes; the work system itself must change in certain ways. Finally, stressors that cannot be changed can be perceived and coped with differently.

The Worker-System Interaction: How Caregivers Burn Out

Since most people work and most are dissatisfied with their work, there is a critical need for more education so persons can alter how they handle work stresses.[15] Also, administration and management need to work collaboratively with employees to reduce work stressors and increase satisfaction. Many of us derive, or would like to derive, feelings of success at reaching our goals through work. Persons who have chosen a human-service field identify with a profession and a particular mission. Their frustrations with the petty problems within a work group, administrative demands, and apparently useless procedures are real. The ways that the work system operates are, and should be, perceived as detracting from delivering services when forms, surveys, and other such operations seem to have top priority.

The individual dedicated to helping others very often continues to stretch personal resources to provide quality care in spite of and in addition to paperwork, understaffing, incompetent coworkers, and unappreciative administration. As this interaction progresses, as the gap between ideals and how things operate widens, the worker burns out. The emotional drain of dealing with people and their problems, of continually caring for others in the face of a nonsupportive, often punitive, work system takes its toll most especially among the best and most dedicated workers. They do not seem to know when to take care of themselves. They cannot resist helping another when a realistic appraisal of the situation would tell them that there are more people needing help than they can possibly help given the inadequate resources where they work. Such a realization is unacceptable to them since it seems uncaring and cold.

Many procedures at work compound the caregiver's individual tendencies to carry too much inside, to keep helping without a pause. Hospitals are prime examples of stress-producing systems. It is common experience to have personnel work two and three shifts in a row to cover for sick coworkers or to have inadequate personnel most of the time along with insufficient supplies. There is no control over patient flow, so it is expected that whoever is working can and will handle all patients. Supervisors are more likely to be doing line work than supporting their line personnel. Many times personnel are performing duties and routines for which they are overtrained and overqualified. Menzies interprets these and other aspects of the hospital nursing system as defenses against anxiety;[16] the apparent overtraining, extreme criticisms for any errors, division of nursing duties so no one has complete patient responsibility, and delegation of responsibility upward are ways that nursing systems cope with the pressures on the individual nurses in the highly emotional and stressful business of life and death.

Defense structures are often themselves painful and anxiety producing. Working within such a system cannot allow one to feel very protective, since the nurses themselves fear criticism as well as feeling considerable self-doubt. When nurses are treated in a stereotypical way and find themselves reacting to their patients with less empathy and individualized caring, they are likely to feel inadequate, unprofessional, cynical, ashamed, and fearful of sharing these feelings. The nurse who suffers silently and resents the lack of understanding is a prime candidate for burnout.

Another way of looking at the individual-system interaction leading to burnout is in terms of the responsibility for providing services without adequate resources. As pointed out earlier, the greater is the gap between ideals and actual practices, the faster and surer is the burnout of the professional who attempts to work harder and longer to reduce that gap. I have observed many work settings where only token services are provided, where personnel accept responsibility for these services as if they were adequate to the task, and sadly, where personnel are blamed by themselves, administration, and clients for the inadequate services. Staffing and organization are clearly administrative concerns, and the responsibility for the service gap belongs to management. Individuals need to examine how they collude with management through overstretching themselves so that the responsibility for solving the problem is not faced.

The guilt and feelings of failure that plague a person who is burning out at work can be avoided or lessened through knowing that many others feel the same way and experience the same problems in their careers. One's perception and experience of work as a stressor undergoes a change as a result of seeing the system's part in the burnout phenomenon. For persons just entering a human-service field, I feel strongly that knowledge of burnout and how to cope with this predictable phenomenon can start new practitioners in a lifestyle at work that will prevent and minimize their own occupational stress.

Some professions seem to have burnout cycles, for example, 5 years for welfare workers and 1 year for free-clinic counselors.[17] Turnover is an indicator, as is the need for extensive time off. Sabbaticals and training or conferences can be built-in means of anticipating the need for a considerable break to recover and become revitalized. I also think that individuals at different stages in their own life cycle are more or less vulnerable to burnout.[18] As with any stress phenomenon, the more stressors within a brief period of time, the greater the likelihood that the individual will not be able to handle the current situation.

The work system can escalate burnout by such means as massive budget cuts, or threats of same, whereby workers face a growing gap between what they should provide their clients and the available resources. I made the point earlier that we cannot maintain an increased output in an acute crisis when the crisis is continuing. It is up to the individual caregiver to assess what is contributing to his or her burnout and to restructure recovery from the emotional drain of providing human services.

For persons already in a work system where burnout is being experienced, a seminar or workshop on burnout and stress in which persons share their experiences immediately reduces the sense of isolation and self-blame for job dissatisfaction. The phenomenon of burnout is so pervasive that talking about it and doing something about it as a work group becomes quite possible. For workers who are themselves patients in a health-care system, patient discussion groups, such as staff support groups, can speed their recovery from work-related stress and provide new tools for stress management once the workers return to work.

Recovery of the Individual and the Work System

One of the first steps in dealing with burnout is to recognize how pervasive it is and to share experiences and feelings with coworkers. Ventilation is especially helpful within an "internal support structure," a regular meeting of coworkers for discussing problems and seeking solutions to whatever is within the scope of the group. There is a great deal to be said for accepting those aspects of the work operations which you cannot change. What is within the ability of each person to change are attitudes, perceptions, and reactions to the stressors that confront us all. Within the group there are some who handle stress better or see alternative solutions to job problems.

Almost before a supportive problem-solving group can work, it is necessary for each individual to develop an awareness of how he or she is handling stress and to change wherever possible. Persons who do not burn-out have regular time and ways each day of taking care of themselves, of recovering from any stresses.[19] In particular, they do not carry work problems home, and they also use an activity at the end of the day, a "decompression ritual," to make the break between work and home. Often some form of exercise or deep relaxation reduces the muscle tension and mental activity that build up during the day. The body, through exercise or relaxation techniques, experiences a calmer state than usual before returning to a physiological baseline. Work worries and problems are not reconsidered later, and there is then time for a satisfying personal life. The break between work and personal life must be made to keep work stress from being a 24-hour-a-day concern.

There are a number of other changes that enable each person to manage stress. Since perception is quite important in whether we react with the automatic stress reaction, what we think and how we interpret a situation can make it easier for us to cope with it. Rather than obsess on what went wrong at work, reflecting on the satisfactions will generate a sense of well-being. Monitoring our individual stress levels and taking minibreaks when we notice our discomfort mounting will help to bring down the level of discomfort and ready us for another demand. It is very important to take breaks, to listen to our bodies when they say we are hungry, tired, not thinking clearly, feeling irritated, or wanting to push through just one more assignment without the energy to do so. Changes of position and walking around help to release the built up muscle tension and get our minds off the present situation.

Discussions with coworkers during breaks and meals should not be about work. This does not allow for relaxation. Sharing gripes is unproductive and makes matters worse by adding stress rather than allowing for relaxation and reduction of stress. A special time must be set aside for problem solving. Each participant in the support group meeting must become as relaxed as possible, so high levels of anger, frustration, and anxiety do not interfere with the group's problem-solving abilities. Any staff meetings that are hostile and nonproductive serve to increase stress and decrease motivation for any sharing.

In preparing for any upcoming stressor, it is helpful to anticipate what may happen and the likely effects, even role-play alternative responses. This is a kind of stress innoculation, which prepares people mentally for a difficult situation. It can be applied to personnel trying to cope with yet another change and to patients who have many anxieties about their lives after recovery.

Pacing oneself and anticipating what will be more stressful and demanding can be a daily process at work. Where assignments can be selected and scheduled, self-pacing is much easier. When locked into a schedule, the individual and group must examine whether the schedule allows for alternating high and low pressure periods and for different kinds of activities, which vary especially in how emotionally draining they might be. On a given day, a staff member who is not feeling well and is feeling rather stressed should be able to request and receive backup for modifying the daily activities to intentionally reduce the pressures. It is most unwise to insist on business as usual if someone has been going through a personal crisis or a recent period of job stress. In the health-care system, what is an emotional event for the patient and the patient's family also has impact on the staff. Some discussion and mutual comforting within the staff at the time of a loss or crisis at work help restore the caregivers so they can continue to give to other patients who will need them also.

Patients' Work Stress

Patients can be viewed in terms of their work and personal roles, not just the "patient role." For many employed persons, much of their identity and satisfaction is tied up in their jobs. Handling pressures can be very ego-enhancing. If the person becomes physically ill, at some level it may threaten this image of self-sufficiency. The taking on of many work pressures without relief could have been the very thing to precipitate the illness. However, the dependency of the patient role is difficult for many to take along with removal from the work role; irritability at hospital personnel and family may be the patient's way of coping with anxieties about competency and self-sufficiency. The patient who feels the need to get back to work as soon as possible and handle the same amount of stress may fight advice about an adequate recovery. The health professional must counsel the individual on how to better manage stress rather than try to control a stress-prone pattern by prohibiting a return to work.

Several points have already been made about stress and burnout that can be shared with patients during their recovery and during outpatient follow-up visits. In exploring how the patient reacts to stress, ask directly about what is demanding and how is it handled, the length of time worked and when breaks occur, and what is done after work. Also inquire about the patients' eating, drinking, exercising, and relaxing habits, their opportunities for sharing problems at work or with consultants, whether they worry at home and discuss problems there, their relationship with their boss and others at work, whether career goals and expectations are being met, what other problems affect work performance and satisfaction, and the quality of work performance.

Health professionals are often asked to assess whether a patient is ready to return to work. If work has been stressful, if the patient is burned out, then the return-to-work evaluation must also consider how work stressors would be handled in the future. The patient may be highly motivated to find new ways of coping with stressors. A good prognosis would be related to changed attitudes and behavior regarding moderation and pacing of present stress levels, taking more frequent breaks from frantic activity, and daily patterns of relaxation and exercise. This assumes the work milieu not to be exceedingly stressful. If work stressors are considerable, the prognosis may be poor for maintenance of well-being in that work environment. Some independent discussion with others in the same work situation can validate working conditions. A change of jobs may be in order and could be facilitated by recommendations to the employer. Once the patient perceives other options besides returning to the same work situation without any new coping skills, the patient may feel less helpless and better able to pursue alternatives. It would be worth exploring feelings about work early in the recovery process in order to speed recovery and to recommend any additional treatment or lifestyle changes.

In the occupational setting, medical leaves can be shortened by such interviews regarding work stress at the onset of the medical leave. It would seem that health professionals who desire to speed recovery also can look into the area of work stress, since it can have quite an influence on the patient's mental health. I hope from the preceding discussion that an educational approach regarding stress would be attempted before a psychotherapy referral. If structured classes and group discussions about returning to work and handling work pressures are not available in either the health service or occupational setting, individual counseling regarding stress and coping skills, along with follow-up discussion, could be an adequate educational approach. Above all, work-stress problems are not easily solved by "rest" and tranquilizers.

The health professional who contemplates a patient's symptom picture should be reminded of how common these signs of chronic stress are among coworkers. Your patient, like yourself, may be experiencing burnout and needs to know how it occurs, even for the most hard-working workers. If you are insensitive to the work aspects of your patient's life and to his or her burnout symptoms, you also may be unaware of these issues for yourself. Health care is a total system, including the caregivers, whose own health affects their ability to care for others. In advocating that health professionals practice stress management, I echo very old advice: "Physician, heal thyself." I believe that better care and a healthy model are provided by caregivers who work on preventing their own burnout.

Notes

1. "Women Workers: Are They Special?" *Job Safety and Health* 3(4), U.S. Department of Occupational Safety and Health Administration, April 1975.

2. Cary L. Cooper and Judi Marshall, "Occupational Sources of Stress: A Review of the Literature Relating to Coronary Heart Disease and Mental Ill Health," *Journal of Occupational Psychology* 49: 11–28, 1976.

3. Patricia Renwick and Edward Lawler, "What You Really Want from Your Job," *Psychology Today* (May 1978): 53–65; Christina Maslach, "Job Burnout: How People Cope," *Public Welfare* (Spring 1978): 56–58.

4. Hans Selye, *Stress Without Distress* (Philadelphia: Lippincott, 1974).

5. Ibid.

6. Cooper and Marshall, "Occupational Sources of Stress," 1976.

7. "Stress, Successs, . . . and Survival," *Harvard Business Review,* (special issue), 1976.

8. Christina Maslach, "Burned-Out," *Human Behavior* (September 1976): 16–21.

9. Thomas Holmes and Richard Rahe, "The Social Readjustment Scale," *Psychosomatic Research* 11: 213–218, 1967.

10. Hans Selye, *The Stress of Life* (New York: McGraw-Hill, 1956).

11. Ibid.

12. Meyer Friedman and Ray Rosenman, *Type A Behavior and Your Heart* (New York: Fawcett, 1974); Lawrence L. Hoffman, "Observations following a Heart Attack," *California State Bar Journal* (Nov./Dec. 1977): 506–513.

13. Maslach, "Burned-Out," 1976; and "Job Burnout," 1978.

14. Renwick and Lawler, "What You Really Want from Your Job," 1978.

15. Ibid.

16. Isabel Menzies, "A Case-Study in the Functioning of Social Systems as a Defense against Anxiety," In *Group Relations Reader* ed. Arthur Colman and W. Harold Bexton, (Sausalito, Calif.: GREX, 1975).

17. Freudenberger, H. "The Staff Burn-Out Syndrome," 1975. Available from Drug Abuse Council, Inc., 1820 L Street, N.W., Washington, D.C. 20036.

18. See Gail Sheehy, *Passages* (New York: Dutton, 1974); and Roger Gould, "Adult Life Stages: Growth Toward Self-Tolerance," *Psychology Today* (February 1975): 74–78.

19. Robert Kahn, "Job Burnout: Prevention and Remedies," *Public Welfare* (Spring 1978): 61–63; and Maslach, "Burned-Out," 1976.

17 Interviewing and Identifying Persons with Alcohol Problems

Seth Ersner-Hershfield,
Mark B. Sobell,
and Linda C. Sobell

Health-care practitioners (hereafter referred to as practitioners) in all areas of practice encounter patients with alcohol problems. These practitioners are not only in a position to identify patients with alcohol problems, but they also can refer such individuals to appropriate treatment providers. This chapter first presents guidelines for identifying individuals with drinking problems and then discusses interview methods that can be used to obtain sufficient and valid information about those problems. The concluding portion of the chapter addresses the processes involved in deciding where and how to refer individuals who have alcohol problems.

Conceptualization of Alcohol Problems: A Historical Perspective

Before discussing how to identify and interview individuals with alcohol problems, a brief historical perspective regarding the alcohol field is warranted. Just a quarter of a century ago, the involvement of health-care professionals in the treatment of alcohol problems was scant. Since that time, however, there have been concerted efforts on both federal and state levels to develop formal medical and psychiatric health-care facilities for persons with alcohol problems. Consequently, most communities now provide at least some type of formal health care for individuals with alcohol-related problems.

Conceptualizations about the nature of alcohol problems have undergone a similarly accelerated development during the last two decades. As recently as 20 years ago, most of our knowledge about alcohol problems derived from the personal experiences of recovered alcoholics and from rather perfunctory clinical observations. Pattison et al. (1977) have summarized this body of phenomenological knowledge as "traditional concepts of alcoholism." These concepts are an accretion of beliefs, values, and ide-

We are grateful to Robert J. Schweikert, M.D., who provided us with a medical practitioner's viewpoint on detection of alcohol problems and referral for services.

ologies that have derived from several sources, the most influential being Alcoholics Anonymous (AA), the disease concept of alcoholism formulated by the late E.M. Jellinek (1960), anecdotal tales of personal struggles with alcohol problems, and popular interpretations of these ideas. This view of alcohol problems can be described as a body of popularly accepted ideas that arose in the absence of scientific knowledge. Briefly, traditional concepts include the ideas that alcoholism is a uniform entity for which only certain individuals in a population are at risk and that the malady is progressive and irreversible. Historically, this set of beliefs seems to have evolved from humanitarian and sociopolitical motivations (Pattison et al., 1977). In fact, a highly significant benefit attributable to the traditional concepts of alcoholism was an increasing public, professional, and governmental concern for the welfare of people with alcohol problems.

Perhaps the most substantial recognition of alcohol abuse as a major national health problem came in 1970 with the establishment of a federal authority—the National Institute on Alcohol Abuse and Alcoholism (NIAAA)—responsible for developing a comprehensive approach to deal with alcohol-related health problems. Furthermore, alcohol was recently recognized as the most abused drug in the United States (Domestic Council Drug Abuse Task Force, 1975). In addition to the NIAAA, several prominent professional health organizations, such as the World Health Organization, the American Medical Association, the American Hospital Association, the American College of Physicians, and the American Psychiatric Association, also have stressed the seriousness and prevalence of alcohol problems. Without question, there is no longer a lack of interest and involvement of health-service providers and organizations in the treatment and prevention of alcohol problems.

Despite the recent upsurge of interest in alcohol problems, definitive answers surrounding their cause(s) remain unknown. While theories abound, the majority of professionals prefer to think of the causes of alcohol abuse as an interaction of physical, psychological, and social factors. Although alcohol abuse is known to be treatable, at this time the state of the art cannot support the use of any single type of treatment for all individuals. Furthermore, efforts to develop secondary and primary prevention programs are just beginning, with hope that such programs may foment a decrease in the tertiary aspects of this serious health problem.

In the early 1960s, prior to the establishment of NIAAA, the scientific community began to seriously study alcohol problems. Some of these early investigations explicitly studied the use of alcohol by alcoholics in laboratory settings. Until that time, most of our knowledge about physical dependence on alcohol in humans had derived from the retrospective self-reports of individuals so afflicted. However, since these pioneering studies, the alcohol field has benefited from enormous gains in knowledge owing to experimental research. In fact, the proliferation of both applied and basic scientific research in this area has forced a reconsideration of traditional concepts of alcohol problems. Since space does not permit a detailed presentation of the prodigious body of evidence disconfirming various aspects of traditional concepts, the interested reader is referred to Pattison et al. (1977).

The new, empirically based conceptualizations of the nature of alcohol problems will probably affect several aspects of the alcohol field, including (1) the provision of services for individuals often considered under the rubric of "alcohol abuser" or "problem drinker" (currently, appropriate treatment programs for such individuals are very few in number), (2) the consideration of alcohol abuse as a multifaceted health problem, and (3) the ways we evaluate improvement from alcohol problems. To briefly summarize the conceptual changes (reviewed in Pattison et al., 1977), the search for evidence of uniformity or homogeneity among persons with alcohol problems has been futile. Rather, the evidence suggests that there is no single entity that can be defined as "alcoholism," but that alcohol problems are multifaceted life health problems defined by drinking patterns and the presence of adverse physical, psychological, and/or social consequences of drinking. Furthermore, there appears to be no clear preexisting difference between persons susceptible to alcohol problems and persons not susceptible to such problems. Instead, it can be argued that any individual who uses alcohol can, under appropriate conditions, develop serious alcohol problems, although a variety of risk factors may differentially contribute to one's susceptibility. The use of alcohol by an individual also can have a broad range of outcomes, from no adverse consequences to severely pathological sequelae and even death. Strong evidence now supports the fact that the developmental sequence of alcohol problems appears to be highly variable over time and does not necessarily progress to chronic or fatal stages.

While evidence supports the fact that continuous drinking of large doses of alcohol over extended periods of time (typically, 2 to 5 days) will result in physical dependence on alcohol, it also shows that ingestion of a small amount of alcohol by even "chronic" alcoholics will not initiate either physical dependence or a physiological need for more alcohol (reviewed in Pattison et al., 1977). Finally, several studies have shown that recovery from alcohol problems bears no necessary relationship to abstinence, although such a concurrence is both frequent and desirable. In this regard, alcohol problems are typically interrelated with other life problems. In view of the strong interrelationship between alcohol problems and other life health problems, it is imperative that treatment address multiple areas of life health and that treatment plans and goals be idiosyncratically developed. Similarly, treatment outcome should measure changes in multiple areas of life health, as well as multiple aspects of drinking behavior.

Identifying Alcohol Problems

Apart from considering their validity, traditional concepts of alcoholism pose other problems. Within the traditional framework, symptoms are usually viewed as the result of a disease and consequently beyond the control of the individual. For alcohol abusers, assignment to the "sick" role may serve to allow the individual to abrogate any responsibility for his or her behavior and thus reinforce deviant drinking (Roman and Trice, 1968). A further consequence resulting from the dogmatic and punitive nature of many traditional treatment approaches may involve the denial of alcohol problems by problem drinkers until their symptomatology reaches crisis or severe pathological stages.

Although a disease model of alcohol problems is certainly appropriate when an individual is physically dependent on or withdrawing from alcohol (Jellinek, 1960), most alcohol problems are more accurately described as a set of health problems that includes a variety of syndromes defined by drinking patterns in the presence of adverse physical, psychological, and/or social consequences of that drinking. Therefore, rather than seeking to identify the stereotypic "chronic alcoholic," practitioners can benefit from looking for evidence of differential adverse consequences often associated with alcohol abuse. This is particularly important when one considers that national survey studies have shown that the greatest proportion of persons with serious alcohol problems have not suffered physical addiction to alcohol (Cahalan and Cisin, 1976; Cahalan, 1970; Cahalan and Room, 1974). The physical or emotional symptoms discussed in this section should be considered as *cues* for investigating the possibility of problem drinking in patients who do not initially acknowledge difficulty in this area.

Practitioners are in a particularly advantageous position for identifying physical health problems associated with excessive drinking. Physical health problems related to alcohol have been found to account for a large proportion of hospital admissions (Waller, 1976; Kissin, 1977) and are a frequent correlate of nutritional disorders (Hillman, 1974). Although we can only briefly mention major alcohol-related physical complications in this chapter, the interested practitioner can obtain more information by consulting two concise summary publications—the *Manual on Alcoholism,* published by the American Medical Association (1978), and the National Council on Alcoholism's *Criteria for the Diagnosis of Alcoholism* (Available from the National Council on Alcoholism, 2 Park Avenue, Suite 1720, New York, New York 10016). When evaluating drinking-related health problems, two points should be kept in mind: (1) persons with alcohol problems often visit physicians or medical clinics for health problems which they do not perceive as associated with their drinking, and (2) in nearly all cases, drinking is simply one of several factors that might account for the observed or reported physical symptoms. Thus, unless a "host" of alcohol complications are present, the symptomatology would suggest only that one inquire further about possible drinking involvement.

It is important that the practitioner recognize medical problems associated with alcohol use. Several medical problems that *may* implicate alcohol problems are summarized in table 17-1. Of course, one should not

Table 17-1
Medical Problems Commonly Associated with Alcohol Abuse

Area of Concern or System	Principle Manifestation
Endocrine	Reactive hypoglycemia
Hematopoietic	Anemia
Pancreatic	Pancreatitis (acute and chronic)
Gastrointestinal	Gastritis Peptic ulcer Esophagitis Duodenitis
Hepatic	Acute fatty liver-elevated liver enzyme levels (for example, SGOT, SICD, γ-GTP) Alcoholic hepatitis Cirrhosis
Nutritional disorders	Varied (multisystem)
Nervous system	Blackouts[a] Short-term memory deficits Cerebellar degeneration Cerebral atrophy Polyneuropathy Wernicke-Korsakoff syndrome
Ethanol withdrawal symptoms	Psychomotor agitation (gross tremors) Autonomic hyperactivity Insomnia Hallucinations (auditory and visual) Delirium tremors Seizures
Physical appearance	Ethanol odor on breath Unexplained bruises, abrasions, and lacerations Marked incidence of cigarette burns on fingertips Puffy edematous appearacne to the skin and subcutaneous tissues Blood alcohol level 0.15 mgm% with no evidence of gross intoxication

[a] The term *blackout* refers to an individual being amnesic for what occurred during portions of a drinking episode although loss of consciousness did not occur. Typically, from simple observation of the drinking, it is quite difficult to ascertain whether a blackout is occurring. Blackouts should not be confused with loss of consciousness and "grayouts" (where there is partial forgetting, but memory of the events that occurred is regained with cueing).

overlook the obvious value of simply asking the patient about his or her drinking pattern and any previous alcohol treatment. This can be accomplished by embedding such inquiries in a series of questions about various health-related behaviors, such as smoking, job-related stresses, and dietary habits. Table 17-1 also includes a listing of the primary symptoms of the acute ethanol withdrawal syndrome that may be present as sequelae to abstinence in individuals who have severe alcohol problems. A particularly useful indicator of drinking problems is obtained from measures of liver enzyme activity; several recent studies have found the serum glutamyl oxaloacetic transaminase (SGOT) and gamma glutamyl transpepdidase (γ-GTP) levels to be related to frequent, continued, and especially excessive consumption of alcoholic beverages (Boone et al., 1977; Luchi et al., 1978; Reyes et al., 1978; Rosalki and Rau, 1972; Wiseman and Spencer-Peet, 1977).

Several other types of complaints also may reflect problem drinking. Patients complaining of depression, insomnia, nervousness, sexual problems, or anxiety or requesting medication to counteract certain of these feelings or states may be drinking excessively to deal with such distress. Such complaints also may signify withdrawal from alcohol.

Finally, major changes or difficulties in the patient's life-family problems, job disruption or dissatisfaction, financial problems—should be explored. Practitioners also should determine how the patient has responded to these pressures. More specifically, has any drinking occurred and how does drinking affect the immediate problem? Does the patient view drinking as a method of emotional coping? Connections between alcohol use and attempted alleviation of emotional distress or interpersonal problems are highly suggestive of a drinking problem.

The relative importance of drinking as it relates to an individual's social or emotional functioning also can signal a problem. That is, is alcohol a usual source of relaxation or reward after a hard day at work? Is it seen as indispensable for filling or structuring the patient's time? Do the patient's social activities revolve around drinking, and do his or her friends drink heavily? To what extent does the patient reveal a preoccupation with drinking—cognitive fixation?

When obtaining information about the patient's past and present drinking patterns, relevant inquiries might include the number of years the patient has been drinking, the greatest amount consumed in one 24-hour period (this can provide evidence of functional tolerance to ethanol), how much the person typically drinks per day, the frequency of drinking occasions (number of times per week), the circumstances under which drinking occurs, the amount of money spent on alcohol per week, reports of alcohol-related blackouts, and reports of frequent thoughts or urges to drink.

When probing for specific amounts of alcohol consumed, vague answers, such as "a few drinks," are not sufficient to evaluate the extent of a drinking problem. Clinical experience indicates that descriptions such as "a few drinks" are subjective terms which, upon further questioning, can range from as few as two or three beers to as much as a pint of hard liquor. More precise estimates of consumption can sometimes be obtained if the practitioner uses a method of exaggeration. For example:

Practitioner: "How much do you usually drink on any given occasion?"

Patient: "Oh, just a few beers."

Practitioner: "Can you be a little more specific? Does a few beers mean two or three, or a couple of six packs?"

Patient: "Definitely less than two six packs."

Practitioner: "Well, is it closer to nine or three beers?"

Patient: "Usually about a six pack."

Physical dependence on alcohol, while most likely to develop in chronic users, can occur even with individuals who report a relatively brief, but intense, drinking history. Therefore, it is also important to establish whether the patient has ever experienced any degree of alcohol withdrawal symptoms. Such symptoms can range from slight psychomotor agitation when coming off a drinking episode to delirium tremens and/or seizures.

The patient's drug history also should be acquired in a similarly careful manner. Beside the obvious interest in what drugs the patient has used or may currently be using, and for what purposes, it is also the case that many people are polydrug abusers, combining various prescription drugs with alcohol. Some individuals who regularly use tranquilizers or sleeping pills also are known to drink alcohol to excess, perhaps because such drugs have central nervous system (CNS) depressant properties similar to alcohol. Using such drugs in combination with alcohol may result in a synergistic and soporific interaction. The synergistic effect of alcohol and barbiturates, for instance, is responsible for many overdoses and deaths in persons who previously only became drunk or "high" when taking the drugs separately.

Some of the preceding clues to alcohol problems will, by virtue of history taking and the nature of the presenting complaints, emerge during the first few visits. Others will appear as a result of the patient's response to treatment. For example, if a generally effective regimen for a gastrointestinal disorder is prescribed and no improvement is seen after a reasonable period of time, the possibility of alcohol abuse should not be overlooked.

Guidelines for Conducting Interviews

While it may seem self-evident, patients should be interviewed when they are sober. Alcohol intoxication, even in small amounts, can impair both the accuracy of information gathered and the general quality of the visit. Although it might appear to be an easy task to ascertain whether a patient is intoxicated, the phenomenon of acquired tolerance to alcohol permits some people to appear coherent and sober even when they have high blood alcohol levels (Maisto et al., 1978; Sobell et al., 1980). The identification of such individuals may even be missed by clinicians who specialize in alcohol problems. If the patient denies having consumed alcohol the day of the visit but is thought to be intoxicated because of certain clues, such as breath odor or a flushed appearance, the practitioner may consider taking a blood sample. However, a less expensive method of obtaining an immediate and direct indication of a patient's level of alcohol intoxication can be obtained using portable breath testers. [One such device, the Mobat (Luckey Laboratories, San Bernardino, CA) provides estimates of blood alcohol levels ranging to 0.30 mg percent at a cost of approximately 70 cents per test (Sobell and Sobell, 1975)]. The use of such testers can be learned rather easily, and the blood alcohol concentration readings are relatively accurate and quite sufficient for clinical purposes (Sobell and Sobell, 1975).

As noted earlier, many medications have a synergistic reaction when combined with alcohol. Therefore, determining whether a patient has a drinking problem is of further importance when the practitioner is considering prescribing medications. Moreover, the effects of certain drugs, such as antibiotics, anticonvulsants, anticoagulants, and monoamine oxidase inhibitors, may be vitiated when paired with alcohol. A handy reference for information about such drug interactions has been published in *RN* magazine and is available as a separate issue (*Drug Interactions,* revised edition, 1975. Available from Medical Economics Company, Book Division, Oradell, NJ 07649. Approximate cost, $2.00).

Interviewing style is also very important when attempting to identify alcohol problems. Many people, fearing the social stigma and sanctions of being labeled "alcoholic," are reluctant to divulge much information about their drinking patterns. Further, even if they trust the practitioner and are not fearful of censure, they may fear the idea that they may be "alcoholic." For these reasons, it is advantageous to *focus on information gathering rather than labeling.* This aim can and probably should be directly expressed to the patient: that the purpose of the questions is not to attach labels, but to look at sources of influence on the patient's functioning, with the nature and consequences of alcohol intake being among those factors.

The practitioner's success at eliciting this sort of information may depend on his or her receptiveness to it. If the practitioner has negative attitudes toward "alcoholics" and communicates these feelings or is hesitant to explore (and perhaps deal with) whether a patient has an alcohol problem, it is probable that little will be gained from any questioning. To this end, it is helpful to understand that alcohol problems are, in actuality, no different than many other health problems, such as high blood pressure, ulcers, diabetes, and obesity.

A useful interviewing method for gathering information about alcohol problems without unduly threatening the patient is to focus on elucidating any alcohol-related *consequences* the patient has suffered. Thus inquiries can focus on whether the patient has experienced legal problems, marital disputes, vocational difficulties (for example, days or hours missed from work, jobs lost), interpersonal problems (for example, frequent quarrels with others), and other life problems often associated with excessive drinking. Such an approach obviates dealing with issues of labeling and denial, which are more appropriately handled in treatment. In fact, after having disclosed several alcohol-related adverse life consequences, it is not unusual for a patient to conclude that he or she may have a drinking problem. In such cases, referral for treatment is obviously facilitated.

Valuable and often overlooked sources of information include a patient's spouse, as well as other family members or significant others. Collateral interviews have the distinct advantage of providing another perspective on the patient's behavior, especially when there is some ambiguity regarding the patient self-reports. Besides providing an evaluation of the patient's drinking from another viewpoint, the collateral usually has a stake in seeing the patient get help and may disclose information concealed by the patient. For this reason, collateral interviews must be tactfully arranged, so as not to put the collateral in the position of betraying the patient. For example, justification for including the collateral may be expressed as a means of furnishing the practitioner with as complete a picture as possible of the patient's health problems.

To reiterate, whenever possible, harsh confrontation of the patient should be avoided. People who have recently developed alcohol problems and are ambivalent about recognizing them may so strongly resent confrontation that subsequent referral is refused. Creating such a state of affairs unnecessarily can hardly be justified as in the patient's best interests. Certain situations might, however, require a direct approach. For example, if a patient who has pancreatitis is suspected of abusing alcohol and fails to benefit from the prescribed and usual treatment regimen, the practitioner might mention the disparity between the expected results and the patient's reaction, noting that such problems can sometimes result from drinking alcohol. This strategy affords the patient the opportunity to concur and to elaborate on his or her alcohol use without feeling attacked or being defensive.

Treatment and Referral

Once the practitioner decides that an alcohol problem probably exists, the patient can be presented with a summary and integration of the information. Again, it is best to *avoid labels*, instead emphasizing the areas of dysfunction connected with alcohol use. Hopefully, when confronted with evidence of alcohol-related damage or the high risk of such consequences, the patient will agree that a problem exists and accept referral to treatment. While many referrals present no difficulties, some patients, in accord with popular stereotypes, will insist, despite the evidence, that their drinking is not a problem: "I can stop any time." The patient can be invited to stop his or her drinking for a specified period of time—and indeed, the patient may well manage to halt drinking or drinking excessively for short intervals. However, if the determinants of the drinking have not changed, the patient is likely to resume abusive drinking shortly thereafter. Therefore, it is important to maintain contact with the patient during this time to minimize the risk that the patient may avoid the practitioner for fear of admitting failure. Should the excessive drinking recur, the practitioner can capitalize on the opportunity to once again refer the patient for treatment.

If treatment seems indicated, to whom should the patient be referred? For most physicians and other health-care practitioners, time is a precious commodity. It is difficult to devote sufficient time to the thorough assessment of an individual's drinking problem, much less engage in a course of treatment. Furthermore, many people who abuse alcohol have associated psychological problems. Adequate treatment in these cases requires the service provider to have training in psychotherapeutic skills and techniques. In our opinion, only those practitioners who are prepared to treat a full range of emotional problems should offer therapy to individuals with alcohol problems. Therefore, referral is usually the most appropriate action for the practitioner to take. If the practitioner is familiar with the patient and has knowledge of the persons's life circumstances, this can often aid in gaining the patient's trust and thus facilitate the referral for treatment.

While our position with regard to referral resources may seem contrary to the popular maxim, "send him to Alcoholics Anonymous," this should not be interpreted as critical of that organization. In fact, in many cases, joining AA may be a part of a patient's recommended treatment plan. Until recently, AA was the favored referral source because abstinence was the exclusive goal of treatment for all alcohol abusers. This orientation derived from the traditional and nondifferential concepts of alcoholism discussed earlier in this chapter. However, abstinence has not been shown to be integral to treatment success in all cases; in fact, some persons with moderate to severe alcohol problems have learned to drink in a nonproblem manner and maintain this pattern (reviewed in Pattison et al., 1977). In considering the preeminence of the consequences of drinking, Sobell and Sobell (1978; and Sobell, 1978) suggest that the most realistic treatment goal for all individuals with alcohol problems is a reduction in drinking to a non-problem level. From the perspective of individualized treatment, the nonproblem level for many individuals will obviously be abstinence; for others, and especially those with less-severe problems, an absence of alcohol problems might be attained within a context of limited drinking.

Given that abstinence will be the most appropriate goal for many patients, should a referral be made to an agency that encourages and supports abstinence but provides no professional psychiatric and/or psychological services? The answer to this question is difficult at best. By learning behavior patterns consistent with nondrinking, the patient can avoid the adverse consequences previously engendered by abusive drinking. These new behavior patterns will, in turn, bolster the maintenance of sobriety (Bandura, 1969). However, persons who have other serious interpersonal and psychological problems probably have a poor prognosis for abandoning their deviant drinking patterns without associated treatment for these other life problems. Such individuals are usually most appropriately treated using psychotherapeutic techniques. For this reason, we believe that the initial referral should be made to a licenced clinician or professionally staffed alcohol treatment agency capable of tailoring the treatment to meet the patient's needs. Of course, while a perfect fit cannot be guaranteed, the practitioner can help enhance the chances of treatment success by arranging referral on an individual basis.

One alternative that can be exercised by the practitioner is to refer the patient to a clinician or agency capable of assessing additional problem areas and willing to make a further referral if this is indicated. Another alternative is for the practitioner to gather information about a number of local resources, so that patients can make their own choice from among several treatment options. Those patients who are confident enough in their ability to select services that would be most appropriate for them may feel a greater commitment to their subsequent treatment than if such a choice had not been offered.

Finally, the professional relationship between the practitioner and the referral source can contribute toward the quality of the referral. With the patient's consent, exchange of information on the patient's progress can both benefit the patient and enhance the practitioner's treatment of the patient's other medical problems. Working in conjunction with alcohol-treatment professionals, health care practitioners are in a unique position to facilitate secondary prevention and treatment of alcohol problems.

References

American Medical Association. *Manual on Alcoholism.* Chicago, 1978.

Bandura, A. *Principles of Behavior Modification.* New York: Holt, Rinehart and Winston, 1969.

Boone, D.J., Tietz, N.W., and Weinstock, A. Significance of γ-glutamyl transferase (GGT) activity measurements in alcohol-induced hepatic injury. *Annuals of Clinical and Laboratory Science* 7:24–28, 1977.

Cahalan, D. *Problem Drinkers: A National Survey.* San Francisco: Jossey-Bass, 1970.

Cahalan, D., and Cissin, I. Drinking behavior and drinking problems in the United States. In *The Biology of Alcoholism.* Vol.4: *Social Aspects of Alcoholism.* ed. B. Kissin and H. Begleiter. New York: Plenum, pp. 77–116, 1976.

Cahalan, D., and Room, R. *Problem Drinking among American Men.* Monograph No. 7. New Brunswick, N.J.: Rutgers Center of Alcohol Studies, 1974.

Domestic Council Drug Abuse Task Force. *White Paper on Drug Abuse: A Report to the President.* Washington: U.S. Government Printing Office, 1975.

Hillman, R.W. Alcoholism and malnutrition. In *The Biology of Alcoholism,* Vol. 3: *Clinical Pathology.* ed. B. Kissin and H. Begleiter. New York: Plenum, pp. 513–586, 1974.

Jellinek, E.M. *The Disease Concept of Alcoholism.* New Brunswick, N.J.: Hillhouse Press, 1960.

Kissin, B. Medical management of the alcoholic patient. In *The Biology of Alcoholism,* Vol. 5: *Treatment and Rehabilitation of the Chronic Alcoholic* ed. B. Kissin and H. Begleiter. New York: Plenum, pp. 53–104, 1977.

Luchi, P., Cortis, G., and Bucarelli, A. Forensic considerations on the comparison of "serum γ-glutamyltranspeptidase" ("γ-GT") activity in experimental acute alcoholic intoxication and in alcoholic car drivers who caused road accidents. *Forensic Science* 11:33–39, 1978.

Maisto, S.A., Henry, R.R., Sobell, M.B., and Sobell, L.S. Implications of acquired changes in tolerance for the treatment of alcohol problems. *Addictive Behaviors* 3:51–55, 1978.

Pattison, E.M., Sobell, M.B., and Sobell, L.C. (eds.). *Emerging Concepts of Alcohol Dependence.* New York: Springer, 1977.

Reyes, E., Miller, W.R., Taylor, C.A., and Spalding, C.T. The activity of γ-glutamyl transpeptidase in the serum of problem drinkers. *Procedings of Western Pharmacology* 21:289–297, 1978.

Roman, P.M., and Trice, H.M. The sick role, labeling theory and the deviant drinker. *The International Journal of Social Psychiatry* 14:245–251, 1968.

Rosalki, S.B., and Rau, D. Serum γ -glutamyl transpeptidase activity in alcoholism. *Clinica Chimica Acta* 39:41–47, 1972.

Sobell, M.B. Alternatives to abstinence: Evidence, issues and some proposals. In *Alcoholism: New Directions in Behavioral Research and Treatment.* ed. P.E. Nathan, G.A. Marlatt, and T. Løberg. New York: Plenum, 1978.

Sobell, M.B., and Sobell, L.C. A brief technical report on the Mobat: An inexpensive portable test for determining blood alcohol concentration. *Journal of Applied Behavior Analysis* 8: 117–120, 1975.

Sobell, M.B., and Sobell, L.C. *Behavioral Treatment of Alcohol Problems: Individualized Therapy and Controlled Drinking.* New York: Plenum, 1978.

Sobell, M.B., Sobell, L.C., and VanderSpek, R. Relationship between clinical judgment, self-report and breath analysis measures of intoxication in alcoholics. *Journal of Consulting and Clinical Psychology* 47: 204–206, 1979.

Waller, J.A. Alcohol and unintentional injury. In *The Biology of Alcoholism,* Vol. 4: *Social Aspects of Alcoholism.* ed. B. Kissin and H. Begleiter. New York: Plenum, pp. 307–350, 1976.

Wiseman, S.M., and Spencer-Peet, J. The effect of drinking patterns on enzyme screening tests for alcoholism. *The Practitioner* 219: 243–245, 1977.

Part III
Delivery of Health-Care Services: Psychological Aspects of Human Sexuality in Health Care

James Thurber and E.B. White once wrote a book called *Is Sex Necessary?* The humor implicit in this title can be taken seriously too, for we know that like most other people, many health-care professionals are able to think with greater ease about their own sexuality than about openly discussing another person's sexuality with him or her. Masters's and Johnson's work was important for some of its objective findings as well as for its merging of the various disciplines of psychology, physiology, and sociology. Their scientific work lifted a subject from the realm of what was previously considered impossible, shocking, and even obscene to the realm of a scientific and yet human objectivity, and this has had many repercussions in the most positive ways. Masters and Johnson maintain that everyone faces the concerns of sexual tensions and that the sexual facet of our lives affects more people in more ways than any other physiological response other than those necessary to our very existence. Sex is impossible to ignore, and whether it is necessary is clearly a question to be answered affirmatively.

We feel satisfied that the space given in this book to chapters on sexuality will not allow the topic to be overlooked or avoided at all. Reynolds and Price (chapter 18) show that a health-care professional's ability to meet the growing need for sex education and therapy will depend on a number of factors, including the professional's time availability, level of training, and degree of interest and comfort in providing sex education and therapy. A model and techniques for providing information and brief treatment as part of a regular office visit are described. This discussion is followed by a review of traditional and emerging treatment approaches for patients requiring more extensive treatment: individual, couple, group, and self-help therapy models are described. Methods for providing patients with an informative and supportive referral for sex therapy are presented.

Cohen and Jospe (chapter 19) focus on sexuality and various medical conditions in which sexual concern is a secondary rather than a primary problem. That is, some aspect of the individual's sexuality becomes involved as a result of medical illness, drug use, or some other event in the individual's life. Medical conditions such as heart disease, spinal-cord injury, cerebral palsy, and cancer are discussed in relation to their effect on the individual's sexual functioning. Issues of hospitalization and the expected "sick role" behavior of patients relative to their expressions of themselves as sexual beings are also presented.

No section on sexuality could possibly be complete without a discussion of nontraditional sexual behavior and the prejudices and concerns that spill over from society in general; gay men and lesbians continue to experience discrimination on all levels and have traditionally received poor health-care treatment. Gonsiorek (chapter 20) focuses on basic information about homosexuality for health-care providers, the impact of the provider-client relationship on the health of gay men and lesbians, particular problem areas prevalent in this population, and general considerations in providing health-care services for lesbians and gay men. Pragmatic suggestions are offered, some theoretical issues are discussed, and a list of recommended readings is added to the bibliography.

Dillehunt (chapter 21) expands on the scope of this section even further. The information presented was gathered from several health professionals regarding the issues concerning sexuality that arise in their practices and how these issues are handled. The issues covered include (1) what happens when the patient displays sexual feelings for the professional, (2) what happens when the professional experiences sexual feelings for the patient, (3) the advantages and disadvantages of frank and open discussions regarding sexuality in the doctor-patient relationship, (4) homosexuality, (5) childhood and adolescent sexuality, and (6) sexuality in older people.

18

Responding to Sexual Concerns in Health-Care Settings: Brief Sex Counseling and Supportive Referrals for Sex Therapy

Barry S. Reynolds
and *Susan Price*

Sexual problems seem to be as prevalent as the common cold. Masters and Johnson estimated that approximately 50 percent of married couples experience significant sexual problems. In a recent study of happily married "normal" (nonclinic referred) couples, 40 percent of the men reported erectile or ejaculatory dysfunction, and 63 percent of the women reported arousal or orgasmic dysfunction (Frank, Anderson, and Rubinstein, 1978). These couples reported even higher frequencies of sexual difficulties that were not dysfunctional in nature: 50 percent of the men and 77 percent of the women reported difficulties such as "lack of interest," "attraction to persons of the same sex," "inability to relax," "partner chooses inconvenient time," "too little foreplay," and so forth. The prevalence of sexual dysfunctions and difficulties in persons without steady partners is likely as high or higher than the incidence of problems reported by couples. In the past, people with sexual problems typically resigned themselves to learning to live with their dysfunctions. However, as people become aware of the highly effective results of brief sex therapy, many will choose to seek help for their sexual problems and concerns. Typically, the first person they will likely turn to for help with their sexual problems is a health-care professional with whom they already have an ongoing, trusting relationship. Unfortunately, patients typically broach their most sensitive questions about sex just when the health professional is half way out the door and ready to see the next patient. This chapter will attempt to identify ways in which health-care professionals might respond to patients' sexual problems and concerns as part of a regular office visit. Since some patients require more extensive treatment than can be offered as part of a regular office visit, this chapter also will include a description of sex therapy treatment approaches and techniques for making an informative and supportive referral for sex therapy.

A health-care professional's ability to meet the growing need for sex education and brief sex therapy will depend on a number of factors, including the professional's time availability, level of training, and level of comfort and interest in counseling patients with sexual problems and concerns. Sex therapy, as it is commonly practiced today, is a brief, time-limited, directive form of counseling that focuses on symptom removal. Sex therapy is comprised of a complex and multifaceted package of many different components including basic information about anatomy, physiology, and sexual response cycles; techniques for increasing sensual pleasure and reducing performance anxiety; techniques for developing effective sexual and communication skills; encouragement to alter destructive interpersonal patterns and lifestyles; and general attitude restructuring (LoPiccolo, 1978). Current reports indicate treatment success rates ranging from 80 to 100 percent for the common male and female dysfunctions (Kaplan, 1974; Lobitz and LoPiccolo, 1972; Masters and Johnson, 1970), but the essential "active ingredients" of this multifaceted treatment approach have yet to be isolated. Treatment typically requires 2 weeks of intensive therapy (Masters and Johnson, 1970) or about 15 to 20 weeks of weekly outpatient treatment (Kaplan, 1974; LoPiccolo and Lobitz, 1972). Annon (1975) was one of the first sex therapists to suggest that not all patients require all the components of sex therapy and that many sexual problems and concerns could be resolved in brief treatment as part of a regular office visit. His treatment approach is practical, realistic, and highly applicable for health-care professionals who do not see sex counseling as a primary focus of their practice.

Annon developed a conceptual scheme for differentiating and treating sexual problems that would require more intensive therapy (Annon, 1974). His model, called the *P-LI-SS-IT model,* involves four levels of intervention for handling sexual problems:

1. *Permission,* which basically involves giving the patient permission to engage in thoughts, behaviors, feelings, fantasies, and so forth that he or she already experiences but is worried may be "weird" or "abnormal."
2. *Limited information,* which involves providing the patient with specific factual information directly relevant to the particular sexual problem or concern.
3. *Specific suggestions,* which involve direct attempts by the health professional to change the patient's and/or the partner's specific problem behavior.
4. *Intensive therapy,* which involves long-term intervention for chronic sexual problems that are often deeply embedded in intrapsychic and interpersonal conflicts. Intensive therapy is most appropriately provided by a highly trained mental-health professional, while the initial three levels of intervention can, at least for some problems, be successfully provided by a variety of trained health-care professionals in one or perhaps only a brief series of office visits.

The PLISSIT model is described in detail elsewhere (Annon, 1974; Annon and Robinson, 1978). We will briefly describe some examples of permission, limited information, and specific suggestions that might be provided as part of a regular office visit, the time involved, and what the health-care professional can do when he or she does not feel comfortable or competent to respond to a patient's questions.

Giving Permission

Despite the so-called sexual revolution, many people continue to experience guilt, anxiety, or concern that they are somehow abnormal if they engage in or even think about certain taboo activities such as masturbation, oral-genital sex, anal sex, fantasizing about other partners or partners of the same sex. They might already have engaged in the behavior either overtly or covertly, but now need to check out with an authority figure that these behaviors or feelings are not "bad," "abnormal," or "sick." For example, many single people who masturbate fear they will get fixated on themselves, will prefer self-stimulation to partner stimulation, will destroy their mental or physical health, and so forth. Married people sometimes fear that masturbation is a sign of marital dissatisfaction or infidelity. Older people often fear that masturbation is a sign that one is becoming a "dirty old person," and parents who observe their child's active interest in masturbation often fear their child may have sex too early or become promiscuous. Similarly, patients may be quite concerned about thoughts and feelings, for example, about sex with other partners or with partners of the same sex (Frank, Anderson, and Rubinstein, 1978; Kinsey, Pomeroy, and Martin, 1948; Kinsey, Pomeroy, Martin, and Gebhard, 1953), and may wonder if these thoughts are a sign of pathology or perversion. Fortunately, simple reassurance from the health-care professional that these activities are "normal," that the great majority of people experience them at some time, and that there is no reason to discontinue what the patient is already doing may be sufficient to resolve the patient's sexual concerns and may prevent further problems from developing in the future (Annon, 1974). In addition, some sexual concerns can be resolved by giving the patient permission *not* to engage in certain behaviors he or she feels pressured to experience, such as partner swapping, a *menage à trois,* multiple orgasms, sex in public places, and so forth. Permission giving tends to be most effective when it is responsive to the individual needs and desires of the patient (Annon, 1974, 1975). Permission giving can be provided for a wide range of behaviors, and the amount of professional time required is typically not prohibitive; a brief discussion of the patient's concern and permission giving from the health professional may require only 5 to 10 minutes. The primary limiting factors are the health professional's breadth of knowledge of the "normal" range of human sexual functioning and the professional's value system and level of comfort with sanctioning certain attitudes and behaviors. The professional's breadth of knowledge can be rapidly increased by reading some of the recent laboratory studies and field surveys that attempt to describe the frequency of a wide variety of sexual attitudes, behaviors, and feelings (Frank, Anderson, and Rubinstein, 1978; Hite, 1976; Hunt, 1974; Kinsey et al., 1948, 1953; Masters and Johnson, 1966). These materials can provide a useful framework for answering patients' questions about the "normal" range of sexual functioning. However, if providing permission to engage in certain behaviors or thoughts conflicts with the professional's value system, a referral to another professional trained in the field of sex therapy would be a more responsible course of action. It is far more helpful to refer a patient than to impose one's own value system on another or attempt to give permission when it is not genuinely meant. The professional could inform the patient, "People have very different ideas about that (for example, anal sex, masturbation). I'd like to refer you to someone who can present all sides of the issue and help you make up your own mind. What's important is for you to have all the information needed to decide what's right for you, and I think this person can help you even more than I can because they're highly trained in this area." If the professional does feel comfortable and competent, permission giving is often combined with the next level of intervention, providing factual information.

Providing Limited Information

Many patients lack basic information about sexual anatomy, physiology, and sexual response cycles, and this ignorance can generate considerable anxiety and, in some cases, sexual dysfunction. Many patients, for example, are concerned about the size or shape of their genitals. Since women's genitals are hidden, women are often ignorant of their own bodies and how they function. Women often express concerns that their clitoris is too small, absent, or in the wrong place, or that their labia minora or majora are too long, too asymmetrical, or strangely colored. In response to these concerns, health-care professionals can use diagrams of female genitals to point out the various structures and normal range of variation in size or color or actually offer the women a mirror and allow the patient to look at her genitals while the professional points out the location of the cervix, clitoris, and so forth. Some professionals routinely include the mirror and self-examination as part of the physical or pelvic examination, while others first ask for the women's permission to include this information: "As part of your pelvic examination, if you like, I can show you your cervix, other parts of your genitals, talk a little about how they function, and answer your questions as we go along.'' Showing the patient photographs of other women's genitals can help illustrate the enormous range of variation in size, shape, and coloration of female genitalia (Blank and Cottrell, 1978).

Similarly, men are often concerned about penis size and the effect of size on female sexual satisfaction. A brief discussion, with diagrams if possible, of the normal variations in penis size can be very helpful (Annon, 1974). Many men may be relieved to learn that although there is considerable variation in penis size in the flaccid state, there is markedly less size variation in the fully erect state (Masters and Johnson, 1966). In addition, a brief discussion of Masters' and Johnson's finding that penis size is not associated with a partner's sexual satisfaction and information that a partner's satisfaction is typically derived from tenderness, a relaxed atmosphere, general body caressing, and direct manual stimulation of the clitoris rather than penis size or the depth and number of thrusts during intercourse may be very helpful in dispelling the common notion that "bigger is better."

In addition to concerns about their genitals, women and men are often concerned that they are not living up to internalized, idealized standards of how men and women *should* perform in sexual situations. Women are often concerned that they are unable to reach orgasm through intercourse without clitoral stimulation, to have multiple orgasms, to feel the vaginal contractions when they reach orgasm, and a myriad of other concerns about how they *should* reach orgasm. One woman thought she was not orgasmic because she had not ejaculated yet. Providing the woman with a brief discussion of the "normal" range of the female orgasmic response can help many patients learn to appreciate their own unique range and intensity of orgasmic response, we well as clear up many common misconceptions, such as the myth of the vaginal versus clitoral orgasm (Barbach, 1976; Kaplan, 1974; Masters and Johnson, 1966).

Men also are often concerned that they are failing to live up to the unrealistic models of male sexuality presented in the media. They expect themselves to always be ready for sex, to be able to prolong intercourse indefinitely, to comfortably initiate sex and easily bring their partner to orgasm, preferably multiple simultaneous orgasm, and so on. For example, a recently divorced middle-aged male who had just begun dating a new partner was puzzled by his inability to get an erection after only one or a few casual dates. A brief discussion of the common myths and unrealistic expectations men tend to place on their sexuality can reduce anxiety and, at times, resolve some sexual problems by helping the man remove unrealistic performance demands and expectations (Julty, 1975; Zilbergeld, 1978).

Health-care professionals, perhaps more than any other professionals, can be particularly helpful in providing patients with accurate information about changes in sexuality associated with aging, illness, drugs, and surgery. For example, as men age, they tend to require more vigorous and lengthy stimulation, their orgasms may feel less intense, and they may not reach orgasm during every sexual encounter (Butler and Lewis, 1976). Without accurate information, the man and/or his partner may interpret this change as a sign of lack of affection and interest or impending loss of sexual function, and they may become depressed and begin to avoid sex. Menopausal women can view the changes associated with the middle years as a calamity or an opportunity for personal growth and increased sexual satisfaction, and the attitude they eventually adopt can be influenced by the information and support provided by health professionals (Goldfarb, 1970). Paraplegics and quadriplegics can benefit from a frank discussion of the sexual options that are still available to them despite their physical disabilities (Mooney, Cole, and Chilgren, 1975). Patients suffering from cardiovascular diseases may experience prolonged periods of abstinence or dysfunction because of misconceptions they have about the potential dangers associated with sexual activity. Rehabilitation efforts, unfortunately, tend to focus on vocational rehabilitation, and the sexual rehabilitation of the cardiac patient is often virtually ignored (Friedman, 1978). Often simple education, encouragement, and reassurance by the health-care professional will be sufficient to overcome the damaging effects of these misconceptions (Abbott and McWhirter, 1978; Scalzi, Loya, and Golden, 1977). Similarly, brief sex counseling has successfully relieved long-standing erectile dysfunction in diabetic men (Renshaw, 1978). Too often sexual dysfunctions associated with chronic illnesses are assumed to be organic and therefore untreatable.

Sexual functioning also can be disrupted by a variety of drugs that alter libido or disrupt the physiological capacity for erection, orgasm, or ejaculation. Unfortunately, very few controlled studies have been done on the effects of various drugs on sexuality. Kaplan (1974) provides a useful summary table of various drugs that may affect sexual behavior. Providing patients with information that their sexual problems are likely a side effect of medication can be greatly reassuring. For example, some of the drugs commonly used in the treatment of hypertension may cause loss of sexual interest, potency problems, and difficulties with ejaculation (Kaplan, 1974). Not all the antihypertensive drugs produce side effects affecting sexual functioning, and the patient and his physician may wish to consider a change in the type or dosage of the medication.

Patients undergoing surgical procedures such as colostomy, illeostomy, or mastectomy commonly experience profound concerns about their sexual attractiveness and sexual capabilities (Dlin, Perman, and Ringold, 1969; Jamison, Wellish, and Pasnau, 1978). The shock of such procedures is often extreme, not only for patients, but for spouses and other family members as well (Wellish, Jamison, and Pasnau, 1978). Frank discussions of sexual anxieties and concerns with the patient and his or her partner, both before and after surgery, can significantly aid in making a successful adaptation to the changes in body image and sexual functioning. In addition, further information and support can be provided by referring patients to various clubs and associations, such as Ostomy Associations. Providing patients with an opportunity to meet and talk openly with people who have already made a successful sexual adjustment to illness and surgery can be extremely beneficial. Some organizations will send a representative to talk to the patient prior to surgery or while the patient is in the hospital. In addition, these associations can provide helpful reading materials that answer common questions about sex, marriage, fertility, and children (Gambrell, 1973; Norris and Gambrell, 1972; Task Force on Concerns of Physically Disabled Women, 1978).

Too often health-care professionals claim that their patients never ask about sexual matters. This typically reflects more about the professional's attitudes and skill in talking openly about sex than reluctance on the part of patients (Burnap and Golden, 1967; Golden, 1976; Lurie, 1978). Many patients, seen for both nonacute care as well as in the follow-up of chronic problems or health maintenance, will have sexual questions and concerns. A professional who can anticipate these questions, respond openly and warmly, and at times initiate discussions about sex with patients can relieve a great deal of unnecessary guilt, anxiety, and hopelessness (Lurie, 1978). Raising questions about sex with patients in order to provide permission and limited information may feel awkward at first as the professional tries to find a comfortable and natural way to ease into a discussion of sexual matters. Some health-care professionals have begun to routinely include questions about sex as part of the medical "review of systems." Others find it more comfortable to raise questions about sex in the context of the patient's specific presenting complaint. For example, one can ask, "How has this constant pain in your lower back affected your sex life?" "You've been depressed for a few months now. Has this affected your sexual relationship?" "How has this affected your partner's feelings about sex?" Rather than seeming to "come out of the blue," questions phrased in this manner tend to communicate that the professional is interested in understanding the full extent of the patient's problems and concerns.

In some instances, patients will raise questions that can be answered in a brief discussion during the office visit. For example, a woman concerned about engaging in sexual relations during the latter part of pregnancy may only require permission and information, such as "Since you do not have a history of miscarriages or problems with bleeding, you can continue to have sex as long as it feels comfortable. There is very little risk of infection, precipitation of labor, or other complications." In addition, the professional can recommend that if intercourse becomes too uncomfortable, she and her partner can continue to engage in various noncoital sexual activities. If the questions raised by the patient would seem to require more time than the professional has available during that office visit, it may be better to urge the patient to return for a brief appointment specifically to discuss his or her concerns. The professional can respond by saying, "That's an important question, and I'm glad you brought it up. I want to discuss it with you, but unfortunately there are patients waiting to see me and I'm afraid I won't be able to give you my full attention today. I'm going to make a note of your question to remind me, and I'd like to set an appointment for us to talk when I won't be so rushed." Some physicians with busy office practices find it helpful to schedule the patient for either the first or last appointment of the day in order to ensure sufficient uninterrupted time.

In other instances, patients will complain of sexual problems that cannot be handled by permission and limited information. In general, sexual dysfunctions such as painful intercourse, lack of desire, lack of orgasm, erectile dysfunction, and premature ejaculation tend to require more extensive intervention. The resolutions of these problems typically require the professional to recommend a number of specific suggestions designed to change the sexual behavior of the patient and his or her sexual partner.

Providing Specific Suggestions

A variety of sexual exercises or "homework assignments" have been developed for treatment of the common male and female sexual dysfunctions. These exercises include redirection of attention, sensate focus techniques, the squeeze and stop-start techniques, self-stimulation exercises, vaginal muscle training, communication skills training, and so forth (Kaplan, 1974; Masters and Johnson, 1970). The suggestions can be given to the patient alone or to the couple. Before specific suggestions can be given, the professional should obtain a sexual-problem history that includes a brief description of the presenting problem, the onset and course of the problem, the client's conception of the factors causing and maintaining the problem, past treatment and outcome, and current expectations and goals (Annon, 1974).

Based on this problem-focused sex history, the professional can then provide specific suggestions directly relevant to the presenting sexual complaint. It is not possible to describe in detail all the specific suggestions that could be provided by health-care professionals, but a few examples will be provided.

Patients sometimes present their complaints in a very global manner, such as "He/she just doesn't turn me on." The brief sex history often indicates that what the patient specifically means is "I like him to touch my clitoris during intercourse," or "I like her to stroke my penis more vigorously before we have sex," but the patient has never communicated this information to the partner. The health professional can suggest that the patient tell, or show, his or her partner the specific ways the patient likes to be stimulated and perhaps suggest that the patient ask the partner to do the same. Many people are unhappy with the way their partners stimulate them, but never openly communicate their preferences. Encouragement from the professional to communicate directly may be all that is needed. Patients also often complain about the time or circumstances surrounding their sexual activities: "We're always so rushed," "We never have any privacy now that we have kids," "I'm too tired," "He always wants it in the morning," and so forth. For some patients, the suggestion that they not have sex when they are tired and tense and instead try to find times when they both can feel relaxed may be very helpful. Others may need the strong suggestion, and permission from the professional, to rearrange their lifestyle to give their sex life a higher priority: "Sometimes after people have been together for a long time they stop doing things that they used to enjoy. They come home tired from work, eat dinner, put the kids to bed, watch TV, and then try to have sex when they're exhausted. Rather than taking time to talk, relax, and caress each other, they just rush into having intercourse and wonder why it's not as satisfying as it used to be. I've found some couples find it very helpful to plan evenings to be together. When they can't afford to go out and hire a baby sitter, some take the kids to relatives while they stay home and spend the evening together. What's important is that you consciously start to plan relaxed, enjoyable times together and make them a priority for once a week, or once every 2 weeks—whatever seems to work out best for you." Many professionals assume that people would think of these suggestions on their own, but they typically do not. Or they never seem to get around to following through on them. The suggestion from the professional, with one or two follow-up visits to discuss their progress, may be all that is needed to motivate patients to change their behavior. In some cases, however, these difficulties are merely the tip of the iceberg. Couples with sexual dysfunctions may require additional interventions.

In general, the female problems of lack of orgasm (primary orgasmic dysfunction) or dissatisfaction with the frequency, range, or intensity of orgasmic response (secondary orgasmic dysfunction) are frequently responsive to brief treatment over a series of brief office visits. A nine-step masturbation program can be recommended (LoPiccolo and Lobitz, 1978), augmented by further suggestions for exercises to be done with the male partner (Kaplan, 1974; Zeiss, Rosen, and Zeiss, 1978). Educational materials are now available that women can read as a useful adjunct to the counseling (Barbach, 1976; Heiman, LoPiccolo, and LoPiccolo, 1976). Similarly, the male problems of premature ejaculation or erectile dysfunction may be resolved by recommending a series of exercises to be done individually and with a partner (Kaplan, 1974; Zilbergeld, 1978). The man can be encouraged to read about the treatment steps (Zeiss and Zeiss, 1978; Zilbergeld, 1978), including the squeeze technique and stop-start technique, practice the techniques, and meet with the professional to discuss any difficulties implementing the procedures with a partner. Although somewhat standardized treatment steps have been developed for female orgasmic problems and premature ejaculation, most patients will need to discuss their own and their partner's reactions to the treatment steps. Ideally, the partner would attend at least some of the office visits. One of the greatest impediments to changing sexual behavior is a general lifestyle in the patient that does not include time to relax and focus on sensual and sexual pleasure. Part of counseling usually involves helping the patient restructure his or her priorities to include time to focus on resolving the sexual problems. Specific homework assignments and weekly appointments with a professional can help provide the necessary motivation and structure (Zeiss, 1977).

There are at least three limitations involved in providing specific suggestions. First, the patient may not be an appropriate candidate for brief sex therapy because of organic involvement, individual psychotherapy, serious marital maladjustment, and so forth. Some guidelines for this assessment have been developed (Kaplan, 1974; Lobitz and Lobitz, 1978; Masters and Johnson, 1970). Second, the professional may lack the training to comfortably and skillfully recommend the various treatment techniques. The specific suggestions cannot be given in a "cookbook manner." Instead, in many cases, they must be tailored to the individual needs of the patient and sexual partner. Most professionals, even those with considerable experience doing patient counseling and psychotherapy, find that they do not feel competent to treat many of the common dysfunctions without first having supervised training in sex therapy techniques (Price et al., 1978). If the professional does not feel that he or she has the skills to provide specific suggestions, then a referral to an experienced sex therapist would be appropriate. Inadequate counseling would only serve to further the patient's feelings of anxiety and hopelessness, and this sense of failure may prevent the patient from seeking further treatment. The last limiting factor is, of course, time. Weekly counseling appointments, even if they are only for 20 to 30 minutes, may simply be too costly. Some professionals find that patients cannot afford to pay the actual cost for professional time, overhead, and so forth required to deliver extended sex counseling services. Sometimes insurance can help ease the financial burden, but in many cases the professional may find that spending a few sessions discussing the patient's problem and making a supportive referral is the most realistic course of action. Once the professional has decided that a referral for sex therapy is the most appropriate course of action for a particular patient, it might appear that all that needs to be done is to provide the patient with the clinic or therapist's phone number or to call the clinic on the patient's behalf. However, since many promising sex therapy approaches have only been developed recently, most patients will likely have many questions and misconceptions about sex therapy at the time of the referral. It is difficult enough for most patients to share their sexual concerns with their immediate health-care provider, and it is even more difficult for many patients to enter something as unknown and potentially anxiety arousing as sex therapy. The likelihood that the patient will follow through on the referral and will benefit from treatment is greatly increased if the referring professional is sufficiently informed about sex therapy approaches to actively solicit the patient's questions, to anticipate possible misconceptions, and to provide accurate information about what the patient is likely to experience in sex therapy. It is the referring health-care professional, with whom the patient already has an ongoing, trusting relationship, who can exert a powerful and positive influence by his or her handling of the referral process. The following description of the major traditional, current, and emerging approaches to the treatment of sexual problems is presented in an attempt to provide the health professional with sufficient information to make an informative and supportive referral for sex therapy. The description of each treatment model will be followed by a discussion of the more frequent misconceptions held by patients concerning that model. Each description will conclude with some examples of ways that the professional might respond to the patient's questions and concerns.

Traditional (Prior to Masters and Johnson) Treatment Approaches

It is useful to begin a review of sex therapy approaches with a look at the theories and treatment procedures that dominated the field of sexual dysfunction prior to the monumental studies of Masters and Johnson. Many misconceptions held by patients about sex therapy reflect the residual influence of theories that were popular prior to the development of brief sex therapy approaches.

Probably the best-known and most frequently practiced traditional treatment approach is classical psychoanalysis and psychoanalytically oriented individual therapy. These psychodynamic approaches begin with the premise that sexual disorders are symptomatic of underlying unconscious conflicts. Some sexual problems are seen as resulting from sexual fear and guilt that can be traced to unresolved conflicts established in early childhood. For instance, the classical psychoanalytic formulation holds that erectile dysfunction is a neurotic defense against the emergence of conflicting and overpowering affects associated with an unresolved oedipal conflict

(Freud, 1910/1953). Sexual excitement and behavior are believed to reevoke both unconscious incestuous wishes and the castration anxiety and guilt feelings engendered by these wishes; the failure to get or keep an erection is viewed as a means of protecting the man from the emergence of this painful conflict. Other sexual problems are seen as motivated more by anger and protective retaliation than by fear and guilt. For instance, premature ejaculation is believed to be caused by an unconscious desire to "soil" or otherwise frustrate the female sexual partner because of unresolved resentments toward a dominating mother. Still other sexual "problems" are viewed as reflecting a fixation at a less mature stage of psychosexual development as a result of unconscious conflict. For example, a woman who is readily orgasmic in response to clitoral stimulation provided by herself or her partner would be seen as less psychologically mature than women who are orgasmic during intercourse without direct clitoral stimulation. In a more recent discussion of a psychoanalytic viewpoint concerning the development of sexual disorders, Bieber (1974) again argued that sexual dysfunctions play a defensive role against irrational beliefs that are developed in response to parental prohibitions regarding sexual expression and to early child-parent interpersonal dynamics. Prohibitions concerning specific sexual behaviors or sexual feeling in general begin in infancy and eventually result in the belief that sex is wrong or evil. Bieber stated that the parental reaction to the oedipal phase is an important interpersonal dynamic associated with later sexual problems. Parents who fear the child's sexual responses to them, who are sexually competitive with their child, or who view the child as a spouse substitute provide a model of rejection, exploitation, or domination. As the child matures, his or her own sexual relationships are perceived as threatening, and the sexual dysfunction develops as a means of resisting the threatening relationship. Although different underlying conflicts are seen as having etiological significance for specific sexual disorders by different writers, psychoanalytic theorists generally agree that the original underlying conflict or irrational beliefs must be brought into consciousness and resolved before any lasting improvement in sexual functioning and satisfaction can occur. According to Bieber (1974) and O'Connor and Stern (1972), the psychoanalytic treatment of sexual dysfunction is not appreciably different from psychoanalytic approaches to other problems; therefore, the patient who enters psychoanalysis or psychoanalytically oriented individual therapy for sexual problems would be expected to work toward substantial underlying personality change over a period of months or years of treatment.

The conception that most people have about psychotherapy has been heavily influenced by media caricatures of psychoanalytic or psychodynamically oriented individual therapy. Therefore, the health-care professional who plans to refer a patient for more intensive sex therapy should remain alert to the possibility that the patient will perceive the referral as an indication that he or she is "crazy," "mentally ill," or otherwise suffering from unconscious emotional conflicts that will require years of therapy to resolve. The tendency to misperceive the referral is increased when the health-care professional, finding no physical cause for the sexual difficulty, merely informs the patient that "the difficulties are psychologically caused" or "it's all in your head." This is not to deny that there are some patients whose sexual difficulties may be related to long-standing unconscious motivations or may reflect more general personality problems. However, a great majority of patients who are essentially psychologically well-adjusted may still be negatively affected by sexual ignorance, misconceptions about male and female sexual adequacy, lack of awareness of their own sexual responses and preferences, difficulty in communicating about sex with their partners, and anxious, inhibitory, or otherwise painful feelings associated with sexual performance and expression. For most people these negative factors develop as a result of absence of, or faulty, learning, reinforced by an inadequate sex education and a stereotypic view of sexuality generally presented in the media. "Psychologically caused" sexual difficulties are experienced by a great many people who are not neurotic, crazy, or inadequate, and it can be very helpful to communicate this information to patients who typically are feeling quite isolated and "defective" when they first seek help for their problems. With these considerations in mind, once the health-care professional has ruled out a physical basis for the sexual dysfunctions, it may be extremely helpful to explain the contribution of psychogenic factors in the following manner: "The physical examination and laboratory tests do not show any physical cause for your problem, and most sexual problems do not have a physical basis. Instead, what I usually find is that a number of factors, other than physical factors, seem to contribute to sexual problems. These include such things as misinformation about male and female sexuality, unrealistic expectations for how a person or his or her partner should function sexually, and a lack of some basic communication skills. Since most people did not receive very much information about sex, or learn to communicate about sex, it is not surprising to find that many couples experience sexual problems. Fortunately, these problems can be greatly reduced or eliminated by brief sex therapy." This explanation provides information about psychogenic factors, normalizes the experience of sexual dysfunction in a way that does not leave the patient feeling "abnormal" or "crazy," and provides a positive expectation for improvement from treatment.

Because of the popularized impressions of psychotherapy that have been heavily influenced by psychoanalytic and psychodynamic theories, patients who are referred for sex therapy also may believe that they will be required to delve at great length into a probing exploration of their early childhood experiences and memories. Such an exploration may seem irrelevant to the patient who is experiencing painful feelings associated with his or her *current* sexual behavior and relationships. When the patient asks the referring professional, "Will I have to talk about my childhood?" the professional can most accurately respond by saying something to the effect that "sex therapy focuses primarily on the problems you and your partner are experiencing, here and now, rather than on the past. You will probably be asked questions about your childhood, your early sexual experiences, and how you first learned about sex at the beginning of treatment, but the majority of time will be spent on talking about, and trying out, various things you and your partner can do at home together to solve the problems you are experiencing right now. The therapist will suggest various ways to increase the pleasure you receive from sex as well as ways to improve communication with your partner."

Patients who are referred for sex therapy also may fear that therapy will take years to complete and will therefore be very costly. If the patient asks "How long will it take?" it may be helpful to respond by explaining: "Although you may have heard of people being in therapy for many years, sex therapy is considered *brief* treatment and usually takes between 2 to 4 or 5 months to complete, depending on the type of treatment and the particular sexual dysfunction. In general, the more motivated a person is to improve his or her problem, and the more time and energy a person or couple puts into improving their sexual relationship, the more rapid and effective treatment will be."

Brief Sex Therapy for Couples

The pioneering research of Masters and Johnson (1966, 1970) in the areas of human sexual response and sexual inadequacy has encouraged the development of brief couple therapy programs for the treatment of sexual dysfunction. Formalized sex therapy programs can frequently be found in the departments of psychology or psychiatry of major universities or university-affiliated hospitals. Although there are significant differences in the treatment format used by the various couple programs, the treatment techniques used in these brief therapy programs are based on the belief that sexual dysfunctions can usually be treated successfully without requiring extensive underlying personality change. Furthermore, these programs usually treat couples rather than individuals, since the treatment focus is on changing the attitudes, communication, and sexual behaviors within the patient's current sexual relationship. Finally, the treatment format of the couple therapies includes the assignment of sensual activities that are carried out by the couple between counseling sessions. These "homework exercises" are regarded as at least as important as the counseling sessions in facilitating change in the sexual dysfunction.

The most well-known example of couple sex therapy is the pioneering program of Masters and Johnson (1970) at the Reproductive Research Foundation in St. Louis. Couples who participate in the Masters and Johnson program attend daily sessions over a 2-week treatment period. The couple is seen by a therapy team that includes both a male and female therapist. Although Masters and Johnson have isolated numerous factors that they regard as having original etiological significance for the different sexual dysfunctions, their treatment program focuses on the more immediate causes within the couple's present sexual interactions. Prominent among these immediate factors are lack of knowledge about the types and amounts of stimulation that are pleasureable and sufficiently arousing for each partner, inability or reluctance to effectively communicate this knowledge to the sexual partner, anxious preoccupation with sexual performance that results from the fear of continued sexual difficulty, and negative reactions by the sexual partner. Masters and Johnson's (1970) treatment format consists of educational presentations, therapy discussions, and couple exercises that are designed to alleviate sexual-performance concerns, dispel sexual misconceptions, and promote new forms of verbal and nonverbal communication. The underlying rationale for this treatment is Masters's and Johnson's strongly stated belief that a redirection of the couple's attention from performance concerns to the reception of erotic input combined with increased communication of preferences and reactions by both partners will result in complete and pleasureable sexual responses that are involuntary, reflexive reactions to erotic stimulation.

The orientation of Masters and Johnson (1970) is perhaps best reflected in the series of "homework exercises" that are carried out by the couple between counseling sessions. In an effort to allow the couple "to think and feel sexually without orientation to performance," the couple is directed to refrain from intercourse attempts during the first days of treatment. Instead, the couple is instructed to engage in a series of "sensate-focus" activities that are assigned in a sequence that involves gradual increases in sexual intimacy. Initially, the partners are instructed to take turns caressing areas of the body other than the genitals or female breasts. The couple is subsequently asked to include the genitals in the sensate-focus activity, and the partners take turns providing manual stimulation to the genitals. The receiver provides verbal and nonverbal feedback to the giver concerning preferences in the positioning, pressure, direction, and rapidity of the genital caresses. Masters and Johnson frequently assign other noncoital exercises that are appropriate for the specific sexual dysfunction experienced by the couple.

Coital activities are then added to the sensate-focus exercises in the second week of treatment. Initially, the couple might be instructed to maintain vaginal containment after intromission without additional stimulation or pelvic thrusting. Eventually the couple is instructed to resume pelvic thrusting in a series of exercises that include changes in coital positions, forms of additional stimulation, alterations in the timing of stimulation, or other procedures that have been found to be helpful in the treatment of the specific sexual dysfunctions. Masters and Johnson never formally instruct a couple to resume intercourse, but they encourage the couple to approach more spontaneous sexual activity with a continued emphasis on mutual pleasuring rather than on performance goals such as erection or orgasm. Masters and Johnson (1970) reported that 81 percent of the couples who participated in their program showed significant improvement in their sexual functioning by the end of the 2-week treatment period.

A number of variations of the basic Masters and Johnson program have been successfully implemented in other major couple therapy programs. Our couple therapy format at the Human Sexuality Program at UCLA allows couples to continue to live at home and to attend therapy sessions on an outpatient basis. Couples are usually seen once a week for approximately 12 to 15 weeks. Masters and Johnson suggested that a vacation from pressures of work and home removed sources of distraction and provided optimal opportunities for the sexual exercises. However, the excellent clinical-outcome results by a number of programs that have used the weekly session variation (Kaplan, 1974; Lobitz and LoPiccolo, 1972; Meyer, Schmidt, Lucas, and Smith, 1975) suggest that there is no loss of clinical effectiveness when couples are seen on a once-a-week basis in their local areas.

Patients who are specifically referred for couple therapy may evidence several additional misconceptions and concerns about what they will experience in sex therapy. One common belief is that the couple will be asked to have intercourse or to engage in other sexual behavior during their sessions at the sex clinic. Actually, couples are never asked to engage in explicit sexual behaviors in the clinic; the sensual activities occur in the privacy of the couple's home. Apparently this misconception has developed in part because of Masters' and Johson's (1966) earlier studies of the anatomy and physiology of the human sexual response. Nonpatient volunteers did engage in various sexual activities including coitus, masturbation, and stimulation from mechanical, response-monitoring devices during this earlier research. However, the treatment model that evolved from this research did not include the requirement of any sexual behavior during the treatment sessions. However, this misconception is sufficiently anxiety arousing for many couples to prevent them from entering therapy, and the health-care professional should directly address this belief. The professional might say, "Many couples have some concerns about *where* sex therapy takes place— at home or in the office. They are afraid that the therapist will ask them to have sex in the office and will either watch them or make movies of them having sex. On the contrary, all the sexual activities will take place in the privacy of your own home, where you can feel more comfortable and relaxed. You might be asked to keep some notes and describe your sexual experiences to the therapist, but you do not have sex with each other, or with the therapist, while you are at the clinic. The therapist is more of a consultant who will suggest various activities for you to try and then meet with you regularly to discuss the activities you enjoyed and to problem solve when any negative feelings or problems arise. All the sexual activities take place at home.''

Patients frequently have other misgivings about entering couple therapy that are related to misunderstandings about the purpose of having both partners attend therapy. When first informed about couple therapy, it is not uncommon for the patient who is directly experiencing the sexual dysfunction to state "But it is just my problem," "My partner is fully responsive and provides me with all the stimulation that anyone could ask for," or "But my problem occurred with previous partners too, so it couldn't be my partner's fault." Such statements reflect several concerns. Some patients may assume that the purpose of having both partners present in therapy is to determine who is "responsible" or "to blame" for the dysfunctions. Other patients may imagine that the partner's role will be that of an additional therapist who will administer the treatment to the patient but will not benefit directly from therapy. Finally, some patients imagine that the therapists will require the partner to engage in discussions during the sessions or sexual activities between the sessions that will make the partner acutely uncomfortable or will challenge the partner's values. All these feelings may reflect a genuine concern for the sexual partner. In addition, these concerns often reflect the patient's own feelings of inadequacy; our society places great value on independent problem solving, and the presence of the partner may be perceived by the patient as evidence that the patient is unable to solve his or her own problems. The referring professional might best respond to these concerns by reassuring the patient that "although one person may feel that he or she initially had the problem, his or her partner usually has feelings and reactions to the difficulty, both positive and negative, and quickly becomes personally and emotionally involved. Sex therapists tend to view sexual problems as a couple's problem rather than an individual's problem, and since overcoming the problems will require the support and commitment of both members, they think it is best to treat the couple together. While your partner may not have a specific problem he or she wants to solve, we have found that nearly everyone can benefit from receiving accurate sex information and learning how to communicate more effectively. Coming in for treatment will also help your partner to enhance his or her own sexuality and to learn how to be most helpful and supportive to you as you try to overcome the difficulties you are experiencing. Basically you will be learning how to communicate and solve problems together, not just sexual problems, and you are likely to get the most benefit if you are both involved. A good sex therapist also will be sensitive to both your needs and values as well as your partner's needs and values and will not force either of you to do or think anything that is unacceptable to you. I am quite sure that the therapist I have in mind will be sensitive to both of you. If any issues should arise, he or she will also be open to your feedback and will be willing to discuss and resolve your concerns, or your partner's concerns, as they come up in therapy.''

Group-Therapy Approaches to Sex Dysfunction

Although couple therapy appears to be an effective and efficient approach to the treatment of sexual dysfunctions, the couple-therapy model is not without limitations. One obvious limitation is that couple therapy cannot be provided to someone with a sexual dysfunction who either does not have a sexual partner or has a partner who is clearly unable or unwilling to participate in therapy. There are other people for whom the participation of the partner may not even be appropriate, at least initially; one example would be a preorgasmic woman who has not yet discovered her own means of reaching orgasm during solitary activities where the likelihood of orgasm is increased. Several group therapy treatment models have been developed and evaluated in recent years, partly in response to the limitations of the couple-therapy model. Patients without partners have been treated in groups of women (Barbach, 1974; Heinrich, 1976; Schneidman and McGuire, 1976), in groups of men (Lobitz and Baker, 1977; Price et al., 1980; Zilbergeld, 1975), or in mixed groups of men and women (Heinrich and Price, 1977; Obler, 1975). The various group-therapy formats have included a variety of treatment techniques, including the assignment of a graded series of sensual exploration exercises, didactic presentations on sexual anatomy and physiology, exploration of myths and realities concerning male and female sexuality and adequacy, discussions of sexual assertion, social skills training, relaxation training, and general reassurance and support. The group meetings are generally held on a once-a-week basis for a period of 8 to 12 weeks. Some of the group treatment programs have utilized one or two therapists who are of the same sex as the group members (Barbach, 1974; Heinrich, 1976; Lobitz and Baker, 1977), while other programs have included a cotherapist of the opposite sex during some or all of the treatment sessions (Heinrich and Price, 1977; Price et al., 1980; Zilbergeld, 1975). Another variation that has been studied is the treatment of two people in a sexual relationship as members of a group of several couples with sexual dysfunctions that are homogeneous (Golden et al., 1978; Kaplan et al., 1974) or heterogeneous (Leiblum, Rosen, and Pierce, 1976;

LoPiccolo and Miller, 1975; Miller, 1974). Golden et al. (1978) found that the couples' group treatment was equally effective as the more traditional couple therapy model, suggesting that the couples group therapy format may be a cost-effective method for treating sexual dysfunctions. The variety of group procedures outlined here have been found to be effective in the treatment of primary orgasmic dysfunction (Barbach, 1974; Heinrich, 1976; Schneidman and McGuire, 1976), premature ejaculation (Golden et al., 1978; Heinrich and Price, 1977; Kaplan, 1974; Zilbergeld, 1975), and erectile dysfunction (Lobitz and Baker, 1977; Price et al., 1980; Zilbergeld, 1975).

Patients who are specifically referred for group therapy for their sexual difficulties may experience misgivings related to misconceptions about group therapy in general and group therapy for sexual difficulties in particular. Some patients may assume that group therapy would necessarily be a less intensive experience than individual therapy and that their own treatment would suffer from the sharing of the therapy session time with other patients. Many patients may doubt that meeting with others who are experiencing similar difficulties could have any beneficial effect. This feeling is often expressed in such statements as "I want to learn some solutions to my problem and not just hear about other people's problems" or "If these people haven't been able to solve their own problem, how can I expect them to help me with mine?" Other patients may have serious doubts about the potential effectiveness of a treatment modality where they are apparently asked to meet with other members of their own sex rather than with members of the opposite sex. For example, many women may respond to the explicit and subtle messages in our society that tell them that they "can't" or "shouldn't" learn about and be responsible for their own sexuality and that men are the ones who "know about sex." Therefore, some women may specifically ask to be seen by a male therapist rather than participate in a women's group. Many men may also view women's reactions to the sexual difficulty as their focal concern, and they may fail to recognize that their own beliefs about male sexual adequacy are at least equally contributory. Based on early learning experiences that place a premium on competition and forbid the expression of feelings of vulnerability or compassion, many men may experience underlying fears that they will not "measure up" to the other group members or that they will be asked to become "too close or involved" with the other men. Both men and women may experience considerable apprehension about the prospect of talking about their sexual experiences and difficulties in front of a group of people. Finally, patients without partners may wonder how their sexual difficulties could possibly be "cured" or their problem's "solved" during the brief therapy period if they are not likely to find a partner during that period.

The health-care professional might respond to the patient's misgivings about group therapy by saying, "Many people initially feel quite concerned about the prospect of talking about their sexuality in front of a small group of people. But there are some real advantages of meeting as a group. I have found that patients in group therapy quickly feel less isolated and alone as they learn that they are not the only person with the sexual difficulty. You can also benefit greatly from hearing about the roadblocks that other people have encountered during treatment and how they overcome them. Very often the other members can provide suggestions of partial solutions to your difficulties that you or your therapist might not have thought of. This is because they have experienced a lot of the same difficulties. It might be helpful for you to know that one of the purposes of the group will be for you to become the expert about your own sexuality, so that you can communicate this knowledge to your partner. If you do not have a partner now, the group experience can provide you with sensual and communication skills that will be especially helpful when you are in a relationship, and the group may also help you with overcoming some of the fears about sexual performance that might be preventing you from enjoying opportunities to get involved in relationships."

Self-Help Approaches

The group treatment procedures result in a reduction in the amount of professional time required to treat sexual difficulties and an increase in the range of populations that can receive sex therapy. The recent development of self-help treatment approaches, in which the professional's time involvement is further reduced or even eliminated, represents further movement toward the provision of inexpensive sex therapy services for a greatly increased range and number of patients.

There are a number of different selp-help models that are currently available for patients with sexual dysfunctions. Some self-help programs are administered at clinical research centers at major universities. In these programs, individuals or couples are initially evaluated by a professional and are then assigned to a self-administered treatment that includes written or audiovisual materials and a programmed sequence of home assignments. In some programs, the patients have no further contact with the professional, while in other programs, the patients have regularly scheduled telephone contacts, regularly scheduled, but widely spaced therapy appointments, or irregularly scheduled, "trouble-shooting" sessions. There are now also a number of self-help guides that have been written by experienced sex therapists and that may be directly purchased by patients at many bookstores. For example, Barbach (1976) and Heiman, LoPiccolo, and LoPiccolo (1976) have self-help guides for women who wish to learn to attain orgasm or wish to increase the range of activities during which orgasm might occur. Zilbergeld (1978) has recently published a self-help guide that is designed to help men understand male sexuality and to reduce the probability of common sexual problems such as erectile dysfunction and rapid ejaculation. Kass and Stauss (1976) have written a step-by-step treatment guide for couples. Many of these books also can be used as additional reading material for patients who have regular appointments with a therapist.

There is one major misconception about sex therapy that has resulted from the increasing availability of the self-help guides. The health-care professional is likely to encounter patients who have already read one or more of these books, attempted to complete the sequence of activities suggested in the book, but continued to experience the sexual difficulty. The patient may conclude that the suggested sensual activities are ineffective and that a referral for treatment with a therapist who uses similar activities will be equally ineffective. In fact, one recent research study indicated that couples who were given a self-help manual with no additional regular contact with a therapist rarely completed the sequence of assignments suggested in the manual and did not benefit from treatment (Zeiss, 1978). However, couples who used the manual and also had weekly, brief telephone conversations with a therapist benefited as much as patients who had regular office visits with the therapist. Regular contact with a therapist may potentiate those therapeutic effects attributable to interpersonal influence. The regular contacts also may provide a greater opportunity to explore misunderstandings and other roadblocks experienced by the patients in the completion of their homework exercises. With these considerations in mind, the health-care professional who encounters a patient who has had a previous unsuccessful experience with a self-help guide may say, "While that book offers many suggestions, I find that most people are not able to change their sexual behavior without some regular contact with a therapist. The therapist can work with you and your partner to tailor the exercises to your unique needs and problems and also discuss your feelings and reactions with you as you go along. The therapist may ask you to repeat an exercise you have already tried, but he or she will also offer many new ones that were not included in the book. In general, most people have difficulty in attempting to solve their sexual problems by themselves. In fact, one study found that none of the couples who used a self-help guide, and did not meet on a regular basis with a professional were successful. I am optimistic that there is still a lot for you to gain from sex therapy."

The prospect of seeking help for sexual problems and concerns can be anxiety-arousing for most people. We find that many patients will cancel or "forget" to show up for their scheduled office visits to discuss sexual problems, and approximately 50 percent will fail to immediately follow through on a referral for sex therapy. The techniques described in this chapter for providing an informative and supportive referral may increase these percentages considerably. Realistically, some people are simply not willing to change any aspect of their behavior, including their sexual behavior. Other patients will first put off working on their sexual problems in the hope that they will somehow magically disappear. We find that these patients will wait anywhere from a few months to a few years before finally making a firm commitment to seek help for their problems. Once they do, we find most of these patients benefit greatly from brief sex therapy. It is unfortunate that many patients take so long to seek help. An informative and supportive referral may help these patients to overcome their initial misgivings, fears, and inertia and to seek the help they know they want and need. Finally, some patients are so encouraged by just one discussion with a health professional that they immediately begin to talk with their partners about sexual problems they have avoided discussing for years, and many times patients are able to solve some of their problems without any further interventions. These patients are, of course, particularly rewarding. The health-care professional's conscientious effort to include sex education, brief sex counseling, and supportive referrals as part of a regular office practice can immediately or ultimately benefit a great number of patients with sexual concern and difficulties.

References

Abbott, M.A., and McWhirter, D.P. Resuming sexual activity after myocardial infarction. *Medical Aspects of Human Sexuality* 12:18–29, 1978.

Annon, J.S. *The Behavioral Treatment of Sexual Problems,* Vol. 1: *Brief Therapy.* Honolulu: Enabling Systems, 1974.

Annon, J.S. Office management of sexual problems: Brief therapy approaches. *Journal of Reproductive Medicine* 15:129–144, 1975.

Annon, J.S., and Robinson, C.H. The use of vicarious learning in the treatment of sexual concerns. In *Handbook of Sex Therapy,* ed. J. LoPiccolo and L. LoPiccolo New York: Plenum, 1978.

Barbach, L.G. Group treatment of preorgasmic women. *Journal of Sex and Marital Therapy* 1:139–145, 1974.

Barbach, L.G. *For Yourself: The Fulfillment of Female Sexuality.* New York: Anchor Press/Doubleday, 1976.

Bieber, I. The psychoanalytic treatment of sexual disorders. *Journal of Sex and Marital Therapy* 1:5–15, 1974.

Blank, J., and Cottrell, H.L. *I Am My Lover.* Burlingame, Calif.: Down There Press, 1978.

Burnap, D.W., and Golden, J.S. Sexual problems in medical practice. *Journal of Medical Education* 42:673–680, 1967.

Butler, R.A., and Lewis, M.I. *Sex after Sixty.* New York: Harper & Row, 1976.

Dlin, B., Perlman, A., and Ringold, E. Psychosexual response to illeostomy and colostomy. *American Journal of Psychiatry* 126:374–380, 1969.

Frank, E., Anderson, C., and Rubinstein, D. Frequency of sexual dysfunction in "normal" couples. *New England Journal of Medicine* 299: 111–115, 1978.

Freud, S. *Standard Edition of the Complete Psychological Works* Vol. 11. J. Strachey, editor and translator. London: Hogarth Press, 1953. (originally published, 1910).

Friedman, J.M. Sexual adjustment of the postcoronary male. In *Handbook of Sex Therapy,* ed. J. LoPiccolo and L. LoPiccolo. New York: Plenum, 1978.

Gambrell, E. *Sex and the Male Ostomate.* Los Angeles: United Ostomy Association, Inc., 1973.

Golden, J.S. How you can help patients with physical ailments to a better sex life. *Medical Times* 104:83–91, 1976.

Golden, J.S., Price, S., Heinrich, A.G., and Lobitz, W.C. Group versus couple treatment of sexual dysfunctions. *Archives of Sexual Behavior* 7: 593–602, 1978.

Goldfarb, A. Sex and the menopause. *Medical Aspects of Human Sexuality* 4: 64–89, 1970.

Heiman, J., LoPiccolo, L., and LoPiccolo, J. *Becoming Orgasmic: A Sexual Growth Program for Women.* New Jersey: Prentice-Hall, 1976.

Heinrich, A.G. The effect of group and self-directed behavioral-educational treatment of primary orgasmic dysfunction in females treated without their partners. Unpublished doctoral dissertation, University of Colorado, 1976.

Heinrich, R., and Price, S. Group treatment of men and women without partners. Paper presented at the meeting of the American Psychological Association, San Francisco, August 1977.

Hite, S. *The Hite Report.* New York: Dell, 1976.

Hunt, J. *Sexual Behavior in the 1970s.* New York: Dell, 1974.

Jamison, K., Wellish, D., and Pasnau, R. Psychosocial aspects of mastectomy: I. The woman's perspective. *American Journal of Psychiatry* 135: 432–436, 1978.

Julty, S. *MSP (Male Sexual Performance).* New York: Dell, 1975.

Kaplan, H.S. *The New Sex Therapy: Active Treatment of Sexual Dysfunctions.* New York: Quadrangle/The New York Times Book Co., 1974.

Kaplan, H.S., Kohl, R.N., Pomeray, W.B., Offet, A.K., and Hogan,

M.A. Group treatment of premature ejaculation. *Archives of Sexual Behavior* 5: 443–452, 1974.

Kass, D.J., and Stauss, F.E. *Sex Therapy at Home.* New York: Simon and Schuster, 1976.

Kinsey, A.C., Pomeroy, W.B., and Martin, C.E. *Sexual Behavior in the Human Male.* Philadelphia: Saunders, 1948.

Kinsey, A.C., Pomeroy, W.B., Martin, C.E., and Gebhard, P.H. *Sexual Behavior in the Human Female,* Philadelphia: Saunders, 1953.

Leiblum, S.R., Rosen, R., and Pierce, D. Group treatment format: Mixed sexual dysfunctions. *Archives of Sexual Behavior* 5: 313–322, 1976.

Lobitz, W.C., and Baker, E.L. Group treatment of single males with erectile dysfunction. Paper presented at the meeting of the American Psychological Association, San Francisco, August 1977.

Lobitz, W.C., and Lobitz, G.K. Clinical assessment in the treatment of sexual dysfunctions. In *Handbook of Sex Therapy,* ed. J. LoPiccolo and L. LoPiccolo, New York: Plenum, 1978.

Lobitz, W.C., and LoPiccolo, J. New methods in the behavioral treatment of sexual dysfunction. *Journal of Behavior Therapy and Experimental Psychiatry* 3: 265–271, 1972.

LoPiccolo, J. Direct treatment of sexual dysfunction. In *Handbook of Sex Therapy.* ed J. LoPiccolo and L. LoPiccolo. New York: Plenum, 1978.

LoPiccolo, J., and Lobitz, W.C. The role of masturbation in the treatment of orgasmic dysfunction. In *Handbook of Sex Therapy*, ed. J. LoPiccolo and L. LoPiccolo New York: Plenum, 1978.

LoPiccolo, J., and Miller, V.H. A program for enhancing the sexual relationship of normal couples. *Counseling Psychologist* 5: 41–45, 1975.

Lurie, H.J. Sexual complaints in family practice. *Medical Aspects of Human Sexuality* 12: 69–83, 1978.

Masters, W.H., and Johnson, V.E. *Human Sexual Response.* Boston: Little, Brown, 1966.

Masters, W.H., and Johnson, V.E. *Human Sexual Inadequacy.* Boston: Little, Brown, 1970.

Meyer, J.K., Schmidt, C.W., Lucas, M.J., and Smith, E. Short-term treatment of sexual problems: Interim report. *American Journal of Psychiatry* 132: 172–176, 1975.

Miller, N.R. The efficacy of using the Masters and Johnson method, with modification, to rapidly treat sexually dysfunctional couples in a group. *Dissertation Abstracts International* 35(2–A): 824, 1974.

Mooney, T.O., Cole, T.M., and Chilgren, R. *Sexual Options for Paraplegics and Quadriplegics.* Boston: Little, Brown, 1975.

Norris, C., and Gambrell, E. *Sex, Pregnancy, and the Female Ostomate.* Los Angeles: United Ostomy Association, Inc., 1972.

Obler, M. Multivariate approaches to psychotherapy with sexual dysfunctions. *Counseling Psychologist* 5: 55–60, 1975.

O'Connor, J.F., and Stern, L.O. Results of treatment in functional sexual disorders. *New York State Journal of Medicine* 72: 1927–1934, 1972.

Price, S.C., Reynolds, B.S., Cohen, B.D., Anderson, A., and Schochet, B. Group treatment of erectile dysfunction for men without partners. *Archives of Sexual Behavior,* 1980, in press.

Price, S., Golden, J.S., Golden, M., Price, T., Heinrich, A.G., and Munford, P. Training family planning personnel in sex counseling and sex education. *Public Health Reports* 93: 328–334, 1978.

Renshaw, D. Impotence in diabetics. In *Handbook of Sex Therapy*, ed. J. LoPiccolo and L. LoPiccolo New York: Plenum, 1978.

Scalzi, C.C., Loya, F., and Golden, J.S. Sexual therapy of patients with cardiovascular disease. *Western Journal of Medicine* 126: 237–244, 1977.

Schneidman, B., and McGuire, L. Group treatment for nonorgasmic women: Two age levels. *Archives of Sexual Behavior* 5: 239–247, 1976.

Task Force on Concerns of Physically Disabled Women. *Toward Intimacy.* New York: Human Sciences Press, 1978.

Wellisch, D., Jamison, K., and Pasnau, R. Psychosocial aspects of mastectomy: II. the man's perspective. *American Journal of Psychiatry* 135: 543–546, 1978.

Zeiss, A., Rosen, G., and Zeiss, R. Orgasm during intercourse: A treatment strategy for women. In *Handbook of Sex Therapy,* ed. J. LoPiccolo and L. LoPiccolo New York: Plenum, 1978.

Zeiss, R. Self-directed treatment for premature ejaculation: preliminary case report. *Journal of Behavior Therapy and Experimental Psychiatry,* 8: 87–91, 1977.

Zeiss, R., and Zeiss, A. *Prolong your pleasure.* New York: Pocket Books, 1978.

Zilbergeld, B. Group treatment of sexual dysfunction in men without partners. *Journal of Sex and Marital Therapy* 1: 204–214, 1975.

Zilbergeld, B. *Male Sexuality: A Guide to Sexual Fulfillment.* Boston: Little, Brown, 1978.

19 Understanding and Treating Medically Related Sexual Problems

Barry D. Cohen
and *Michael Jospe*

All people will probably, at some time in their lives, have sexual problems. These sexual concerns may be of short duration, or perhaps they will be present for a much longer period of time. It should be no surprise, then, to realize that various medical conditions can result in sexual difficulties for people who suffer them. There are times when sexual dysfunction is the primary problem (information relative to this aspect is discussed in chapter 18). Sexual difficulty also may arise secondary to a medical condition. That is, some aspect of the individual's sexuality becomes involved as a result of medical illness, drug use, or some other health-related event in the individual's life.

If we assume that everyone has sexual concerns from time to time (a fairly safe assumption), then persons with medical conditions have all the usual concerns, plus some specific ones based on their illness. Maintenance of the sexual relationship becomes particularly valuable to persons whose self-esteem is already suffering because of their illness and the isolation and limitations that it imposes (Golden, 1975). It is the responsibility of the health professional to explore such concerns and to assist patients in resolving their sexual difficulties so that this important area of relating can be maintained. This chapter will highlight various medical conditions in which sexual concern is a problem and will discuss the role of health professionals in attempting to assist patients to change this situation.

Enormous change has occurred in our knowledge and understanding of human sexuality during the past 15 years, in large part owing to the pioneering work of Masters and Johnson (1966, 1970, 1979) and to the many who have followed (including Kaplan, 1974, 1979; LoPiccolo and LoPiccolo, 1978).

For many years, "knowledge" about human sexuality came from psychoanalytic theory and not from scientific experimentation. The notion of having to make complex dynamic formulations of sexual problems may have scared many physicians and other health professionals away from the area. Now that different understandings of both the etiology and circumstances that perpetuate sexual concerns exist, health professionals may be

283

able to be more comfortable and convinced that there are pragmatic, usable techniques available to them. There is little doubt that the theoretical jungle hiding most attempts to understand human sexuality was one that obscured any reasonable framework for an understanding of both function and dysfunction. As impressive as Freudian or Reichian (and other analytic and neoanalytic) views were to theoreticians, it remained extremely difficult to draw connections between the supposed causal processes (largely unconscious) leading to any observed manifestation and that behavior itself. This was particularly true when attempting to be what was in fact technological: applying theories in practical ways to problems that needed to be solved. Persons not trained in psychiatry thus found themselves facing an extremely complex system, with little knowledge of how to translate theory into therapy. This dilemma, in addition to the prejudices and biases of health-care practitioners themselves about dealing with any aspect of sexuality, doubtless led to a situation in which many practitioners simply ignored their patients' sexuality altogether, even in circumstances where the need to address the subjext was obvious. Practitioners did not just ignore their patients' sexual *problems,* they ignored and denied that patients were sexual at all. It was simply easier to not put oneself in a discomforting situation in that way. What the work of Masters and Johnson and their followers did, was to allow good empirical connections to be made between concepts and what was observed, thus bringing the whole matter of sexuality back into the realm of scientific systems, albeit rather elementary ones at this early stage of the research. As a consequence, we were able to begin gaining an understanding of human sexuality that allowed us to be aware of physiological, behavioral, cognitive, and affective processes and their complex interactions; therapy then became a matter of applying in practice what had been learned in principle from initial empirical investigations in the area. For the first time it was possible to formulate answers to questions of the relationships among physiology, behavior, affect, cognition, and experience and to apply these formulations in retraining patients to experience their sexuality in new and different ways that would not perpetuate their dysfunction.

At about the time that these advances in knowledge of human sexuality were just beginning to find their way to both professional and lay audiences, Burnap and Golden (1967) surveyed physicians in a large Western city. The purpose of the survey was to estimate the incidence of sexual problems in their patients. The results were what was expected at that time. Family practitioners, gynecologists, and urologists estimated about 15 percent of their patients had sexual problems. Psychiatrists reported 77 percent, and internists reported 6 percent. However, most physicians in very specialized or surgically oriented practices reported no significant incidence of sexual problems in their patients. Even among the primary-care physicians, reports of sexual problems associated with acute and chronic diseases, physical disabilities, and surgical procedures were negligible. Golden (1979) reports that this finding seemed reasonable at that time. However, in subsequent work, he and his associates questioned patients directly about sexual matters. Patients similar to those in the 1967 survey reported that they, in fact, did experience sexual problems after surgery, immobilization, or other aspects of their illness. Golden (1979) concludes that the apparent discrepancy was due to the fact that the physicians in the original survey had never asked their patients about sexual problems.

At this point, one may question why patients do not take responsibility for initiating the discussion of difficulty in sexual functioning. Even with increased awareness about human sexuality, most people are reluctant to discuss sexual issues. The old taboo that "sex is something you do, not something you talk about" lingers on. Thus the scene is set for a lack of attention to sexual concerns in medical settings. Both the patient and the physician or other health professional are reluctant to initiate a sexually oriented discussion. Perhaps the health professional assumes that if sexual problems were present, the patient would volunteer the information. At the same time, the patient, viewing the physician or other health professional as the "expert," assumes that if sexual difficulties were a part of the illness, then the health professional would ask about such problems. Thus, when the health professional fails to include sexuality in the discussion, the patient assumes it should not be discussed. The result, as Golden (1979) describes it, is that health professional and patient are deadlocked in a "conspiracy of silence." Golden continues by stating that patients are correct in their expectations. Since the health professional, in all other areas, takes a review of systems and includes a history of complaints, there is no reason to exclude the area of sexual functioning. In fact, a main goal of this chapter is to stress that all health professionals should be open to the possibility that because of the presence of a medical condition, any patient might have sexual problems, until one seeks and obtains (rather than assumes) proof to the contrary.

If it is the responsibility of the health professional to initiate discussions of sexual concerns with patients, a position that we are advocating, (see also Crewe, 1979; Wallston, Calhoun, and Cohen, 1977), then the next issue is evident: *How can the health professional become more comfortable in talking with patients about sexual problems?* This is discussed elsewhere in this book (see chapters 18 and 21), but several important points can be stated here. Knowledge is an essential element for increasing one's comfort in approaching sexually oriented discussions. More and more, health professional training programs are including human-sexuality courses in the curriculum. Recent legislation in several states requires that health professionals have human-sexuality training in order to be eligible for licensure or relicensure. Comfort in sexual discussions can then be increased merely through practice. Health practitioners often worry that raising the subject of a patient's sexuality will lead to an embarrassing silence. It is interesting to discover in practice that most patients will not, in fact, be offended or embarrassed, and this discovery can assist the health professional in raising sexual questions. With basic knowledge and increasing comfort, the next fear most often is "What will I do if the patient says there are sexual problems? It is like opening up Pandora's box." Many health professionals do feel that they lack training in the treatment of sexual problems once they are diagnosed. For the physician who feels untrained in talking to patients about nonmedical aspects of sexuality, it is important to realize that he or she can begin the discussion with medical aspects of sexuality. This is especially relevant to our topic, since the etiology of the sexual concern stems from the primary medical problem. It is appropriate to provide basic information and give patients permission for experimentation and broadening of the sexual repertoire. The health professional therefore must be in touch with his or her own strengths or weaknesses and be ready to refer to more skilled and knowledgeable colleagues at the appropriate time.

For those health professionals who decide to refer, it is obviously very important to know the most appropriate referral resources in the home community. In chapter 18, Reynolds and Price discuss the basic issues involved with the "when to refer" question. In order to make the decision to refer, the health professional must be aware that the condition exists, which is particularly a problem with sexual difficulties secondary to medical conditions. Thus the reader who is certain he or she would refer such cases is encouraged to continue reading, so that the likelihood of recognizing and acknowledging sexual concerns in medical patients is increased.

Once the decision has been made by the health professional to get involved in a discussion of the patient's sexual concerns, then an effort must be made to include the patient's spouse or significant other. If a person with a medical condition has a sexual problem, then so does the partner. All too often the partner, and hence his or her sexual needs, are neglected by the health professional (Cohen, Wallston, and Wallston, 1976). For example, a woman whose husband has suffered a myocardial infarction may be terrified at the prospect of resuming sexual relations. She may be fearful that this activity would bring on another attack and may also feel selfish and guilty for imposing on someone who is "sick." Her spouse, having heard only that he should "take it easy," is also afraid to initiate sexual activity. At this point, both these people have a sexual problem, and both require the attention of their physician or other health professional. In working with couples, one should also recall the Masters and Johnson (1970) model for dual sex therapy teams. Whenever possible, a male-female health-professional team should be utilized for discussion of sexual concerns in heterosexual couples. Biggs and Spitz (1975) put this well when they said, "In any sexual dysfunction, there is no uninvolved partner. No male distress lacks female contribution; the converse also pertains. Furthermore, since no male can ever fully comprehend femaleness (nor the converse), we endorse therapy for sexual inadequacy by both a female and a male serving as cotherapists."

Sexuality and Physical Illness

The capacity to function sexually may be impaired by physical illness and by significant physical disabilities. This may occur not only from the organic difficulties associated with chronically debilitating diseases, but also from the psychological problems arising because of the presence of any significant illness. Whether the disease process interferes directly with the functioning of the sex organs or only indirectly by producing psychological impediments does not matter. The point is that there may well be a disruption in sexual functioning (and thus in sexual health). One study of 34 men and 21 women adapting to chronic illnesses reported that 78 percent of the subjects showed a decline in the frequency of sexual activity (Sadoughi, Leshner, and Fine, 1971). These individuals were attempting to cope with emphysema, arthritis, stroke, or amputation. Nearly half these subjects indicated that they would have benefited from discussing their sexual concerns prior to their medical discharge. There are ways for patients, even those with severe organic disruption in their sexual functioning, to enjoy sexual relationships (Golden and Milne, 1978). Physical illness or disability does not mean loss of sexuality. Increasingly more attention is being paid to the sexual concerns of various medical populations. Spinal cord injury (Higgins, 1979), cardiac disease (Scheingold and Wagner, 1976; Cohen et al., 1976), diabetes mellitus (Renshaw, 1978), and chronic renal failure (Abram et al, 1975; Golden and Milne, 1978) are medical areas that have been receiving more attention in relation to secondary sexual problems. Since it is beyond the scope of this chapter to explore these areas in depth, the reader is referred to the stated references as good beginning sources for obtaining more detailed information.

Many people who seek health services are "at risk" for experiencing sexual problems. Potential threats to sexual health include anatomic disruptions, changes in one's physiology, and body-image distortion (Woods, 1979). In order to provide an overview of the possible sexual problems resulting from various medical conditions, tables 19-1, 19-2, and 19-3 are presented. Table 19-1 looks at anatomic disruptions, which are perhaps best represented by spinal-cord injury. The cord-injured person has sustained irreversible neural damage and thus has some level of disruption with

Table 19–1
Anatomic Disruptions and Their Hypothesized Interferences with Sexual Health

System	Hypothesized Mechanism of Interference
Central and peripheral nervous systems	
Spinal-cord injury Spinal-cord tumors Herniated disk Multiple sclerosis Spina bifida Amyotrophic lateral sclerosis	Disrupts integrity of peripheral nerves and spinal cord reflexes involved in sexual response, for example, erection
Tumors of the frontal or temporal lobes Cerebrovascular accident Trauma to the frontal or temporal lobes	May interfere with function of the centers controlling sexual drive
Cardiovascular system	
Thrombus formation in vessels of the penis Leriche syndrome Sickle cell disorders Leukemia Trauma to vasculature supplying sexual organs	May interfere with the blood supply to the penis, thus interfering with erection
Genital system	
Radical perineal prostatectomy Abdominal perineal resections Lumbar sympathectomy Rhizotomies	May destroy nerve supply, interfering with sensory and motor aspects of sexual response May result in disturbed ejaculation May result in impotence as well as disturbed ejaculation
Absence of the penis or penile injury Imperforate hymen Congenital absence of the vagina	Precludes or discourages intromission
Obstetric trauma or poor episiotomy Damage to pubococcygeus	Leaves gaping vaginal opening or painful scarring, discouraging intercourse

Source: N.F. Woods, Problems of sexuality. In *Medical-Surgical Nursing,* ed. W.J. Phipps, B.C. Long, and N.F. Woods (St. Louis, Mo.: Mosby, 1979). Adapted from H.S. Kaplan, *The New Sex Therapy* (New York: Brunner/Mazel, 1974). Reprinted with permission of the publisher.

Table 19–2
Physiologic Interferences with Sexual Health

Interferences	Hypothesized Mechanism of Action
Systemic diseases	
Pulmonary disease Renal disease Malignancies Infections Degenerative diseases Some cardiovascular diseases	Debility, pain, and depression probably interfere with sexual libido as well as expression

Table 19-2 continued

Interferences	Hypothesized Mechanism of Action
Metabolic disruptions	
Cirrhosis Mononucleosis Hepatitis	Hepatic problems in the male result in estrogen build-up due to inability of the liver to conjugate estrogens; similar processes occur in the female along with general debility
Hypothyroidism Addison's disease Hypogonadism Hypopituitarism Acromegaly Feminizing tumors Cushing's disease	By depression of CNS function, general debilitation, and depression libido may be decreased, and impaired arousal in the female and impaired erectile abilities in the male may result
Diabetes mellitus	With diabetes there is a hypothesized relationship between neuropathic and vascular damage and impotence or impaired sexual response in women
Diseases of the genitalia	
Priapism Peyronie's disease Balantitis Phimosis Genital herpes Trauma to the penis Vaginal infections Senile vaginitis Vulvitis Leukoplakia Bartholin cyst Allergic response to vaginal sprays, deodorants Vaginitis following radiation therapy Pelvic inflammatory disease Fibroadenomas Endometriosis Uterine prolapse Anal fissures, hemorrhoids Pelvic masses Ovarian cysts	Each of these problems involves damage to the genital organs, which may result in painful intercourse
Prostatitis Urethritis	Local irritability, damage to genitals, and consequent interference with reflex mechanisms involved in erection and ejaculation
Medical or surgical castration	
Orchiectomy Radiation therapy Ovariectomy, adrenalectomy	Lowered androgen levels depress libido and lead to impotence, retarded ejaculation, and/or impaired sexual responsiveness

Source: N.F. Woods, Problems of Sexuality. In *Medical-Surgical Nursing,* ed. W.J. Phipps, B.C. Long, and N.F. Woods (St. Louis, Mo.: Mosby, 1979). Adapted from H.S. Kaplan, *The New Sex Therapy* (New York: Brunner/Mazel, 1974). Reprinted with permission of the publisher.

Table 19-3
Some Health Problems Resulting in Body-Image Changes that May Raise Sexual Concerns

Surgically Induced	Traumatically Induced	Others
Mastectomy	Burns	Dermatologic disorders
Ostomy	Lacerations, scarring	Obesity
Hysterectomy	Amputations	Congenital anomalies of the sexual organs, such as absence of penis, hypospadias
Amputations of limb(s)		Unusual breast size, including immaturity or hypertrophy

Source: N.F. Woods, Problems of sexuality. In *Medical-Surgical Nursing*, ed. W.J. Phipps, B.C. Long, and N.F. Woods (St. Louis, Mo.: Mosby, 1979). Adapted from H.S. Kaplan, *The New Sex Therapy* (New York: Brunner/Mazel, 1974). Reprinted with permission of the publisher.

his or her usual method of sexual functioning. Table 19-2 presents physiological disturbances. Physiological disturbances, such as those associated with diabetes, probably change the person's ability to respond sexually by interfering with the vasocongestive and sensory-motor conduction that are essential in human sexual response. Table 19-3 present body-image distortion problems that may affect sexual functioning. Such problems may occur after surgery or traumatic injury. Some conditions may involve disruptions in more than one area, so the tables should not be read as mutually exclusive. For example, chronic renal failure, a physiologic disturbance, also may involve body-image distortion, and both these factors must be taken into account when considering sexual-functioning concerns.

Drugs required for proper treatment of a primary medical condition may have secondary effects on sexual functioning. Many drugs, including hypotensive agents, antibiotics, and the mood-altering drugs such as tricyclic antidepressants and the phenothiazines, may interfere with sexual functioning. Physicians caring for patients when these or other drugs are administered should be on the lookout for sexual side effects. At times it is possible to alter the dosages or to substitute others of similar classes so that the likelihood of negative effects on sexual functioning is either reduced or eliminated.

When a medical condition becomes severe enough to warrant hospitalization or to cause a person to feel "sick" much of the time, then these factors must be considered in light of that person's sexual functioning. As Woods (1979) points out, from the time of admission to a hospital until discharge, the person identified as "patient" is subjected to a wide variety of intrusive experiences that have the ability to minimize sexual integrity as well as human dignity. Hospitalization will mean separation from one's sexual partner, and when the partner is present, the lack of privacy will inhibit most expressions of warmth and sexual caring. These environmental problems will all compound whatever other effects the medical condition is having on the patient's sexual functioning.

Even without hospitalization, "sick" people may experience a variety of environmental infringements on their sexual functioning. Fatigue, weakness, and/or reduced activity may lead to social isolation, increased dependency, and decreased feelings of sexual worth or ability. Whether a patient is seen in an inpatient or outpatient setting, the health professional must remember that the patient is still a sexual being. Thus the health professional has an integral role in attempting to prevent the environmental influences that might lead to secondary sexual dysfunction.

It is an interesting experience to talk with both health-care professionals and patients about their experiences when sexuality has not been dealt with. Two examples from our own clinical experience might help reinforce some of the points we have made. A nurse with whom one of us worked was a woman who for many years was in charge of the main (day) shift on a spinal-cord-injury unit in a large hospital. As is commonly the case, most of the patients were young, vigorous males in the age range of late adolescence to the midtwenties. Very few of the patients were females. The nurse talked about how, in their discomfort with even thinking about their patients' changed sexuality, medical personnel either never mentioned it at all or else gave the topic a superficial glossing over. It was not uncommon for the only mention of sexuality to be made at times when it was seen as a problem, such as when the nurse would become embarrassed if, in the course of daily toileting of a paraplegic or quadriplegic man, the patient would become erect, either apparently spontaneously or through direct stimulation of the genitals. The nurse, reacting with embarrassment or discomfort, would reinforce the patient's already low self-image and distorted body image, leading to even more distortion on the patient's part and more feelings of disgust with his changed sensuality and sexuality. The nurse, in turn, would reinforce precisely the "conspiracy of silence" that Golden (1979) talks about and that we mentioned earlier in this chapter. The situation on the unit was not rectified until a new physiatrist came to the hospital and, seeing what was going on with regard to the subject of sexuality, immediately introduced a series of workshops, weekend-long seminars, and attitudinal-change educational materials for the nurses and for his physician colleagues. The opening up of the area did not occur overnight, but it did occur, much to the relief of all concerned, who were now able to deal with patient's changed sexuality in much the same way that they dealt with any other changes consequent to the traumatic injury. Significantly, the psychiatrist, nurses, and consulting psychologist also began dealing with patients' significant others, including them in the discussion, assessment, and treatment planning of sexual difficulties. This was done in much the same way as the spouses, lovers, or mates were routinely included in such aspects of the patient's pre- and postdischarge functioning as self-help skills, ambulation, education, mobility, or whatever special needs had to be attended to.

Adults who have cerebral palsy (CP) have often described to us that, because their condition often manifests itself in a variety of physical problems that are very conspicuous to other people, it is not at all unusual for non-CP people to have an astonishing array of responses when they find out that CP people are sexual too. Such responses range from disgust to sheer amazement. A particularly bright patient with whom one of us was in contact for about a year described the way in which men would react to her relatively mild speech slurring by immediately setting up barriers when she said anything. Another woman whose severe athetoid posture of the extremities was not amenable to orthopedic surgery but who nevertheless learned an extremely wide repertoire of maneuvers to increase her mobility, described how even CP males would be frightened of approaching her in ways even remotely sexual. She asked her physician to arrange a referral to a psychologist so she could learn how to be more socially and sexually asser- tive. Her physician was aghast at her request, not only because "women are not supposed to do that sort of thing" (that is, be sexually assertive), but also because it never occurred to the physician that just because he might not find her sexually attractive did not mean that she was not capable of being sexual, or that other people would not find her attractive. Neverthe- less, the patient was referred, and her goals for coming to therapy were met.

Looking at tables 19–1 through 19–3, we can see that the effects of medical conditions can be quite varied. In spinal-cord-injured males, there is a direct disruption of peripheral nerves and spinal cord reflexes involved in erection. In cerebral palsy, the innervation might be quite intact, so that there is no interference at all with sexual functioning per se. Rather, prob- lems might arise because of problems with body posture, mobility, spasticity, and appearance. What the conditions can have in common, though, are the things that every health-care professional should attend to in the case of every patient presenting with a medically related sexual dif- ficulty. First, the matter of the patients' view of himself or herself as a sexual being must be attended to. Such views can be radically different depending on when the condition arose: a person born with cerebral palsy will probably view his or her sexuality in a more integrated way than one who has suffered a sudden, traumatic injury. Whatever the case, though, the helping professional needs to be very sensitive to the patient's particular needs. Second, the way in which the person will practice his or her sexuality might be quite different from the usual, societally accepted ways in which people without physical disability, injury, or illness will practice theirs. The treatment for the man with spinal-cord injury involves essentially learning how to maximize the functioning that remains. The treatment for the woman with athetoid cerebral palsy involves discovering the many ways in which she needs to learn to utilize positions other than the stereotyped ones of romance, dirty jokes, or traditional sex manuals. Treatment of both involves a clear perception on the part of the health-care practitioner that any way in which patients can achieve sexual gratification can be satisfying—whether it be masturbation, with a partner, or any variation thereof. Such a view therefore must be clearly and unequivocally presented to the patient as being good for that patient, something not to be judged by what other people do, say, or think.

Sexuality throughout the Lifespan

Much of the discussion in this chapter has approached sexuality as an adult concern. This reflects the general state of the literature on human sexuality. That is, much of it deals mostly with adult sexuality and problems of sexuality specific to the older population. This seems to ignore the sexual nature of infants and children and denies the developmental patterns of human sexuality. The sexual concerns of children and adolescents must be addressed by the health professional, particularly when there is a medical condition that may influence sexual functioning. For example, certain anatomical problems (for example, hypospadias, spina bifida, cerebral palsy, spinal-cord injuries) may affect psychosexual development. In addition, the parents may not be comfortable with thinking about their child as a sexual being. Thus the health professional must work not only with the child, but also with the parents.

On an inpatient service, the staff must be sensitive to the child's sexual desires. There may well be much sexual acting out, a "normal" part of that stage of growth, which is compounded by long hospitalization. Staff feelings often are quite strong in such cases and must be discussed.

We have frequently encountered situations in which we have been called to attend to a sexual "problem," only to find that what is going on is something quite innocuous, such as a child masturbating or two or three children "playing doctor." Such problems arise in any situation and bear no particular relationship to the health-care setting. More problematical can be a situation such as the one encountered by one of us recently. A 15-year-old boy with an inguinal rhabdomyosarcoma was referred to us after initial treatment in the oncology service of a hospital in another state. Following surgery and extensive radiation (and continuing chemotherapy), the boy is doing fairly well. The problem in relation to his sexuality is twofold. First of all nobody told him he would have to undergo a unilateral orchidectomy. Second, he was not informed at all that after surgery he would show retrograde ejaculation. The boy had been quite sexually active prior to the diagnosis and initial treatment for his cancer. Needless to say, the shock and tremendous adjustment to living with cancer were compounded when he discovered he had only one testicle and that he could no longer see his ejaculate. Since nobody at all in the other treatment facility had broached the subject of his sexuality, he kept his part of the conspiracy of silence and went through untold emotional anguish. One of the things we do quite routinely is discuss patient sexuality (at age-appropriate levels, of course) with every child and adolescent on our oncology service. When the patient discovered that someone was going to be able to discuss his sexual concerns with him, he was at first very resistant, but once a trust level had been established, he was enormously relieved to be able not only to just talk, but also to ask many questions. The sexual sequelae of this treatment and surgery were explained by the oncologist, a urologist, and the psychologist, and the patient expressed amazement that the previously taboo topic was approached at all, much less discussed at such length. His concerns about retrograde ejaculation were allayed to a significant degree, and a testicular prosthesis allowed most of his deep-seated fears about the awful symbolism of being castrated to disappear. Many other aspects of his sexual functioning were discussed with him over the course of the following few months. The case illustrates how very wrong we can be when we do not deal with children's and adolescents' sexuality and how great an extent of suffering can be caused by such a shortsighted and incomplete approach to young people.

The other end of the lifespan, namely, aging persons, also warrants discussion here. It is often the case that older people are stereotyped as not being sexual (see chapter 15). Masters and Johnson (1966) found that the process of human sexual response in all phases slows with aging, but at no point does sexual responsiveness stop in either males or females. It may take longer to reach orgasm, the sexual experience itself may be shorter and less intense, and certain physiological changes may occur, but sexual responsiveness definitely continues as the individual ages. The stereotype of the aged as nonsexual is further compounded when medical conditions exist. The health professional may make every effort to deny that his or her older patients could possibly have sexual concerns secondary to their medical conditions. Although many do not expect it, the aged, even when ill, are sexually active at times.

This brings up the issue of the role of expectations in sexual functioning. With regards to aging, if there is an expectation that sex stops at age 50, then persons over 50 years of age may not question their sexual responsiveness or lack thereof. If there is an expectation that a paraplegic or quadriplegic is a nonsexual being, that person does not function sexually. When there is a vague societal expectation, the effect on sexual functioning may be serious. However, when there is a health professional's negative expectation, effects may include sexual dysfunctioning; this is the notion of the iatrogenic or "doctor-caused" dysfunction. With increasing education and heightened awareness of these issues, all persons with medical conditions—children and the aged, spinal cord injured, and those with renal failure, to name just a few populations—may no longer be denied the opportunity to function as sexual beings.

Conclusion

The purpose of treating sexual concerns in persons with or without primary medical conditions is to try to improve the quality of life. In discussing sexual concerns, every effort should be made to do things that give these patients a sense of being worthwhile, a sense of positive self-esteem. If something can be done to improve the sexual functioning of patients with varying medical conditions, then it makes simple sense that these patients will benefit. To the extent that they recapture the ability to function sexually or maintain the ability that might be threatened, the patients could feel more adequate (Golden and Milne, 1978). Thus there is the likelihood not only of maintaining the relationship that might have existed prior to the onset of the medical condition, but also of being able to enjoy the pleasure that comes from sexual contact with a partner. In addition, one generally feels less "sick" if one is able to do what "healthy" people can do.

As outlined in this chapter, there are varying medical conditions, as well as aspects of hospitalization and sick role behavior, that may result in patients' secondary sexual concerns. It is the responsibility of the health professional to initiate the discussion about sexual functioning. In order to be able to do this, health professionals may have to work hard to gain comfort in having such discussions, in revising their sexual expectations of others, and in broadening their notions of what is normal and appropriate sexually.

It is very important for health-care providers to raise the issue of their patients' sexuality; to not ignore that everyone is sexual; to not perpetuate the conspiracy of silence; to recognize the value of being able to talk about sexuality via the medical facts; if need be, to include the patient's significant other in discussion and treatment; and to be sensitive to the individual patient's special needs. Only in these ways will we acknowledge that almost everyone has the capacity to function sexually and that all people are entitled to as fulfilling a sexual life as is possible.

References

Abram, H.S., Hester, L.R., Sheridan, W.F., and Epstein, G.M. Sexual functioning in patients with chronic renal failure. *Journal of Nervous and Mental Disease* 160:220–226, 1975.

Biggs, M., and Spitz, R. Treating sexual dysfunction: The dual-sex therapy team. In *Human Sexuality: A Health Practitioner's Text,* ed. R. Green. Baltimore: Williams & Wilkins, 1975.

Burnap, D.W., and Golden, J.S. Sexual problems in medical practice. *Journal of Medical Education* 42:673–680, 1967.

Cohen, B.D., Wallston, B.S., and Wallston, K.A. Sex counseling in cardiac rehabilitation. *Archives of Physical Medicine and Rehabilitation* 57:463–464, 1976.

Crewe, N.M. The psychologist's role in sexual rehabilitation of people with physical disabilities. *Sexuality and Disability* 2:16–22, 1979.

Golden, J.S. Sexuality and the chronically ill. *Pharos of Alpha Omega Alpha* 38:76–79, 1975.

Golden, J.S. How you can help patients with physical ailments to a better sex life. *Medical Times* (September 1976).

Golden, J.S. Sexuality and physical illness: Breaking the conspiracy of silence. *Sexual Medicine Today* 3:38, 1979.

Golden, J.S., and Milne, J.F. Somatopsychic sexual problems of renal failure. *Dialysis and Transplantation* 7:879–890, 1978.

Higgins, G.E. Sexual response in spinal cord injured adults: A review of the literature. *Archives of Sexual Behavior* 8:173–196, 1979.

Kaplan, H.S. *The New Sex Therapy*. New York: Brunner/Mazel, 1974.

Kaplan. H.S. *Disorders of Sexual Desire*. New York: Brunner/Mazel, 1979.

LoPiccolo, J., and LoPiccolo, L., eds. *Handbook of Sex Therapy* New York: Plenum, 1978.

Masters, W., and Johnson, V. *Human Sexual Response*. Boston: Little, Brown, 1966.

Masters, W., and Johnson, V. *Human Sexual Inadequacy*. Boston: Little, Brown, 1970.

Masters, W., and Johnson, V. *Homosexuality in Perspective*. Boston: Little, Brown, 1979.

Renshaw, D.C. Impotence in diabetes. In *Handbook of Sex Therapy*, ed. J. LoPiccolo and L. LoPiccolo. New York: Plenum, 1978.

Sadoughi, W., Leshner, M., and Fine, H.L. Sexual adjustment in a chronically ill and physically disabled population: A pilot study. *Archives of Physical Medicine and Rehabilitation* 52:311–317, 1971.

Scheingold, L.D., and Wagner, N.L. *Sound Sex and the Aging Heart: Sex in Mid and Later Years with Special Reference to Cardiac Disturbance*. New York: Human Sciences Press, 1974.

Wallston, K.A., Calhoun, G., and Cohen, B.D. The nurse's role in counseling patients about sexuality. In *Social Perspectives in Nursing: Current Trends.* ed. M. Miller and B. Flynn. St. Louis: Mosby, 1977.

Woods, N.F. *Human Sexuality in Health and Illness*. St. Louis: Mosby, 1979.

20 What Health-Care Professionals Need to Know about Gay Men and Lesbians

John C. Gonsiorek

Even using the conservative figure of 5 percent, there are an estimated 11 million gay men and lesbians in the United States. If one accepts less conservative estimates, the figure approaches or exceeds 20 million. In many of the most basic aspects of health care, the needs of this minority population parallel those of the general population. However, in a number of crucial areas, this group presents many unique health-care needs.

For example, some epidemiologists estimate that gay males may account for as much as 50 percent of new cases of gonorrhea. In various cities that have concentrations of gay men, there are virtual epidemics of hepatitis in these gay male populations. Intestinal disorders such as amebiasis and shigellosis, which have low base rates in the general population, have substantially higher base rates in gay male populations of certain cities.

These unique health-care needs extend particularly into psychosocial areas. Many lesbians and gay men are denied the support and comfort of their friends and lovers in times of sickness by insensitive hospital personnel who, overtly or covertly, exlude all but "family members." Lesbian mothers in particular, but also gay fathers, fearful of potential legal repercussions, often find health-care and social-services agencies lax and insensitive about volatile confidentiality issues and overtly hostile to such parents. These agencies and their services are therefore often inaccessible. Many lesbians must often endure a double insensitivity to their status as unmarried and female from health-care professionals who provide gynecological and related services.

Faced with prejudice and insensitivity from many traditional agencies, gay men and lesbians across the country have been creating and turning to alternative agencies for health-care, advocacy, mental-health, social-welfare, and chemical-dependency services. These agencies are typically unfunded or underfunded. In areas where established professionals avoid such agencies, these agencies and their clients suffer from lack of professional expertise, relying instead on well-meaning but more limited paraprofessionals and laypersons. This, then, creates a situation ripe for exploitation by health-care providers, both gay and straight, with weak skills and weaker ethical standards, but a convincing "sympathetic" pitch.

In the wake of the recent backlash against gay civil rights, physical and sexual assaults by heterosexual males against gay men and lesbians (or those they perceive to be gay or lesbians) have increased dramatically. Emergency rooms and crisis centers are typically poorly informed about this problem, heavy-handed, and insensitive to such clients and lacking adequate aftercare provisions for assault victims. The discrimination and social-economic problems faced by aging Americans can be especially strong for older lesbians and gay men, who have few family members to serve as their advocates and who may be exceedingly distrustful of existing agencies.

While many of these problems require some measure of broader political solutions, most can be at least ameliorated by educating health-care professionals in the direction of greater sensitivity to the needs of lesbians and gay men. While some of the specific topic areas just noted will be detailed later in this chapter, a few basic facts and principles will first be presented in the hope of being generally useful.

Core Information on Gay Men and Lesbians

First, there is no inherent relationship between sexual orientation and psychological adjustment or psychopathology. Despite the removal of homosexuality in 1973 from the American Psychiatric Association's official list of mental disorders, the American Psychological Association's support of this resolution in 1975, and a preponderance of evidence repeatedly suggesting that personality differences between homosexual and heterosexual populations (when found at all) are in the normal range, a number of writers (usually of a psychoanalytic persuasion) continue to advocate an illness model of homosexual behavior (for example, Bieber, 1976; Socarides, 1975). Given what is currently known about homosexual behavior, this stance borders on the professionally irresponsible.

There are literature reviews available (for example, Gonsiorek, 1977) that summarize the relevant literature in this area and that clearly support a nonpathological view of homosexuality. A number of studies are as reasonably controlled as one could hope for given the considerable problems of obtaining representative gay or lesbian samples (for example, Dean and Richardson, 1964; Hopkins, 1969; Hooker, 1957; Siegelman, 1972a and 1972b). The interested reader is referred to such primary sources and others in the just-mentioned literature review.

It is important to realize that this concept does not imply that there are no disturbed gay men or lesbians, but rather that the base rates of psychological disturbance should minimally parallel those of comparable heterosexual samples and that such disturbance is not an inherent quality of a homosexual orientation.

Moreover, it would be reasonable and consistent with this concept to assume that the base rates of some varieties of psychological disturbance should be at least somewhat higher in some gay and lesbian populations, given the psychological impact of societal intolerance of homosexuality. For example, Saghir and Robins (1973) found greater alcohol abuse in their lesbian sample as compared with their group of heterosexual women.

Allport (1954), writing about the effects of prejudice primarily on Jews and blacks, described the psychological effects of social oppression, which he termed *traits due to victimization*. These include obsessive concern and preoccupation about minority or deviant group membership, feelings of insecurity, denial of membership in the group, withdrawal and passivity, selfderision and protective clowning, strong in-group ties coupled with prejudice against out-groups, slyness and cunning, self-hate owing to identification with the value system of the majority group, aggression against one's own group, sympathy for other minorities, militancy, enhanced striving and symbolic status striving, neuroticism, and acting out self-fulfilling prophecies about one's own inferiority. Allport stated that a minority group member might develop any combination of such traits in response to social oppression. It is ironic to note that these traits comprise a fair match to those which Bieber et al. (1962) believed to be the inherently neurotic characteristics of homosexual men.

What emerges, then, from the literature on psychological adjustment and homosexuality is the conclusion that sexual orientation is not intrinsically related to psychological disturbance. Some gay and lesbian populations may experience higher rates of some forms of disturbance, most likely the result of higher levels of environmental stress and societal intolerance and oppression. No person who is gay or lesbian requires a psychiatric evaluation merely because of a homosexual orientation, but many may need counseling and supportive services as a result of their victimization as gay and lesbian citizens.

Second, homosexual behavior is unrelated to most major demographic variables. Most demographic studies on lesbians and gay men have consistently found little or no relationship between homosexual behavior and most major demographic variables (see Gebhard, 1972, for a review of this literature). Homosexuality cuts across racial, ethnic, social class, educational, occupational, age, and regional variables. Homosexuals are raised in all religious backgrounds and vary in degree of religious observance. Gay men and lesbians can be found at all points of the political spectrum and level of involvement. Lesbians and gay men are widely diverse in their attitudes toward sexual expression, relationships, finances, use of leisure time, work and career, and virtually every other attitude of interest.

While some spokespersons for the gay and lesbian communities may speak of "the gay community" or "the lesbian community," this is more a political fiction (at times useful) than a social reality. Gay men and lesbians are not monolithic, but are variable and heterogeneous. While this concept can be comforting and demystifying, it makes lesbians and gay men difficult to weld together in all but small groups of relatively similar individuals. This population has little in common except their sexual orientation, society's reaction to their orientation, and a few institutions developed to insulate members from that reaction.

These institutions can periodically pull people together around a common cause, more often when societal oppression increases. Some of the social institutions created by gay men and lesbians—organizations, cohesive friendship networks, bars, support groups, and so forth—can exert a binding influence, usually when the members of the institution have other factors in common, such as social class, student status, or a common goal. Viewed as a whole, however, lesbians and gay men are considerably more diverse than similar. Many lesbians and gay men report that this diversity is one of the more interesting aspects of gay/lesbian organizations, bars, and so forth, in that they meet individuals quite different from themselves whom they would otherwise not meet.

What this means for the health-care professional is that knowing that a client is lesbian or gay is a relatively uninformative fact. Any other assumptions about the personal characteristics of the individual that the health-care provider may create are likely to be erroneous and stereotyped, perhaps condenscending, and possibly insulting.

Third, treatment focused on "changing" a homosexual orientation is rarely successful in the long term and of questionable ethics. As Coleman (1978) found in his review of the literature on changing a homosexual orientation, a long-term change to more or less exclusive heterosexuality is very rarely achieved. In addition, the treatments attempted tend to be long, arduous, expensive, psychologically disrupting, and alienating. Further, the ethics of such a change have generated heated controversy (see *Symposium on Homosexuality and the Ethics of Behavioral Intervention*). Perhaps the most insensitive thing a health-care professional can do is to assume that the presenting complaints of a gay or lesbian client are related to dissatisfaction with homosexuality and a desire to change.

In the few studies that report any change of orientation, the change occurs almost exclusively in those individuals who are already bisexual and who shift to more or less exclusive heterosexuality. This is true even in the work of those who retain optimism about and a favorable disposition toward this change (Bieber et al., 1962).

For clients who are dissatisfied with their sexual orientation, a careful assessment should be made of whether the desire for this change is due to external pressure, social oppression, or inappropriate or unproductive interpersonal behavior patterns on the part of the client. These will likely comprise most of such cases and can probably best be treated by assisting the client to enlarge his or her social-support system, change unproductive patterns of interpersonal behavior, clarify goals and values, and generally provide the client with a supportive, nonjudgmental sounding board for creating his or her own ethical place in an often hostile society. For those remaining clients who continue to desire change, some writers have suggested an approach more geared toward expanding the client's repertoire of sexual behaviors to encompass the desired goal, as opposed to eliminating same-sex behaviors and desires (for example, see Binder, 1977). This rationale for approach stems both from the recognition that empirically, long-term change of orientation is usually elusive and also from an attempt to create a middle ground on the ethical controversy.

A number of researchers, practitioners, and gay/lesbian mental-health organizations have been developing new treatment approaches focused on same-sex relationship counseling, assertiveness training, behavioral rehearsal, individual growth, and other techniques designed to help lesbians and gay men lead full productive lifestyles of their choosing (see Coleman, 1977, for a review of this emerging model).

It is noteworthy that the scant literature that does exist suggests that those gay men and lesbians who have affirmed their homosexuality tend to be psychologically healthier than those who have not (Hammersmith and William, 1973; Weinberg and Williams, 1974). Further, Weinberg and Williams (1974) found that psychological adjustment in their male homosexual samples was positively related to having a social support system of other male homosexuals. It is interesting to note that many writers (for example, Bieber et al., 1962; Hatterer, 1970; Socarides, 1968) who advocate "curing" the "illness" of homosexuality believe it is important for such a cure that their patients avoid social contacts with other homosexuals. One wonders if such practitioners, in so doing, end up contributing to poor psychological functioning in their homosexual patients.

Fourth, sexual orientation is best conceived of as a continuous, not bipolar, variable. Kinsey et al. (1948) introduced the notion of a continuum of heterosexual-homosexual behavior and produced considerable data to support this concept, which has become increasingly accepted over the years. Basically, this formulation maintains that individuals can be rated on the extent to which they report differing proportions of homosexual and heterosexual behavior and fantasies. Kinsey's figures for males, for example, suggest that about 50 percent of the adult male population is exclusively heterosexual and 4 percent are exclusively homosexual. This leaves a sizable portion of the male population with a more complex sexual orientation.

Recently, Shively and DeCecco (1977) have expanded this notion to include separate rating scales for homosexual and heterosexual orientation, arguing that a single, bipolar scale is insufficient to explain sexual behavior and orientation. In their system, for example, an individual could be rated both as strongly heterosexual and strongly homosexual. On the Kinsey scale, there is an implication that the bisexual positions are watered-down mixtures of the two components and that one form of sexual expression is at the expense of the other. This intriguing concept needs further research to support its validity and utility. It is also important to note that both Kinsey and later researchers differentiated between sexual behavior and fantasies. It cannot necessarily be assumed that these are congruent in a given person. Further, knowledge of an individual's sexual orientation is uninformative as to the kind of social sex role he or she may present, both in general and in specific situations.

Moreover, these scaled ratings of sexual orientation are measurements taken at one point in time. It is unknown how changeable sexual orientation may be over time. It is this author's clinical experience that at least a few individuals do experience apparently spontaneous changes in heretofore stable sexual orientation over time. These changes seem to occur in a variety of directions. However, research on the stability of sexual orientation is virtually nonexistent. The health-care practitioner should be aware not only of the variability and complexity of sexual orientation, but also of the apparent flux and fluidity of sexual orientation in some individuals.

Finally, the pattern and meaning of sexual experience changes over time for most individuals. Some of the changes are likely related to aging, maturing, personal experiences, and the "natural history" of the individual. This also is an area that is essentially unresearched.

With these basic considerations in mind, specifics of the health-care needs of lesbians and gay men can be discussed. Perhaps the best starting point would be the provider-client relationship.

The Provider-Client Relationship

Health-care providers can reasonably assume that their gay and lesbian clients have, to some extent, negative expectations of the health-care system in their initial contact. This attitude may have been verified by the client's past experience or vicariously, through the experience of others in his or her social circle. From the outset, this creates a situation that may range from merely awkward to absolutely forbidding.

Many health-care professionals make an assumption that from the start exacerbates this tension, namely, that the client is heterosexual. While this is a reasonable base rate guess, it often communicates to gay or lesbian clients that their sexual orientation should best remain unspoken. If knowledge about a client's sexual orientation or sexual lifestyle is at all appropriate to the professional service the client is seeking, it should be inquired about—

never assumed. Practitioners also should keep aware that heterosexual marriage does not at all guarantee that the individual is exclusively—or even predominantly—heterosexual. Despite a variety of attempts to "measure" or "detect" sexual orientation, by far the easiest and most accurate method is to simply ask.

Simply asking, however, is not simple. When dealing with a client who has been sensitized to rejection or prejudice for any reason—sexual, racial, ethnic, religious—and who may be fearing or anticipating a negative response, the manner in which this asking is done is likely to set the tone of much of the following interaction. If the professional is prejudicial, fearful, tense, awkward, condescending, confused, or ignorant, this will probably be communicated. Likewise, genuine acceptance, warmth, understanding, competence, and a professional demeanor are likely to be communicated by the same nonverbal routes. The attitude of the professional toward a gay or lesbian client will in most cases be apparent to that client. Perhaps more than any other minority group, gay men and lesbians are more sensitive to and experienced with "detection games" and their implications—probably more so than most professionals.

There are some health-care professionals who should immediately refer a gay or lesbian client to a more tolerant colleague, because their own attitudes toward homosexuality and change are too negative. There are some who will have no problems at all in establishing a good working relationship. Many professionals, however, have a good deal to learn in this area and are willing to examine their previous attitudes.

There are a number of ways to create a learning process: educating oneself through readings, consulting with gay or lesbian professional colleagues, making the acquaintance of lesbians and gay men living a variety of lifestyles, becoming familiar with resources in local gay and lesbian communities, and obtaining training and consultation from a gay/lesbian community service center or similar organizations. Anyone who knows 100 people knows at least 4 or 5 gay men or lesbians, probably more. Professionals who claim they know no lesbians or gay men are probably making more of a statement about their own accessibility and perceived openness than about their social circle.

It is this author's belief that the single most effective way of changing attitudes is to become acquainted with a variety of lesbians and gay men on a personal basis. A list of suggested readings in the area, in addition to the bibliography, can be found at the end of this chapter. Clients themselves can be an excellent source of feedback as to whether the interaction was both caring and competent. However, professionals cannot expect their gay or lesbian clients who are in need of service to provide them with an education on homosexuality. Obtaining this knowledge is the responsibility of the professional.

If an initial positive communication has been established, there will rarely be impediments to the professional obtaining whatever information may be relevant to the service or treatment desired and in gaining the cooperation of the client. A few lesbian or gay clients may remain distrustful, evasive, or uninformative. If reasonable attempts at reassurance, clear statements of the professional's attitude about homosexuality, and attempts to understand this negativism are not helpful, it should be remembered that some gay men and lesbians have been seriously scarred by societal intolerance. Also, there are as many neurotic or dysfunctional individuals in this population as in the general population.

Once rapport has been established and relevant information has been obtained, further discussion about the client's sexuality and lifestyle should be at the client's initiative. Occassionally, well-meaning professionals put too much emphasis on the client's homosexuality in their efforts to be reassuring. This may embarrass or irritate some lesbians or gay men. Needs for privacy and optimal social distance are the same for individuals of all sexual persuasions.

The careful reader may notice that no special dispensation to the preceding suggestions has been made for lesbian or gay health-care professionals. This is deliberate. While many lesbian or gay clients may be reassured by health-care professionals of the same orientation, and even seek them out, the fact that a health-care provider is lesbian or gay does not necessarily give any assurance of sensitivity toward gay men and lesbians. Some gay and lesbian health-care professionals, particularly those who have felt the need to remain "closeted," may themselves have judgmental and unhealthy attitudes toward their own and their gay and lesbian clients' sexuality. The suggestion that gay men and lesbians seek health-care needs from only gay and lesbian health-care practitioners is a naive one. Since gay men and lesbians are a minority of the population, there may not be many gay or lesbian professionals in all areas. Further, sexual orientation has nothing to do with general competence, ethical standards, sensitivity, and the ability to establish a positive and mutually respectful professional relationship.

Efforts to establish rapport with lesbian or gay clients are not merely liberal or humanitarian gestures. They will have a clear impact on the ultimate competence of the service rendered. Establishing a trusting and workable relationship is necessary to provide efficient and quality service. This is not to demean a civil libertarian or socially conscious motivation, but merely to point out that there are reasons that are purely professional and pragmatic.

An example can illustrate this point more clearly. A gay male goes to a physician complaining of urinary-tract symptoms and general fatigue. If the sexual orientation of the client is ignored, the physician may neglect to screen for pharyngeal and rectal gonorrhea, in addition to screening for penile gonorrhea. Examination for possible prostatitis also may be in order. Knowing the client is gay also might clue the physician to rule out hepatitis as a source of the general fatigue. The ability to ask the client a variety of questions about sexual habits—which presupposes that the physician does ask, and in a manner that elicits cooperation and valid information—will be a sine qua non for proper diagnosis and treatment in this case. Further, the physician will need to have specialized knowledge about diseases more common in gay males (for example, pharyngeal gonorrhea is usually asymptomatic; rectal gonorrhea often does not respond to dosages of antibiotic effective for penile gonorrhea, and so forth). Failure to build a cooperative and mutually respectful relationship, to ask the right questions, and to have the specific relevant knowledge will create a sense of failure, frustration, and resentment in the health-care professional and feelings of distrust, low self-esteem, and anger in the client, in addition to the poor-quality care.

Medical Information about Gay Men and Lesbians

The area of specialized information on diseases and disorders that are more common in gay men and lesbians is an important one. Until quite recently, knowledge about sexually transmitted diseases in these populations was scant and often inaccurate. However, more medical attention has been focused on these areas in the past 10 years or so, and there have been resulting increases in information. There are at least two books devoted to this topic (*The Gay Health Guide* by R. Rowan and P. Gillette, Little Brown, Boston, 1978; and *The Advocate Guide to Gay Health,* by R. Fenwick, Dutton, New York, 1978), and the Center for Disease Control, Venereal Disease Control Division in Atlanta now publishes an updated schedule of recommended treatments. Physicians have a clear professional responsibility to use such sources to inform themselves about proper treatment and to continue to keep themselves updated on this information as knowledge increases and new treatment schedules are devised. It is not possible in this chapter to include all relevant medical information, particularly since this information is rapidly changing. Interested readers are referred to the preceding sources as a starting point for such information.

The gonorrhea and hepatitis epidemics current in the gay male communities of certain cities are probably related to some lifestyle factors, such as certain sexual practices (for example, oral-anal contact is a possible mode of transmission for hepatitis A and certain intestinal diseases such as shigellosis and amebiasis), and promiscuity in some segments of the gay male community. However, a greater share of responsibility rests with the medical community, whose indifference to the health-care needs of this population, misinformation, inaccurate diagnoses, and inadequate treatment (usually in the direction of undermedication) led to the development of high rates of untreated or undertreated diseases in pockets of gay male communities. This condition, interacting with lifestyle factors, has led to the current epidemics.

In contrast to gay males, lesbians tend to have considerably lower rates of sexually transmitted diseases such as gonorrhea. However, lesbians have a number of special health concerns. Specialized knowledge about women's health care is necessary for any physician who treats women. Vaginal gonorrhea, for example, is often asymptomatic. The incidence of certain diseases and conditions is different for women who do not bear children or who never or rarely engage in heterosexual vaginal intercourse. This has obvious implications for many lesbian women. For example, women who never bear children likely have, as a group, a higher risk of endometriosis, galactorrhea, and perhaps other conditions. Women who never have vaginal heterosexual intercourse, or who engage in it only with circumcized males, appear to have lower rates of cervical cancer. In general, there are many open empirical questions about the long-term effects of sexual lifestyle variables on the incidence and form of various medical conditions and diseases, for both women and men. Longitudinal research in this area is sorely needed.

Obtaining competent and sensitive gynecological care can be a difficult experience for lesbians, particularly since questions about birth control practices are definitely linked to sexual orientation. Further, the need for sensitive, competent, and professional health care for women is a pressing issue in its own right, requiring reeducation of many professionals. Readers are referred to chapter 14 in this book as well as to the chapters on health care in G. Vida's *Our Right to Love*. If a health-care professional has followed the general principles on establishing a working relationship discussed earlier, it is unlikely the practitioner will lack the competence and sensitivity to push for birth control when it is unnecessary—or overlook the birth control needs of women who may prefer sexual activity with both sexes.

Issues of Privacy and Confidentiality

Personnel in medical and social service agencies should be aware of potential confidentiality problems for their gay and lesbian clients. Before entering sensitive information in any written record—even a simple statement as to the sexual orientation of the client—the health-care professional should question the necessity and advisability of entering such information in a record and should know who has access to such records. If there is any question as to whether such recorded information might be deleterious to the client, or if it may be accessible to inappropriate sources, it should probably best be kept as a mental note.

The issues of privacy and confidentiality are especially salient for lesbian mothers and gay fathers. Any number of relatives, former spouses, neighbors, or outside agencies and organizations can transform the relationship between a lesbian or gay parent and her or his children into a personal, social, legal, and economic nightmare. Given the unpredictability of the legal process in this area, the invasion of privacy, the often sensationalistic media coverage, and the general disruption, it is generally wise for gay parents to avoid legal involvement, unless there are no other alternatives. Parents and children who do get caught in legal situations will require major support services and the most sound legal counsel available.

Other Issues

The close friends and lovers of gay and lesbian patients should be accorded all the information, privileges, and respect given the family members of a heterosexual patient. All persons who are ill need the healing value and support of those closest to them for their complete and quick recovery. Some lesbians or gay men, particularly older individuals, assume that hospital and nursing-home personnel will make them unwelcome. It will require tact, sensitivity, and patience to communicate to these persons that they are welcome without making a major and embarrassing issue about sexual orientation. Health-care professionals should take responsibility to be certain that their clients are not harassed, subtly or overtly, about their sexual orientation and lifestyle, whether by other professionals, secretarial, maintenance, or other support personnel, or judgmental chaplains. Nursing and social work staff have a particularly crucial role to play for their lesbian and gay clients in mobilizing the support of their friends and lovers and making them welcome.

Again, assumptions should not be made about the sexual orientation of clients when this is not clearly known. For example, the best instruction in heterosexual sexual technique will be of little use to a gay or lesbian spinal-cord-injury patient and may communicate powerfully to them that their sexual needs are unimportant or unmentionable to the staff.

Hospitalized or ill children whose parenting is being shared by a lesbian or gay male couple need the support of both members of this unit. In general, when family involvement is an aspect of health care and the client or parent of a child client is gay or lesbian, the "family" as it exists for that client, not as it "should be," ought to be involved. Counseling centers for lesbians and gay men have been using established couples and family therapy techniques when indicated with few major alterations and as much success as can be expected from the techniques.

Older gay men and lesbians often have not experienced the greater tolerance and freedom which their younger counterparts have and may be quite reluctant to be open with health-care professionals. It should be remembered that as young adults, they experienced considerably more repression, ostracism, legal harassment, and outright violence. For some of these persons, there may be no way to reveal their sexual orientation in a nonthreatening manner. Health-care professionals will often have to exercise considerable patience and gentleness with these individuals and let them pace the disclosure and information giving. If certain information is vital and necessary immediately and they remain reluctant, lovers or close friends can be helpful sources of information. With this exception, the individual's need for privacy and feelings of vulnerability should be respected.

To assume that lesbians and gay men have little or no social support and structure because they often do not live within a traditional family system is erroneous and biased. Many gay men and lesbians often live their adult lives with little traditional family support and have created alternative support networks, which health-care professionals can utilize as they would a traditional family. The social structure and support systems of many gay men and lesbians are not weaker, just different.

Physical and sexual assaults by heterosexual males against lesbians and gay males, particularly the latter, are endemic in many areas of the country and appear to have increased with the recent political backlash against gay and lesbian rights. Only a handful of American communities have gay/lesbian civil rights ordinances. Of those which do exist, most remain untested in the courts and often offer only limited protection. More important, it is difficult or impossible for many lesbians or gay men to use these ordinances or file complaints and charges in assault cases because this may well expose them to more discrimination, suffering, and harassment.

There is considerable distrust of the police by many lesbians and gay people, given the violence of many police departments toward sexual minorities and overt political efforts by some police organizations to block gay/lesbian rights. Often assaults occur in isolated "cruising" areas, which tend to be frequented by those gay men who feel they cannot go to gay organizations or bars for fear of exposure, especially since many are likely to be heterosexually married. These victims are extremely unlikely to report the incident or seek assistance. For a lesbian, a heterosexual rape can be especially devastating.

A few gay/lesbian agencies, such as Gay Community Services and the Minnesota Committee for Gay Rights in Minneapolis, have begun programs to respond to the needs of gay and lesbian assault victims. Their efforts have included providing educational and training programs for crisis-intervention center and emergency room staffs, attempting to inform and educate local officials and police departments, providing training in self-defense techniques, as well as providing direct service to the assault victims and educating lesbians and gay men about their rights, how to mobilize against these violations, and how to cope with such stresses.

While such agencies are still developing a model based on their clinical experience for handling such cases, it appears that gay and lesbian assault victims are best treated in a fashion similar to rape victims. Massive short-term crisis intervention is needed. Long-term aftercare is often required to handle the emotional sequelae to the assaults. Victims often report phenomena similar to rape victims for a considerable time afterwards: social withdrawal, loss of libido, phobias and fears, depression, anxiety attacks, somatic complaints, and avoidance of anything related to the assault (for example, time, place, and circumstances of the assault).

While exact figures are difficult to determine, it appears that many gay and lesbian populations may have higher rates of chemical dependency than comparable heterosexual populations. Many gay men and lesbians find established chemical-dependency programs to be hostile, unsupportive, threatening, insensitive, or judgmental. An excellent analysis of the heterosexual bias in chemical-dependency programs is provided in articles by Schoener (1976, 1977). Finally, many chemical-dependency programs have religious and moralistic overtones that gay men and lesbians often find relegate them to a position of sinners and second-class citizens.

In recent years, a number of chemical-dependency programs for gay men and lesbians have developed in a few large cities. Gay and lesbian AA groups are more numerous. However, these do not begin to meet current needs. Virtually all chemical-dependency treatment formats emphasize the involvement of those who are significant to the chemically dependent individual. In order to be useful to gay and lesbian clients, any chemical-dependency program must be accepting of same-sex relationships and be willing to work aggressively within the social network of the client. Programs must, of course, first be sensitized to working with gay and lesbian clients. Further, chemical-dependency programs should be sufficiently in contact with the local gay and lesbian community resources to provide aftercare and follow-up services, and they should obtain regular consultation for competent gay or lesbian mental-health professionals.

It is hoped that these limited examples will give readers a sense of the health-care needs of lesbians and gay men. In summary, health-care professionals are initially encouraged to carefully examine their own attitudes to determine if they should work with lesbian and gay clients at all. This writer strongly encourages health-care professionals who do choose to work with gay and lesbian clients to (1) become knowledgeable about the full range of human sexual expression, as well as obtain specific information relevant to their practice with gay and lesbian clients; (2) examine further their own attitudes toward homosexuality and work toward a genuine acceptance of gay and lesbian clients and a sensitivity to their health-care needs; (3) scrutinize treatment strategies, programs, and clinical-practice techniques for heterosexual bias and eliminate this bias when it exists; (4) obtain consultation from relevant gay/lesbian organizations and professionals; and (5) incorporate this knowledge, openness, attitude reexamination, and sensitivity into training programs for health-care professionals.

References

Allport, G.W. *The Nature of Prejudice.* Reading, Mass.: Addison-Wesley, 1954.

Bieber, I., et al. *Homosexuality: A Psychoanalytic Study of Male Homosexuals.* New York: Basic Books, 1962.

Bieber, I. Homosexuality: The ethical challenge (Discussion). *Journal of Consulting Clinical Psychology* 44: 163–166, 1976.

Binder, C. Affection training: An alternative to sexual reorientation. *Journal of Homosexuality* 2(3): 251–259, 1977.

Coleman, E. Toward a new model of treatment of homosexuality: A review. *Journal of Homosexuality* 3(4): 345–359, 1978.

Dean, R., and Richardson, H. Analysis of MMPI profiles of 40 college educated overt male homosexuals. *Journal of Consulting Psychology* 30: 558–560, 1964.

Gebhard, P. Incidence of overt homosexuality in the U.S. and Western Europe, In *NIMH Task Force on Homosexuality: Final Report and Background Papers.* DHEW Publ. No. (HSM) 72-9116. Washington: USGPO, 1972.

Gonsiorek, J. Psychological adjustment and homosexuality, *JSAS Catalog of Selected Documents in Psychology* 7(2): 45, 1977.

Hammersmith, M., and William, C. Homosexual identity: Commitment, adjustment, and significant others. *Sociometry* 36: 56–79, 1973.

Hatterer, L. *Changing Homosexuality in the Male.* New York: McGraw-Hill, 1970.

Hooker, E. The adjustment of the male overt homosexual. *Journal of Projective Techniques* 21: 18–21, 1957.

Hopkins, J. The lesbian personality. *British Journal of Psychology* 115: 1433–1436, 1969.

Kinsey, A., Pomeroy, W., and Martin, C. *Sexual Behavior in the Human Male.* Philadelphia: Saunders, 1948.

Saghir, M., and Robins, E. *Male and Female Homosexuality: A Comprehensive Investigation.* Baltimore: Williams and Wilkins, 1973.

Schoener, G. The heterosexual norm in chemical dependency treatment programs: Some personal observations. *Stack Capsules* 8(1). 1976.

Schoener, G. *The Heterosexual Norm Revisited, 1977.* Available from G. Schoener, Walk-In Counseling Center, 2421 Chicago So., Mpls., MN 55404.

Shively, M., and De Cecco, J. Components of sexual identity. *Journal of Homosexuality* 3(1): 41–48, 1977.

Siegelman, M. Adjustment of homosexual and heterosexual women. *British Journal of Psychology* 120: 477–481, 1972*a*.

Siegelman, M. Adjustment of male homosexuals and heterosexuals. *Archives of Sexual Behavior* 2: 9–25, 1972*b*.

Socarides, C. *The Overt Homosexual.* New York: Grune and Stratton, 1968.

Socarides, C. *Beyond Sexual Freedom.* New York: New York Times Book Co., 1975.

Symposium on Homosexuality and the Ethics of Behavioral Intervention. *Journal of Homosexuality* 2(3): 195–259, 1977.

Weinberg, M., and Williams, C. *Male Homosexuals: Their Problems and Adaptations.* New York: Oxford Univ. Press, 1974.

Additional Readings

Bell, A., and Weinberg, M. *Homosexualities: A Study of Diversity Among Men and Women.* New York: Simon and Schuster, 1978.

Churchill, W. *Homosexual Behavior Among Males.* New York: Hawthorn, 1967.

Clark, D. *Loving Someone Gay.* New York: Signet Books, 1978.

Ford, C., and Beach, F. *Patterns of Sexual Behavior.* New York: Harper & Row, 1951.

Jones, C. *Homosexuality and Counseling.* New York: Fortress Press, 1974.

Journal of Homosexuality (published by Haworth Press, N.Y.).

McNeill, J. *The Church and the Homosexual.* Kansas City: Sheed, Andrews and McMeel, 1976.

NIMH Task Force on Homosexuality: Final Report and Background Papers. DHEW Pub. No. 1 (HSM) 72-9116. Washington: USGPO, 1972.

Silverstein, C. *A Family Matter: A Parent's Guide to Homosexuality.* New York: McGraw-Hill, 1977.

Tripp, C. *The Homosexual Matrix.* New York: Signet Books, 1976.

Vida, G. (ed.). *Our Right to Love: A Lesbian Resource Book.* Englewood Cliffs, N.J.: Prentice-Hall, 1978.

Weinberg, S. *Society and the Healthy Homosexual.* New York: Doubleday, Anchor, 1973.

21 Sexuality and the Health Professional

Harold Q. Dillehunt

What is of critical importance in any kind of sex counseling is that the health professionals attempt to understand the situation from the patient's point of view and empathize with the struggle to become a sexually functional individual. This means examining and abandoning our own prejudices, misconceptions, and illusions about our sexuality as well as that of the person with whom we are working. Otherwise, we are likely to condemn and reinforce old maladaptive patterns for ourselves and our patients. As Edmund Bergler puts it, "Sex 'tastes' better when combined with tender love. This is an experience that has nothing to do with moral attitudes" (Bergler, 1948).

For the health professionals to be more effective in dealing with sexuality, we must all become more comfortable with sexuality in general and our own in particular. To do this there are numerous books and professional courses available in nearly every metropolitan area. The point is not for every health professional to become an expert in sex counseling, but rather to be comfortable enough to at least explore the area with a patient in order to determine the necessity for some kind of appropriate intervention.

Sexuality in the health professions historically has been, and continues to be, a difficult issue for many professionals. There are a number of reasons for this phenomenon, the major one being our societal attitudes regarding sexuality. The situation, however, does seem to be changing, in part as a result of the work of Masters and Johnson and others and the establishment of centers for the training of professionals in the various aspects of human sexuality.

The intent of this chapter is not to provide a detailed sex manual, since these are readily available, but rather to illustrate the importance of dealing with sexuality in our practices and our own lives.

The notoriety that some professionals receive when sexual experiences between practitioner and patient are made public continues to demonstrate the difficulty with which the health professions and society at large have in dealing with the whole question of human sexuality. Further evidence comes from antiquated laws regarding human sexuality and organizational opinions on various forms of human sexuality. Sigmund Freud, in his extensive writings on the psychosexual stages of development, stressed the importance of individual restraint and repression of sexual urges and instincts. He identified the social role that education could play in ensuring

313

that the individual expression of sexual desires was consistent with the needs and demands of society (Freud, 1920).

Freud and many more contemporary thinkers and investigators of human sexuality have felt that overt sexuality, especially among the young, was not in the best interests of society. These views have received quasi-widespread acceptance among most educated segments of Western society. However, maybe it is time for us to rethink our positions on human sexuality, sexual development, and the implications for the health professions.

There are probably three major groupings of health professionals. There are those dealing with the physical health of patients, such as physicians and all their various subspecialties; those dealing with the emotional health of patients, such as psychologists, social workers, psychiatrists, and counselors; and those dealing with a combination of nonmedical modalities involving both physical and emotional health of patients, such as acupuncture, structural reintergration, and other more experimental forms of treatment. The specific issues related to human sexuality are likely to vary for each of these different groupings of health professionals owing to the varying roles each assumes and the divergent settings in which each may practice. However, all health professionals are confronted with certain general aspects of human sexuality. For the purposes of this chapter, several health professionals were interviewed to obtain their personal experiental data regarding sexuality in the health professional's practice. While the outline of this chapter presents six different topics to be covered, the topics are by no means mutually exclusive, nor do they exclude a number of other issues that may tangentially affect the health professional in his or her attempt to provide services to the community.

The Health-Care Professional and Sexuality

There is probably not a single health professional who has not at some time encountered either an overt sexual advance from a client, worked with clients who expressed sexual feelings for the professional, or personally experienced sexual fantasies about a client during his or her career. How we handle these situations is likely to have enormous implications for the well-being of our patients and ourselves. A number of health professionals interviewed indicated that at some time during their years of practice they had been propositioned by at least one patient. For the male professionals, these patients tended to be depressed women who were either unmarried or unhappy in their marriages. The female patient's proposition was seen as an attempt to reach out to someone who might fill the void she was experiencing in her life. By in large, the physicians among the group tended to respond anxiously to the proposition, attempting to avoid any direct confrontation, and tended not to refer the female patient for counseling. Those professionals within the mental-health field tended to be more relaxed in dealing with these issues, viewing the proposition within the context of the therapeutic situation. The women physicians who were interviewed, however, tended to be more understanding of a male patient's proposition and more likely to both discuss the implications of such a relationship and to make a referral to a psychotherapist or some counseling setting. Female mental-health professionals tended to respond to this kind of situation in much the same way as their male counterparts.

It would appear that whenever patients make sexual advances toward a health professional it generally stems from a desire to fulfill a sense of emptiness or dissatisfaction with their lives. This would suggest that these people are in need of more than just sexual information or a sexual experience. They are generally isolated and lonely and need help in rearranging their lives and understanding themselves. My bias is that they do not need a brief affair with their physician or health professional. Difficulty in dealing with sexuality is not limited to physicians or health professionals. Suffice it to say, difficulty in dealing with sexuality permeates our entire society.

The health professional needs to become sensitive to the ways in which patients present sexual feelings, the majority of which are nonverbal. A physician may encounter a patient who is either suggestive or exceedingly embarrassed within the examining room. A mental-health professional may encounter a direct verbal proposition or suggestive posturing. In either of these situations, the health professional has the opportunity to respond in a warm and accepting manner, which may help the patient understand the needs that are not being met in his or her life. The following example of a former client of mine is meant to be illustrative of this point.

When this patient first sought psychotherapy, he was a young man in his midtwenties. He was in graduate school at the time and, from all external evidence, quite functional. His presenting complaints were that he wanted to know and understand himself better and become more accepting of his sexuality. He had become sexually active around the age of 12 or 13 and experienced tremendous guilt over his sexual interests as well as his masturbation. Shortly after he became sexually active, he suffered an intestinal obstruction that required surgery. He recalled that he suffered the attack for some time before telling his parents because he was sure that God was punishing him for having masturbated. After the operation, he saw his physician to have the stitches removed and received a proctological examination. During the examination, his penis became fully erect. The physician responded by covering the boy's genitals with a paper towel, which evoked tremendous guilt and shame in the young adolescent. The patient stated in therapy that he had not wanted to get an erection, and had even fought it, but it just happened. Clearly the physician did not want to deal with the situation, which only served to intensify the patients' guilt about sexuality and shame about his body. As an alternative, the physician may have made a casual remark such as "Don't worry, boys your age are always getting uncontrollable erections," or "I see you have become aroused, would you like to tell me how you are feeling?" The first comment would have provided reassurance without inviting open discussion, while the second comment could have opened discussion. Regardless, as health professionals we need to become knowledgeable about human sexuality and comfortable with our own sexuality in both our personal and professional lives.

Coping with Sexual Feelings toward Patients

There have been a number of stories in recent years about health professionals, particularly psychotherapists, engaging in sexual relationships with patients. This situation again seems to reflect a general lack of understanding of sexuality and how it effects the doctor-patient relationship. While most of the incidents that have come to light have been heterosexual in nature, undoubtedly homosexual experiences of this kind also occur. The fact that most of these cases involved psychotherapists is really not very surprising in light of the intensity of many psychotherapeutic relationships as well as the degree of intimacy that frequently occurs. Many people enter psychotherapy because they have had difficulty in establishing intimate relationships in the general society. The psychotherapist, however, makes his or her mistake by thinking that the establishment of a sexual relationship with the patient will aid the patient in establishing an intimate sexual relationship outside the psychotherapy relationship. A very learned and wise psychotherapist, Dr. Ludwig Lefebre, once said that the only possible reason for a psychotherapist to engage in sexual relationships with a patient is if the psychotherapist is a very bad sexual partner. What he meant by this comment was that if the psychotherapist (or health professional) were a bad sexual partner, the patient's fantasies would be discarded and thus the person would be possibly free to go on to develop an intimate relationship with someone other than the professional. Otherwise, the psychotherapist would be encouraging the fantasies of the patient, which would inhibit growth, maturity, and the establishment of external relationships, and would be misleading the patient into expecting more of a relationship than was possible. Psychotherapy, in order to be effective, must be primarily a one-way street. Otherwise, the psychotherapist's own personal dynamic interferes with the process. The same situation applies to other health professionals, because society as a whole imbues us with an aura of authority and we are taught from very early on to "respect" and "please" authority. This situation, when it occurs, presents the patient with a classical "double bind" that seriously compromises emotional growth. Afterall, how can you tell your "lover" your inner most thoughts and feelings if you are trying to "please" that "lover authority" at the same time? Again, this is why we, as health professionals, must understand sexuality and our own sexual motives.

The health professional, regardless of the area of specialization, should be concerned whenever sexual feelings are evoked within himself or herself, particularly if the situation is unfamiliar. Consultation with a fellow professional is nearly always appropriate in this regard. Consultation will often help the health professional gain a better understanding of the doctor-patient relationship as well as bolster the necessary courage for the health professional to deal with the situation in an open constructive manner with the patient. This is particularly important if the professional is to give accurate, unbiased information to the patient.

Broaching Sex-Related Issues with Patients

Many questions about sexuality do not come up in practice simply because the patient is too embarrassed to confront the situation directly and the professional does not know how to make the patient feel comfortable and ask the right questions. There was general agreement among the professionals interviewed, with some exceptions by those in the mental-health area, that they were generally not confronted with questions of unusual sexuality in their practices. Their exposure to any unusual sexual behavior among patients came during their internships, residencies, and when covering emergency rooms. Without exception, they indicated that in settings where they saw these patients there was never an attempt made to provide counseling for these patients. If the sexual behavior was harmful physically, the patient might receive an admonition from the physician, but rarely a description of why the particular sexual behavior should be avoided and never an interview to find out from the patient why the particular sexual practice was appealing to the patient. There are many sexual practices that occur frequently within various subcultures of society. The health professional must know where to get information on these practices and subcultures as well as on the concomitant ailments and treatments that accompany these situations. There are many different ways to approach the subject, and they would vary depending on the patient. It is usually best to begin with some comments such as, "I would like to ask you some personal questions that people occasionally find somewhat difficult to answer. If you feel too uncomfortable now to answer them, just let me know and maybe we can deal with them at a later time when you are feeling more comfortable." Then begin the questioning by taking a sex history. History is usually easier for a patient to relate than current status. You will want to cover the following areas at least: age when patient became aware of sexuality, how and from whom they learned about sexuality, perceived parental and sibling attitudes about sexuality, age when masturbation occurred (including frequency and concomitant feelings), extent, if any, of homosexual experiences or fantasies, age of first intercourse and associated feelings, cultural practices regarding sexuality, other significant sexual experiences that have occurred, and finally a description of current status of sexual relating. This last area should cover the frequency of sexual relations, the fluidity of sexual relating, the feelings associated with sexuality, and the patient's perceptions of their partner(s) responses. This last question is particularly important, as illustrated by one professional's experience interviewing a couple individually about their marriage. He asked the same question of both, "How's your sex life?" The wife responded, "Oh, it's great, we do it once or twice a week." The husband responded, "Not so good, we only do it once or twice a week."

In interviewing several physicians of differing specialties, there was unanimity in their lack of formal education in sexuality. They all indicated that their training focused exclusively on the physical/biological aspects of the person. They also indicated that they felt inadequate to identify sexual and/or emotional difficulties in their patients, let alone treat these problems. While this chapter is not designd to teach the physician how to treat sexual and/or emotional difficulties, it is designed, hopefully, to aid the physician and other health professionals to identify these difficulties. Most physically oriented health professionals tend to avoid dealing with any sexual attitudes, values, and experiences of their patients. This is largely due to lack of training, but also may stem from a sense of discomfort with their own sexuality. One physician indicated that prior to taking a course in human sexuality, he avoided dealing with almost any aspect of sexuality in his patients. After taking the course, he felt more confident, although somewhat reluctant to discuss sexuality with a patient. He also indicated that he felt better prepared to make an appropriate referral in relation to sexual difficulties.

There are many kinds of sexual difficulties that may mask deeper psychoemotional problems. Consequently, it is important to remember that simple exposure to information about sexuality may not serve the needs of the patient. A patient's way of relating sexually may likely reflect the way in which he or she deals with others in a nonsexual relationship, and therefore, other aspects of their life may likely need attention in addition to their sexuality. For example, a woman who is nonorgasmic may have a need for control that permeates her relationships and may masque deeper fears. A man who is premature in ejaculation or impotent may fear success and the concomitant responsibility of pleasing his partner. He may view his partner with disdain. These people need help in understanding their own dynamic both in and out of the bedroom, in order to develop their sexuality as a person.

Working with Gay-Male and Lesbian Clients

The majority of health practitioners interviewed indicated that they tended to become anxious when working initially with gay and lesbian clients. This anxiety seemed to dissipate after the professional had a chance to get to know the client as a "complete, whole person" over the course of time. However, homosexuality continues to present difficulties for many health professionals and society at large. In years past, identifiable homosexuals tended to adopt culturally sanctioned, stereotypic careers and lifestyles. More recently, gay men and lesbians have been "coming out" (meaning to disclose one's sexual and personal lifestyle to friends, family and/or coworkers), and they represent all races, religions, occupations, and social backgrounds. Moreover, the question of what "makes a person homosexual" is as unanswered as the analogous question of what "makes a person heterosexual or bisexual."

The health professional is subject to the same prejudices as the society at large, and yet the prejudices regarding sexuality are frequently not incorporated into professional training. Again, the crucial issue is that the health professional should become informed and aware of personal biases that may affect and interfere with treatment. If the health professional had little or no prior contact with healthy homosexual men or women, he or she might label behavior that he or she views as unfamiliar as "unusual" or "deviant" as a means of reducing his or her own discomfort. Rather than adversely judge an individual's choice of sexual expression with another consenting adult, the professional should carefully examine his or her own biases and stereotypes, seek professional consultation, and/or refer the client to another professional who can work with the patient in an unbiased fashion.

The question of similarity of sexual orientation between health professional and patient has been raised on a number of occasions in recent years. From the community of homosexual counselors, psychotherapists, and physicians has come the notion that if the patient is homosexual, then he or she should seek a homosexual health professional. This has been particularly true within the area of mental health. While there may be some truth to this position from the standpoint of the homosexual health professional having had some first-hand experience with what the patient is dealing with, there is a basic fallacy in this assumption. Adopting the position that the patient and the health professional must be of the same sexual orientation is similar to the position that only a female patient should be treated by a female professional, or a Catholic by a Catholic, or a black by a black, or paraplegic by a paraplegic. By casting the analogy to the extreme, we quickly see the absurdity of the assumption. There are many homosexual patients who have been successfully treated by heterosexual health professionals and many heterosexual patients who have been successfully treated by homosexual health professionals.

Childhood and Adolescent Sexuality

Another area that generally proves to be difficult for the health-care professional as well as society at large is sexually active children. Society as a whole has attempted to postpone the development of sexuality in children, at least on a conscious level. Traditionally, educators have sought to impose the values of self-restraint on the young in order that the values of the Judeo-Christian tradition might be instilled with commensurate intellectual maturity so as to carry on the society as it has existed.

Consequently, almost all infantile sexual activities are forbidden or made distasteful to the child. The goal has been to make the child's life asexual. Freud (1964) supported this notion in his descriptions of patients and their early sexual experiences. In describing early sexual experiences of patients, he said: "They make it responsible for all their troubles and we have the greatest difficulty persuading them that they are mistaken. In fact, however, we ought to admit to them that they are right, for masturbation is the executive agent of infantile sexuality, from the faulty development of which they are indeed suffering" (Freud, 1964). Haim Ginott has the following to say about childhood sexual development: "Childhood masturbation may bring comfort to children, but it certainly causes conflicts to parents" (Ginott, 1952). He feels that many children may utilize masturbation as a response to loneliness, rejection, and boredom. Parents, however, often feel anxious about such practices. "The sight of her five year old boy waling around holding his penis in public arouses embarrassment and anguish even in the most progressive mother. Of course, parents have heard, read or even experienced that masturbation is harmless; that it does not cause insanity, sterility, impotence or any of a dozen other plagues" (Ginott, 1952). It would appear that even the reassurances about the harmlessness of masturbation are a source of anxiety for parents. Ginott continues his discussion of masturbation by saying, "Intellectually, parents recognize that masturbation may be a phase in the development of normal sexuality. Emotionally, it is hard to accept. And perhaps, parents are not altogether wrong in not sanctioning masturbation. Self-gratification may make the child less accessible to the influence of parents and peers" (Ginott, 1952). He seems to feel that if one masturbates, it is a short cut because one is only concerned with self-pleasuring. In a society as goal-oriented and imbued with the work ethic as ours, it is easy to understand the negative value placed on self-pleasuring. It also may be true that some people at various times in their lives use masturbation as a way of avoiding problems and/or dealing with failure. However, there has been little statistical data to support this notion.

Ginott not only indicates a belief that something is wrong with masturbation, he also implies that it can lead to social isolation as well as an inability to form relationships. I would contend that it is not masturbation that may lead to social isolation; rather, if sexuality is at the root of social isolation, then it is the guilt stemming from masturbating that inhibits social development. The parent who adopts Ginott's notions will pass on to the child that there is something wrong with masturbation, sexuality in general, and his or her body in particular.

Sexuality and Older People

The phenomenon of self-pleasuring is not exclusively related to young people. Self-pleasuring continues to be an issue throughout our lives and again becomes an issue in older adults. Our culture, with its worship of youth, seems to think that sexuality ceases at age 50. In part this may relate to most women's inability to bear children after that age, as signified by menopause, and to our own connections between childbearing and sexuality. The link between childbearing and sexuality is well described clinically in a case presented by Masters and Johnson (1970). They described a couple in their midfifties to early sixties who had not had sexual relations for several years. When their children were finally married, the wife announced that it was no longer appropriate for a woman her age to engage in sex. They consulted a clergyman for marriage counseling, and he supported the wife's views, which inhibited any attempts by the husband to seek professional help for some time. Needless to say, there was definite resistance from the wife when the couple went to see Masters and Johnson. Obviously, myths perpetrated out of ignorance can be very damaging.

The response to menopause in women is not always to feel that their sexual life is over. Some women react with a renewed interest in sexuality because they need no longer associate it with motherhood. Some men respond to this renewed interest with intimidation. This obviously may result in problems of impotence for some men and consequently indicate the need for reeducation of both partners. Health professionals need to be aware of these phenomena, and they must understand how these sexual concerns change over the course of a lifetime.

There are well-documented physiological changes in sexual response with aging; however, these should not inhibit sexual activity or interest. As with everything else related to aging, we all seem to *gradually* slow down. There is, however, growing knowledge of the physiological changes of aging and how these changes affect the sexual response. Even more important are the development of various means to alter these changes, such as sex-steroid replacement. In any event, it is important that health professionals recognize the legitimacy of sexuality in older adults and help patients develop socially acceptable and personally satisfying ways of expressing their sexuality.

One of the more common difficulties of aging is loss of a partner through death or ill-health. This raises for many adults, for example, unresolved conflicts around masturbation. Many people may need direct encouragement and approval to rekindle or even begin masturbatory activity. The health professional's ability to accept sexuality in the older patient will aid him or her in exploring sexuality with patients. The health professional who is not comfortable with his or her own sexuality or the patient's sexuality, regardless of age, has a responsibility to at least be aware of appropriate referral sources in the community.

References

Bergler, E. *Divorce Won't Help*. New York: Harper & Row, 1948.

Freud, S. *A General Introduction to Psychoanalysis*. New York: Boni and Liveright, 1920.

Freud, S. *New Introductory Lectures on Psychoanalysis*. New York: Norton, 1964.

Ginott, H.G. *Between Parent and Child*. New York: Macmillan, 1952.

Masters, W.H., and Johnson, V.E. *Human Sexual Response*. Boston: Little, Brown, 1970.

Part IV
Delivery of Health-Care Services: Cross-Cultural Factors and the Health Professions

The importance of considering cross-cultural factors in health care is probably appreciated by most practitioners only in the context of markedly obvious cultural differences, such as the practice of African tribal medicine or the practice of some of the ancient folk medicines of North America. It is more difficult to appreciate the impact of cultural differences when we are dealing with a medical and health-care system which, in North America at least, is fairly homogeneous insofar as most of its technological practices are concerned, subscribing to modern developments in Western medicine. We know, however, that different groups of people are affected by, and respond to, illness and disease in different ways. It is essential that we view illness as a state that occurs as a function of many factors, not least in importance among which is the role of background and personal factors, as well as social environmental factors (all mentioned in the introduction to this book in the model of adjustment to illness). The myths and symbols surrounding illness are inextricably intertwined with the cultures within which they arise. This part of the book will look at four prominent subcultures in North America, blacks, Hispanics, Native Americans and Asian Americans, and will attempt to allow the health practitioner an initial understanding of issues to which one must become sensitive. Medial sociologists and anthropologists are aware of the issues and have conducted a considerable amount of enlightening research in the area. Many health-care practitioners are not aware of such work simply because they have never had any exposure to it. The aim of this part is to expose health-care practitioners to issues that arise when subcultures interface with the medical-care system of North America, issues that will make practitioners more understanding of how members of those subcultures perceive illness and interact with a health-care system that is frequently culturally quite different from themselves.

22 Psychological Factors in Providing Health Care to Blacks

Robert Mahon

Introduction

The question before us deals with delineating the psychological factors that may exist in providing health care to black people. The question itself appears relatively straightforward; however, there are some hidden assumptions that are important to consider. The first assumption is that some formula can be derived that will benefit both the health practitioner and the black patient in terms of the quality of treatment provided. Its corollary is that one can productively generalize the needs, thoughts, and behavior of over 20 million people in a fashion that will allow one to deal with the distressed individual who may be one of that 20 million. There also might be present the fear that blacks will be different or more difficult for the white practitioner to treat than other groups, most especially whites. A second, and in some ways more harmful, assumption is that in addressing this question we need only look at the concerns, traits, and values that black people bring to a medical setting without, at the same time, considering the backgrounds and personalities of practitioners. Given the proportions of whites to blacks in medicine, with the emphasis on physicians, most practitioners will be white, and it is to this group that many of the comments in this chapter are directed.

Doctors, nurses, aides, and technicians all bring with them into their work various aspects of their personalities that deal directly with race. Many believe that they can make a separation between their own feelings about a particular patient and the quality of care given. Yet there are innumerable circumstances where nonmedical factors strongly influence medical care. For example, medical research is dependent on the availability of both private and governmental funds, which in turn are subject to political and economic forces. Issues such as abortion, euthanasia, birth control, medical costs, and professional lobbies encompass political, social-economic, and moral concerns. The medical practitioner is not isolated from social currents and values, even though he or she may believe, or wish, it to be so. The goal of this chapter will also be to examine and hopefully stimulate further discussion of how race and racial attitudes influence medical care and the manner in which it is provided.

Racial Identity

A crucial observation to test and keep in mind is that blacks are not a totally homogenous group. There are many factors that interact with race to produce a variability that at times defies easy generalizations. In that black people are dispersed throughout the 50 states, there will be a variability based on geographical characteristics attributed to each region. A proportion of blacks have immigrated from the British and French West Indies. Their social and cultural habits may be divergent from those whose origins are in the continental United States. There are also dark-hued people who see themselves as Latino, who do or do not identify with Afro-Americans, and who may or may not maintain separate traditions from those which are most evident in the states. Age and religious differences exist and affect behavior. Economic status may be a factor that, at times, overrides racial commonality. Most black people are not poverty stricken, although they do earn less than their white counterparts. For the physician to assume the life-style of the patient is a serious error. However, within any given treatment program, there may be issues related to the patient's economic status that must be taken into consideration, for example, diet, living conditions, resources, and the ability to follow through with aftercare plans. These factors will elude the practitioner who relies on generalities and stereotypes and does not take time to learn about the patient he or she plans to treat.

This diversity among black people has periodically been seen as problematic, both for those of the race who wish to present a united front in redressing grievances and those not of the race who, out of their own social-psychological makeup, wish to perceive all black people as being alike. Nevertheless, there are strong ties that bind. There is a common heritage that dates back to Africa and is evident today, in some ways overtly, such as the arts, and in other ways more subtly, such as in a sense of "peoplehood." This speaks to a bond that exists as a result of racism and the necessity to develop strategies to both protect oneself and family members from its insidious effects and to overcome it in the struggle for personal, social, and racial advancement.

This common heritage involves, primarily, a sense of "blackness," a term that has only come into popular usage in the past 10 to 15 years, yet which describes an emotional identification that has always been there, no matter what term has been applied. It is a recognition and self-identification with the history of displaced Africans in this hemisphere. It is the sense that one is not totally alone in confronting the basic issue of food, clothing, shelter, and health in a society that historically has been hostile to one's race. It implies, at times, a consciousness, an identification with each other that excludes those who are not black. It means that in areas such as art, literature, music, religion, speech patterns, childrearing, family composition, and political values, one can begin to see characteristic adjustments that have been mechanisms of cultural survival and enrichment.

The Black Family

The primary institutions of social survival for black people have been the family and the church. Much has been discussed regarding both, yet it is not too often that one hears of the strengths of black families. Within the confines of the family, however, blacks have found the emotional support and buffer against the hostility of the larger culture. The black family has had to withstand many assaults on its integrity, from the horrors of slavery to the misrepresentations of some contemporary theorists. A case in point has been the stereotype of the black family as being a matriarchy where the predominant force has been an emasculating woman. This contradicts the fact that the majority of black families have both parents in the home and that power is shared and delegated among the adults along what might be considered traditional lines—father as the "breadwinner," mother as the "childrearer" (Hill, 1972). If, however, these roles were adhered to rigidly, it would have been counterproductive in the face of economic realities. Those families in which various members could interchange their roles, without a subsequent blow to self-identity, were those which survived and prospered. At times, for example, it has been necessary for the female to assume more responsibility for the economic well-being of the family. A large proportion of black middle-class families attain their economic position by virtue of both parents working. Given the disparity between the incomes of whites and blacks in the United States, it would be very difficult for black families to advance economically solely on the earnings of one parent. As a result, children are often asked to assume more responsibility for themselves and their siblings. Hence, a great value is placed on the interdependence of family members and their ability to adapt to situational needs.

A further illustration of the adaptability of the black family that has bearing on medical services is the concept of the extended family. The extended family involves those individuals related by blood or friendship who can be viewed as part of a unit which in many various ways performs the functions of what is generally seen as the traditional family. This may include neighbors, distant relatives, and companions who provide support in a manner that would seem more characteristic of family members. In my work as a psychotherapist, some black clients have mentioned having "play brothers," "play mothers," and so forth who act as surrogates or confidantes, sometimes in place of traditional family members, but more often as a complement to biological family members. Very often these individuals can be extraordinarily important in a patient's health care. For example, in excluding them from a patient on a ward that is accessible only to family members, one may be eliminating a prime source of comfort and support, thereby jeopardizing the patient's recovery. In any interview with a patient, it would be important to ascertain who are the individuals closest to him or her regardless of their familial relationships and to enlist their aid in the patient's treatment, especially if this "family member" has accompanied the patient to the office, clinic, or hospital (and if the patient feels they can be of help). They may assist by reminding the patient to take the medication, helping them in following any prescribed regimen, and assisting the patient in returning for follow-up visits (if they are necessary). In addition, this "family member" may more clearly remember the diagnosis and instructions or advice given the patient by the health-care practitioner, particularly if the patient is too anxious or ill to fully comprehend the meaning of what was said. This would seem to be good standard practice for any practitioner. In working with black people in this manner, one is, however, relying on an African orientation of the group, tribe, or family being primary, especially in providing support and sustenance, and deemphasizing the more American, traditional value of relying on the individual to provide for himself or herself.

Of course, all these survival tactics succeed or fail to varying degrees on the basis of the individuals and the circumstances in which they live, but to characterize the black family as a matriarchy is negligent of how blacks perceive themselves, ignorant of the diversity of black people, and at times grossly abusive of empirical data. Researchers such as Robert Hill (*The Strengths of Black Families*) have helped to counter the pathological image of the black family. Hill (1972), using data available in the early 1970s, summarizes some important findings about the black family as follows:

1. Authority and decision making are shared along egalitarian lines.
2. The husband is the principal source of family income regardless of the family's socioeconomic status.
3. A majority of black infants born out of wedlock are raised by parents or relatives, while (in 1969) most white infants born out of wedlock are put up for adoption.
4. Almost 60 percent of the black women who do head families work—a majority of them full time.
5. A common belief is that there is a widespread male desertion rate among Black families. Yet, according to DHEW figures (for 1969), this was true of only one-fifth of the families receiving AFDC.
6. A strong sense of social mobility and achievement is encouraged in many Black families. For example, 75 percent of Blacks attending college were raised by adults who, themselves, had no college education.

This all-too-brief discussion of the family is relevant to the practitioner in helping him or her to counteract some widely held prejudices and to help establish a positive foundation for interaction with black patients. The attitudinal stance of the caregiver toward the patient often affects treatment. To patronize, ignore, and demean others does not make for a therapeutic relationship. To approach a patient with the necessary respect for him or her as an individual and crucial partner in his or her treatment is extraordinarily difficult when one devalues him or her for any reason as vacuous as racial background. It is the mutual respect of patient for practitioner and vice versa that is the basis for a good working relationship.

Racism and Vulnerability

Blacks have had to deal with racism all their lives. Racism involves believing and acting on certain stereotypes of ethnic or racial groups that are often lies, distortions, or rationalizations that foster the identification of another individual or group as being different (in this case, as black) in order to deprive them of power and the opportunity to achieve and enjoy their full potential as human beings. The general public is probably aware of the gross issues of discrimination in education, jobs, and housing. However, it is in the daily interactions between individuals and within institutions that these gross issues become personal crises. Racial slurs, insensitive comments, misunderstandings, assumptions, and ignorance can be the subtle, or often not so subtle, forms of racism that will never be the subject of discussion in legislative chambers or court hearings, but remain incidents which the victim of such a process must resolve on some level. One can actively express the pain and anger that ensues or one can take out those feelings on the perpetrator in an indirect manner that can be both gratifying and self-defeating. Another associated reaction may be a self-accusation of stupidity, naiveté, or blindness for having been so trusting or open as to believe that one would be dealt with on the basis of one's qualities as a human being. The most vicious result of racism is the victim's belief that the negative treatment he or she receives is somehow correct and the way things should be.

Most blacks bring with them into any interaction an extensive history of working with white people, a background that is generally more involved and varied than most whites' experience in working with blacks. Black people have had to deal with whites in many situations where they have less situational power and authority, such as with teachers, police, social workers, employers, and physicians. Any situation or interaction where one party has less power than another involves a certain amount of vulnerability, one is placing one's welfare in someone else's hands. Few situations pull for this sense of vulnerability as much as illness and the need for treatment. To become ill, be it with a cold or cancer, is a statement that one is not invincible, that forces which can be sensed and experienced but which often are not seen (with the exception of physical trauma) have a great effect over what you can do and how you feel. Some illnesses allow for more control by the patient and therefore decrease this experience of vulnerability. For a common cold, one can usually taken one's treatment into one's own hands, the same with minor cuts or injuries. To go to a doctor, however, is a statement of the extent to which one feels unable to maintain one's own physical well-being. The more one has to depend on others, especially "strangers," the greater that sense of vulnerability can become. Cancer, for example, is so frightening not only because it can be fatal, but also because the process by which it incapacitates the individual often results in an overwhelming sense of helplessness. With some illnesses, and possibly with cancer, it may be that reasserting the patient's sense of control over the disease process can be a critical factor in remission. Biofeedback, for example, is one method of treatment for which patient monitoring and control is a foundation of treatment.

In contrast to such a patient's vulnerability, a doctor is an individual whose position and status in the community is generally very high and whose judgment is seldom questioned (notwithstanding the rising number of malpractice suits). The American doctor represents one of the most highly educated and trained professionals in the world and is therefore seen as the authority. Doctors hold within their grasp a wealth of knowledge that is supposedly much too vast and complicated for the simple layperson. The doctor chooses which information he or she wishes to dispense, although the effect of consumerism on the medical field has been for practitioners to dispense more of their knowledge to patients than has been done in the past. This image of the omniscient, omnipotent physician and his or her staff assistants is somewhat of an exaggeration given the state of medicine today. Yet there is enough truth in it to alert one to the actual danger of the practitioner believing his or her own press releases and the patient surrendering all responsibility for his or her care, much to the detriment of both parties and the treatment.

This whole issue of vulnerability can become considerably heightened when racial factors enter the picture. This is not to say that racial issues will be in the forefront with all black patients. Generally, people are looking for competent, thorough care. Sometimes, the treatment difficulties that may arise are similar to what the physician should expect regarding the nature of the illness and the manner in which most patients have reacted. But given that this is a racist society, where race is a major determinant in how people are perceived and treated, it is certainly unlikely that the caregiver will not be confronted by these issues in his or her professional capacity.

There have been some historically generalized tactics that have characterized stereotypically the ways in which black people have dealt with racism and vulnerability. Within a medical context, a patient, at one end of the spectrum, may uncritically accept all that he or she is told by virtue of the fact that the individual providing care is white and/or is a doctor or a nurse. Their responses in other situations may or may not be so acquiescing, but the vulnerability and sense of helplessness that may attend an illness causes them to be less than active participants in their own health care. At the opposite end of the spectrum, one may have a patient who is angered about being ill and needing to rely on anyone, much less a white physician, for assistance and treatment. He or she may be demanding, hostile, and resistant to treatment. He or she may undermine the best efforts on the part of the medical staff. Both these patient stances may or may not be the result of experiences, both immediate and remote, that have little to do with past or present medical treatment or racial factors.

In both these cases, it is important for the practitioner to clearly state what he or she sees as his or her responsibility to the patient and how he or she can best meet that responsibility. It is equally necessary to state what role the patient must play in his or her own treatment and recovery, emphasizing the need for mutual cooperation. The practitioner will most likely experience the greatest discomfort with those patients he or she views as being angry, hostile, and/or potentially violent. This perception is more likely if the patient is male. Often the doctor or nurse will react solely to the affect or emotion being expressed and ignore the content of what is being said. Any assertiveness, no matter how appropriate, on the part of the black patients is often seen as a potentially explosive situation. One of the many lessons that black people have learned is that one will be treated as an "invisible man" until one gets angry. Requests, questions, and statements that are made calmly often get ignored by whites. At times this extends to one's very presence—such as being overlooked when one is next in line. These are not uncommon experiences for blacks, and the healthy, appropriate response is anger. The practitioner can prevent many difficulties by *listening* and *responding* before a situation escalates. He or she should acknowledge both the content and affect of what is being expressed. If the anger is justified, then acknowledge it as being so. If the patient (or patient's family or friends) believe that someone is concerned enough to pay attention, then there is no need to raise voices or become threatening. When emotions are getting in the way of the treatment, clearly stating that fact also may help calm the situation. If the situation continues to escalate, it may be necessary to withdraw from the scene until tempers cool, to remove from the scene any parties who are agitating the situation, or finally to call for other support personnel. As often as not, the response of the practitioner is the catalyst for confrontations. Concurrently, there will be patients who are characteristically threatening. The practitioner need not endanger himself or herself if the patient refuses to respond to reasoning, at which point treatment should be suspended until both staff and patient can proceed safely. There are times when anger becomes the acceptable way for patients to express other concerns, such as the social or economic effects of illness. Empathizing with the patient's concerns might be helpful. At the same time, any note of pity should be avoided. Anger also may be the strategy with which an individual deals with authority. These instances may be difficult for the practitioner to sort out and address, but again, the first step is to listen.

As mentioned previously, there have developed some stereotypic tactics for blacks in dealing with whites, especially when racism or the difference in race between practitioner and patient is seen as important (by either party). A common strategy is to be withholding of information. Often the diagnostic questions that may be asked may appear to be prying to the patient. Black people, as a means of self-protection, generally have learned to share only certain information about themselves with whites. As diagnostic questions begin to deviate from those focused on physical, biological processes and begin to probe into the patient's social and economic life and well-being, the interviewer might find that some people give less information or overtly exhibit annoyance. This response stems from the fact that these questions appear to be unnecessary and an example of "snooping" for purposes unrelated to what brought them to the physician in the first place. To counteract this and to lessen the feelings of vulnerability, it is helpful to explain to the patient the rationale behind the questions. This is especially evident in stress-related diseases, where environmental and psychological factors play a crucial role. To assure the patient that the information is of use for the proper treatment and to communicate why it is important (beyond generalities) may mitigate the resistance that might be evident in the interview.

Other patients may attempt to gain control or express anger regarding their treatment by not following suggestions or plans. Physicians and others who have patient contact invite this response when they are brusque, rude, or exhibit no more concern for the patient than they would for a culture in a petri dish. Black patients may view this as racism, as it well may be, most especially if it is perceived that white patients receive more time, care, and consideration. Assuming that this is not the case, the physician may increase the chances of a patient following through on treatment plans if he or she makes sure that the patient not only understands what those plans are (possibly by having the patient repeat in his or her own words his or her understanding of the rationale for the plans, which includes any medications), but also by taking a few minutes to discuss with the patient the difficulties the latter may expect to have in complying. This includes sorting out with the patient those difficulties which are avoidable and establishing with him or her the priority his or her treatment has as compared with the demands life makes on us all in general and the patient specifically. If possible, one should avoid placing the patient's medical treatment in direct conflict with other needs the patient feels are important. The mother who needs to care for her children while at the same time care for herself is helped best by the practitioner who aids her in resolving what might be seen as conflicting demands in a manner that does not put the medical treatment against the children. The more the treatment can be incorporated into the patient's daily life, the more likely the patient is to accept an active and positive role in his or her care.

All this increases in importance as hospital emergency rooms and medical clinics (particularly in the inner city) supplant the role of the family physician. The personal relationship that developed between family practitioner and patient is rapidly disappearing and, with it, one of the reinforcements that patient's develop toward institutions, for better or for worse, generally, the latter. The staff with whom one interacts one day may be different the next. Many big-city clinics and emergency rooms are overcrowded and understaffed, which encourages noncompliance, withholding of information, or overt expressions of anger. It is important to reemphasize that most black patients do not present themselves in a fashion that differentiates them greatly from other patients. However, the staff members who take time to interview carefully and provide to the patient some understanding of the process in which he or she is involved is counteracting what can be a depersonalizing trend in medicine.

Racism and the Practitioner

Up to this point, this discussion has focused primarily on the patient characteristics and how the practitioner might respond in any number of situations. However, it is important that some attention be directed toward examining some of the issues that practitioners, specifically those who are white, might bring to an interaction with black people. All too often the difficulties that minorities experience in this culture are seen as their problem—"the black problem," "the Indian problem," "the Mexican problem"—examples of blaming the victim. Very seldom are these difficulties referred to as "the white problem." When this does occur, as in the Kerner Commission Report of the sixties, many find it baffling or offensive. They examine themselves cursorily and absolve themselves of racism.

Often some personal positive experience with a black person or people in general is seen as an indication of their innocence. Yet in a society where the means of communication, production, and political power is controlled by one racial group, that group will project its norms, beliefs, and values as being preeminent. The society's institutions operate in a manner to confirm the validity of those values. They do not reward the constant reexamination of those values, the result being that one need not look at one's own role in an interaction when one is in the majority and holds the power. The medical profession and the individuals within it have been no exception. All the evils of segregation and discrimination that black people have experienced in general have been experienced within the confines of medicine—segregated facilities, substandard care, and neglect, on the one hand, and discrimination in medical school admissions, employment, and professional organizations, on the other. The cloak of science is often used as a defense for certain social attitudes, including racism, allowing many in the medical profession to believe that they are somehow immunized from what is a major American social illness. A prime example of this is when social decisions are made by medical personnel, as in coerced sterilization of women for the purpose of limiting the size of families. A client of mine reported that a physician recommended a hysterectomy to her after he overdramatized the potential harm of some fibroid tumors present in her uterus. She acquiesced to his advice. When a second doctor examined her records at a later date, his opinion was that the hysterectomy was totally unnecessary—much to the anguish of the patient. The first doctor acted on feelings that were unrelated to the practice of good medicine. He was more concerned with issues of social policy, politics, and possibly his own racist attitudes than with the health of his patient. He clearly abused his power by misrepresenting the medical information he had and denying the patient the opportunity to make an informed judgment regarding an irrevocable medical operation. Yet this doctor might not have experienced his decision as malicious. As already mentioned, our society does not encourage a self-examination or reassessment of values as long as one's role and power are sanctioned by that society. The individual may be castigated some time in the future for gross abuse or negligence, but the values that encourage that type of behavior receive scant attention, especially within the medical profession.

Racism and prejudice may best be examined within a context where they are seen as social illnesses; and one of the first steps to recovery that a patient must undertake is to acknowledge the presence and effect of an illness. How does the practitioner initiate this process, in terms of both himself or herself and the setting in which he or she works? Some self-examination is in order. What does his or her own ethnic background mean to the practitioner? When is he or she most conscious of being white (if that is the case)? What feelings are associated with that consciousness? It has been my experience that these three questions are very difficult for many white professionals to actively consider, excluding, of course, the rabid racist who is easy for most of us to readily identify. A white physician once related an incident to me in which a very angry black patient called her a white "so and so" quack doctor, which upset her very much. It was not being called a quack that bothered her, nor was it the obscene adjectives that preceded it, it was being called a *white* "so and so." Being called white, in anger, conjured up feelings of guilty inadequacy about her ability to work with this patient and, by implication, any black patient. Yet the decision she made that set off the patient's tirade was medically correct and ultimately in the patient's best interests. It is obvious that coping with her own sense of racial consciousness had not been achieved, and though her insecurity did not effect her decision (as it might in other cases), it certainly was an unsettling, if not painful, experience.

Other questions must be addressed. For example, what experiences has he or she had with other ethnic and racial groups? What associations come to mind when one thinks of black or other Third World people? How do these experiences and associations enhance or limit one's ability to provide care? How does one's political identification enter into treatment considerations? Feelings about federal- or state-funded medical insurance programs may influence the manner in which one views particular patients. Finally, there are a set of issues related to the setting in which one works. What are its characteristics and treatment philosophy? Doctors, clinics, or hospitals that are primarily concerned with high patient flows and serve that end by cursory examinations, shoddy treatment practices, and prescribing of ill-advised medications are guilty of racism, if not by motivation (which may be pure ignorance or greed), then certainly by effect. This is all too often the standard of health care that many of the poor have come to expect. Granted, there are times when the personnel in these settings are acting heroically, doing their best with what the system gives them; yet that is a terrible indictment in a nation as wealthy in financial and human resources as this one. It is a devastating message to actual and potential patients that there are higher priorities than their health.

The Minority Professional

Some words need to be addressed to the minority professional, who faces special issues in the performance of his or her work. This is especially true for physicians, given their standing in the pecking order of medicine. Pressure emanates from the social isolation that may be present in predominantly white institutions, the often strong internal and external demands to succeed as an individual and as a member of a particular racial group, and the sense of privilege and accomplishment that is accorded them by their racial brothers and sisters. At the same time, others may question or castigate the professional's achievements as being the product of a sellout to the larger culture's values at the expense of their own racial identity. Whites often expect the black professional, for example, to either be an expert commentator on all black people and issues or totally ignore his or her experiences as being a valid and important contribution toward a given situation. Patients may sense a special ally in the minority practitioner and see him or her as someone they can especially trust. Or they may resent his or her achievements, believe that he or she cannot be qualified as his or her white counterpart, or feel chagrined in confiding some embarrassing detail to another member of their own minority group. This set of negative reactions happens with diminishing frequency as the number of minority professionals increases, although it still may take place when minority practitioners work with white patients. In that instance, the best stance is to rely first on one's sense of knowledge, professionalism, and self-confidence. If that fails to elicit the necessary cooperation from the patient, it may be more fruitful to address the issue squarely and calmly confront the patient with the belief that his or her attitudes are interfering with what you, *the professional,* feel is their best interest, that is, quality treatment. At that point, some decision must be made regarding continued contact with that patient. Depending on the situation, one might transfer the patient's care to another doctor or nurse with whom they would feel more comfortable or insist that you intend to follow through with the assignment.

Additional questions emerge. How does the minority professional respond to the needs of poor or ethnic communities that lack services, particularly when it might be to his or her economic disadvantage? Does one become the special advocate of minority patients, or should one assume a "colorless" stance toward patients and deny any bond the patient wishes to establish based on a common racial background? Again this situation may dictate the response. The junkie who sells a line based on the "both of you being brothers" in order to get some pills calls for one type of response. The Latino patient who speaks poor English and is grateful for a doctor who understands not only Spanish, but also the patient's lifestyle calls for a different response. The bottom line in all these situations remains quality medical care, and each individual needs to assess how best they can serve their patients as well as their own sense of professionalism. The minority professional, however, is in a position to monitor, inform, and educate both his or her colleagues and patients. In some manner, that responsibility should be considered and met.

Summary

This chapter has attempted to speak to some of the psychological issues involved in the treatment of black patients. A number of points bear reiteration. Blacks are a diverse people, and as such, one must be cautious in generalizing their experiences. Each individual needs to tell his or her own story, and to this end, the patient and practitioner are best served by careful listening and questioning. Both white and minority medical personnel need to examine and assume responsibility for their own interactions with patients. Finally good medical treatment is a cooperative effort between the help seeker and the caregiver and has a foundation in a mutual respect for each other's knowledge, skills, and humanity.

References

Hill, R.B. *The Strength of Black Families.* New York: Emerson Hall, 1972.
National Advisory Commission on Civil Disorders. *Kerner Report.* Washington: USGPO, 1968.

23

Overcoming Barriers to the Treatment of the Hispanic Patient

Carmen Carrillo

A varied and complex population, Hispanics number 11.2 million people in the United States. Socioeconomic, cultural, and linguistic barriers have determined Hispanics to be a medically underserved population. Effective treatment of individuals of Hispanic heritage is predicated on the health practitioner's ability to communicate effectively, approach the patient with an understanding of her or his world view, and reduce her or his ethnocentric stereotypes. This chapter explains the roots of cognitive/affective processes that influence interactional behavior among Hispanics. The harsh realities that form a backdrop for Hispanic behavior are described. Prevalent ethnocentric views of Hispanics and their negative consequences are explored. Suggested approaches for successful treatment are delineated.

The Hispanic Population

According to the 1975 Census *Current Population Reports,* there were 11.2 million persons of Spanish origin in the United States (U.S. Bureau of the Census, 1976). This figure is a conservative estimate when the factors are taken into consideration; the population figure estimates double to 23 million Hispanics owing to census undercount, legal and undocumented aliens, and increases from births. It is estimated that Hispanics will be the largest ethnic minority group by the year 2000.

The largest Hispanic subgroup is of Mexican origin (59 percent) and lives primarily in Arizona, California, Colorado, and Texas. Puerto Ricans constitute 16 percent of the Hispanic population, many of whom live in New York State. Following are Cuban Americans, who are concentrated in Florida and represent 6 percent of the Hispanic population. The remaining 19 percent are either of Central/South American origin or are identified as "other," including such groups as the Filipinos (U.S. Bureau of the Census, 1976). Eighty-four percent of Hispanics reside in urban areas. Medium age for Hispanics is 20.7, the youngest of all ethnic groups, compared with 28.6 years for the general population (U.S. Bureau of the Census, 1976).

As with other ethnic minorities, Hispanics are overrepresented among the poor. Ten percent of all American families are classified as poor. Only

8.7 percent of white families are poor, while 21 percent of families of Hispanic origin fall into this category. Thirty-seven percent of Hispanic American families with seven or more members are below the poverty level (U.S. Bureau of the Census, 1976).

Hispanic as a Medically Underserved Population

Hispanics are not only overrepresented among the poor, they generally experience a higher degree of unemployment, poor housing, discrimination, poor education, and inadequate nutrition than the dominant population group. Poverty not only limits the ability of Hispanics to afford adequate health care, its resultant effects predispose the Hispanic population to illness.

Discrimination and poverty contribute to inner stress, internal conflicts and, repressed anger, which have had severe effects on the physical and mental health of Hispanics. Drug abuse, alcoholism, and suicide have increased among Hispanics.

Despite greater health-care needs, Hispanics either underutilize available services, seek treatment for disabling illness at later stages than other groups, or are offered inferior-quality health care than that offered the Anglo community. Additionally, Hispanics lack the opportunity for adequate health education or access to the technical advances of public health.

Even the known health needs of Hispanics have not been adequately addressed. Services to Hispanic communities are deficient in many respects: availability, accessibility, comprehensiveness, continuity, and appropriateness. Furthermore, the quality of service available to Hispanics is often inferior to that available to other groups. The resources to Hispanic communities are inadequate in number for certain services, such as alcoholism treatment, long-term care, and home-health services. Thus, available programs are insufficient to meet the needs of Hispanic communities. For example, community mental-health or mental-retardation programs, residential half-way houses, or alternatives to hospitalization are not commonly available to Hispanics.

Finally, Hispanics are served more often by paraprofessionals or others with limited training, rather than by licensed professionals.

Toward Effective Treatment

Effective treatment of individual of Hispanic heritage is predicated on the health practitioner's ability to communicate effectively, approach the patient with an understanding of her or his world view, and reduce her or his ethnocentric stereotypes. There is a lack of sensitivity to racial, cultural, and ethnic factors or preferences of cultural groups. This may explain why some services are utilized and others not. For example, there is a lack of health-education materials for minorities. For Hispanics in particular, this means an absence of culturally relevant materials and, in some cases, of Spanish language information. Furthermore, there is a reliance in fields such as mental health on the traditional medical model rather than on an understanding and application of a psychosocial model, which adapts itself more readily to the special needs of Hispanics.

The severe lack of minority health professionals has a special impact on the Hispanic population. Currently, there are 136 physicians for every 100,000 Americans. Yet there are only 250 Mexican-American physicians for Hispanics, the second largest minority group. There is even a shortage of professionals qualified to provide service to the Hispanic population, that is, professionals who also have a thorough understanding of or sensitivity to the linguistic and sociocultural characteristics of patients.

Knowledge about the health needs and practices of Hispanics is woefully sparse. There is a lack of culturally sensitive researchers whose findings and interpretations are free of the biases and stereotypes that have characterized previous research.

Last, but not least, Hispanics are underrepresented among those who make policy, control budgets, or operate programs. Thus changes beneficial to Hispanics are infrequent and slow to take effect.

Suggested Approaches for Successful Treatment

In working with Raza groups, it is necessary to be familiar with specific behaviors, values, and belief systems. Following is an attempt to outline and describe behaviors that have special connotations to Raza groups. The underlying assumption here is that there is a great risk of innacurate evaluation, particularly in mental health, of a Raza person or family if the evaluator is unfamiliar with Raza culture. The information to be presented is complex and sometimes seemingly contradictory. The seeming contradictions emerge because culture is a changing phenomenon, with Hispanic culture being a mosaic of rich and shifting characteristics. Raza groups will naturally vary according to generational status, socioeconomic level, educational level, and regional identification.

Observations and points for the reader's consideration in understanding Raza culture are organized into the following categories:

1. Sex roles
2. Childrearing practices
3. The extended family

Sex Roles

One of the most outstanding features of the literature on Raza groups is the agreement among authors concerning the theme of rigid adherence to sex roles and gender-appropriate behavior. Researchers note that sex roles among Raza groups tend to be more clearly defined than in other cultures.

At this time, it will be helpful to name some commonly accepted stereotypic attributes to describe some of these specific gender-role models. The reader must keep in mind that these descriptions are not to be considered general rules of conduct applicable to all Raza groups, but rather merely as a basis for understanding stereotypic ideals.

The Raza male stereotypically can be described as proud, authoritarian, controlled, vengeful when dishonored, and possessive in relationships. The Raza female stereotypically can be described as protected, submissive in relation to the male, sexually pure, and seen as vulnerable to seduction by the sexually aggressive male.

Currently, both men and women are far less insistent upon strict separation of sex roles. Based on recent changes within Raza culture, it has been established that these traditional sex roles have been changing drastically. The impact of political and social movements for greater personal freedom and self-expression has altered sex-role behavior, especially that of the "submissive female." The woman's movement and the *movimiento* of the Chicanos are examples. Additionally, the more urbanized Hispanics become, the greater is the opportunity for Raza women to reach economic independence from men. Economic dependence on men has contributed greatly in nurturing and maintaining their submissiveness. Nonetheless, one may expect to encounter a higher of adherence to sex-role behavior within Raza culture than among non-Raza groups.

A major point affecting the incidence of rigid sex roles is the practice of childrearing within Raza culture.

Childrearing Practices

Parental authority is highly valued among Raza groups, and historically, the final authority rested with the authoritarian father. The mother, in contrast, has typically been portrayed as protective of her children, favoring male independence, and encouraging female children to be "cooperative" and "respectful." Typical styles of relating to children include indulgent affection mixed with severe discipline.

Again, it is important for the reader to note that these descriptions are traditional and might not be representative presently in light of the impact of sociopolitical movements. It is nevertheless safe to say that any major changes occurring at different social levels are reactions against a strictly adhered to system of childrearing practices.

Since the disciplinary responsibility usually falls on the father, the value of male dominance becomes a learned concept for children as they grow up. The concurrent behaviors in relating to male children consequently affords them social privileges not afforded to females.

Boys are discouraged from participating in activities which might be interpreted as "submissive" and unmanly, such as helping with the dishes. These tasks are "traditionally" female and should be left to the female. Boys are encouraged to be "little men," to come and go as they please, to play with other boys, and to gradually grow into their adult roles as "authority figures." Therefore, they are discouraged from demonstrating weakness and should instead strive to be "in control" of their feelings and to expect that most of their physical needs will be handled by the female. Little boys, for example, may be specifically trained not to make their beds, since this would be contrary to their roles as men and would furthermore indirectly affront the male supremacy of the father.

The mother may relate to her son with ambivalent attitudes of veneration in catering to his needs and resentment of her own social position in not being afforded the same privileges. It is important to note that despite the emphasis on being "strong," boys are raised with a spirit of enjoying friends, especially male friends, and of valuing warm and expressive interpersonal relations.

The rearing of females, on the other hand, is very different. The daughter is raised to see the father as the ultimate authority who can determine her fate by either permitting her of prohibiting her from realizing her plans. When she asks her mother's permission, she is presented with *"Preguntale a tu papa, lo que diga tu Padre"* (Ask your father; whatever he says). Already at a very early age she is trained to believe in the supremacy of the male. Being a female, she must learn how to please the family and be cooperative, thereby avoiding conflicts. She is to be respected because she is a female and is taught to conduct herself as a "lady" in order to maintain that respect. Because women are expected to be ideally "pure" and "chaste," they are frequently protected from men and expected to live more sheltered lives than men.

Clearly, we appear to be moving away from such strict concepts of role and authority within the family and, with this move, approaching new normative behaviors for males and females. A word of caution is necessary here. It is important to clarify the possibility of misdiagnosis in the light of these observations concerning sex roles. Viewed within a cultural context, male domination is not necessarily an indication of psychopathology on the part of either sex. A Raza man who prefers the company of other men and who behaves in an authoritarian manner with his wife may be manifesting his *machismo* rather than indicating personal pathology. Such behavior among other cultural groups may imply "latent homosexuality" or an "inferiority complex" or that the woman prefers to be a "martyr." Such is not the case necessarily among Raza groups.

It is imperative for persons working with Hispanics in the helping professions to be able to identify behavior that is "normal" or accepted in the culture from that which is "abnormal" in other cultures. The crucial point is that health professionals must be informed of cross-cultural sex-role differences before rendering verdicts concerning psychopathology or appropriateness and inappropriateness among Raza groups.

For example, there seem to be a number of "emotional" behaviors characteristic of Raza men that occur less frequently among men of other cultures. Raza men appear more "open" in their expression of emotion and seem to demonstrate extremes of joy and anger more freely. Furthermore, affection toward other males is expressed without embarrassment by hand-shaking, an embrace upon meeting, and frequent touching during conversation. Misunderstandings can arise if these behaviors are elicited during an interview. Considering this, such behaviors should not be misconstrued as denoting "lability," "hysterical response to stress," or "latent homosexuality."

The Extended Family

A characteristic of Raza groups is strong adherence to the tradition of an extended-family system. The system has been described as a tightly knit organization of family members who would provide support and acceptance to one another. A basic point to be considered is that because of the function of the family, a Raza individual may not refer himself or herself to a clinic that may be percieved as "alien." That individual may be more likely to seek out the advise and support of the family and close family acquaintances.

Such a strong reliance on family members may denote a certain degree of overdependence on parents and underdevelopment of self-autonomy in other cultures, but this is not necessarily the case among Raza groups. On the contrary, reliance on the family may be a very adaptive response to stress. Furthermore, when interaction with the family is involved, caution must be exercised in not pathologizing differing psychological and social interactions. For example, a male who calls his mother once or twice weekly cannot be legitimately accused of oedipal conflict without thorough and sensitive examination of other factors in his life. Such behavior must be viewed within the context of respect and devotion to the mother. Conversely, to behave aloofly and indifferently toward a parent might be interpreted within Hispanic culture as indicative of serious pathology.

A vital point to consider at this time is that as Raza groups become less rural and move to the cities to find work, and as admissions to the higher-learning institutions increase, the extended-family tradition appears to be changing. Certain trends indicate that the extended family is weakening and diminishing. As Raza groups move from rural areas where tradition is emphasized more than in the cities, they tend to loose some of their older customs. This is a point that requires more research. Preliminary indications are that the divorce rate for Hispanics is reaching parity with that of other groups, the percentage of single-parent households is close to that of other groups, and Hispanics are beginning to develop alternative lifestyles.

Finally, surrogate extended families are increasingly emerging. For Hispanics who no longer enjoy the advantages of a genetic extended family, the definition of *family* has broadened. Thus a surrogate family can be sculpted with friends who become *tias y tios* (aunts and uncles), children are adopted, and older persons are invited to be acting grandparents.

General Suggestions

Health programs must be made relevant to Hispanics. Thus consideration of Hispanics must be made in planning, training, recruitment, and integration of services to make programs relevant to the Hispanic population. Moreover, in the development of supportive services, coordination with community support systems as they exist in the Hispanic communities is crucial. Continuity of care, preventive care, and health maintenance must be approached from a culturally sensitive perspective.

Government can assist us in these efforts. Federal data collection relevant to minorities, particularly Hispanics, would assist planning for regional national policy that emphasize the specific health needs of Hispanics. Program planners at state and local levels could promote and institutionalize pilot projects that have proved effective. Some ways of achieving this are to make available training grants to hospitals, medical schools, and research institutions for programs relevant to Hispanics. Above all, the appropriateness of services to needs must be gauged. Health professionals must recognize the special health problems of Hispanics and assist in articulating the need for health and demographic data, as well as program development.

24 Cultural Background of Native American Health Behavior

Luis Kemnitzer

For the purposes of this chapter, we can separate components of "health behavior" into (1) deciding that an illness exists, (2) choosing a healer, (3) interacting with the healer, and (4) following the advice of the healer. These sets of behaviors are influenced by historical, social, and cultural factors, as well as individual psychological and situational factors. I shall not refer explicitly to these categories of behavior again; rather I shall discuss what seem to be the most salient influences on these behaviors, especially behavior associated with healers. It should be remembered that the discussion that follows rests on generalizations, explicit and synthetic cultural rules, and cross-tribal cultural comparisons, and that members of widely different traditions have undergone different kinds of experiences, with Euroamerican culture. Accordingly, each patient is an individual, with more or less adherence to the picture outlined here.

Perception of one' illness and the usefulness of the medical system for treatment is based on the individual's personal history of relating to health and illness as well as the manner in which their referent group conceptualizes the role of illness and medical treatment. This includes not only the diseases and their effects on his or her people, but also the quality of medical care they have received and the ways in which Native Americans have received medical care. A full discussion of these topics is beyond the scope of this chapter, but a sketch of the biological and historical background of health behavior is essential. The belief that disease is more than a biological process, but also part of a cosmological and moral system is not unique to Native Americans. However, the pervasive nature of this belief in Native American cultures is striking and strongly influences interpretation and response to symptoms. In some cases, this belief may influence the onset and development of symptoms. Ideas about spiritual power, its source, and its expression are allied to moral interpretations of disease and also influence the perception of Western medicine and its practitioners. Finally, all these ideas, as well as ideas about the relations of humans to each other and to the universe, are expressed in the way people behave toward each other and expect others to behave toward them—in our interest, in encounters of medical significance.

Disease Patterns in Native Americans

The most accessible statistics concerning disease patterns in modern Native Americans are those published by the Indian Health Service (IHS) of the U.S. Public Health Service. These figures are derived from IHS hospitals and clinics and reflect only those reportable conditions which are presented to IHS agencies on reservations. Since half the estimated 1 million Native Americans live off the reservations, in small towns near reservations or in larger cities, and are thus not eligible or conveniently located to these services, there is no way of knowing whether the reservation patterns reflect those of the Native American population as a whole. In addition, the unreported and undiagnosed disease entities remain an enigma, and conditions that reflect states of health rather than disease entities only show up when someone makes a specific survey to determine them. This happened in very few places. Keeping these cautions in mind, we shall make a quick survey of what is available.

In 1974, accidents were the leading cause of death, causing one out of five deaths on and around Indian reservations (compare one out of sixteen deaths in the United States as a whole). These were followed in importance by diseases of the heart, malignant neoplasms, and cirrhosis of the liver. The last has increased 221 percent since 1955, the year responsibility for medical care to Native Americans was tranferred from the Bureau of Indian Affairs to the Public Health Service. Deaths from suicides, diabetes mellitus, and homicides also have increased since that time. While the death rate from tuberculosis has declined considerably since 1955, it is still 4.6 times that for the United States as a whole, and one-fourth again larger than that for blacks. Arteriosclerosis hits Native Americans harder than it does U.S. whites and others, while cerebrovascular disease and hypertension present lower mortality rates in Native Americans than in whites or blacks. In sum, the age-adjusted death rate for Native Americans is 35 percent above that for U.S. whites and 11 percent below that for other nonwhites.

Otitis media, strep throat and scarlet fever, gastroenteritis, pneumonia, influenza, and gonorrhea are the leading causes of nonfatal illness. Incidence of both otitis media and gonorrhea increased almost threefold between 1962 and 1971. While incidence of trachoma has declined considerably from pre-World War II epidemic figures, about one-half of 1 percent of Indians were so diagnosed in 1971, most of these in the Southwest. Similarly, the morbidity rate for tuberculosis in Indians remains almost 9 times that for U.S. all races.

Not only is the disease pattern different in Native Americans from that in Euroamericans, some diseases present different clinical features. This has been best documented for diabetes (Rimoin, 1969). In a comparison of Navajo and Amish responses to glucose tolerance test, it has shown that

Navajo controls responded similarly to Amish diabetics, while one form or Navajo diabetic responded like Amish controls and a second form of Navajo diabetic displayed only a slightly lower level of plasma insulin than Navajo controls. Diabetes is usually mild in Navajos, the juvenile ketotic form is unknown, and vascular complications are rare.

Nevertheless, reservation populations are less healthy than official figures imply, and reservation residents have less opportunity to do anything about it. The results of a multiphasic screening test on three southern California reservations are an example of this (Wood, 1970). Of ninety-six persons examined, twenty (including six under the age of 12) had previously undiagnosed urinary tract infections. In addition, thirteen indicated elevated eosinophilia, sixteen had abnormal lactid dehydrogenase, and twelve showed hyperglycemia. In other words, conditions are undetected, undiagnosed, or ignored, because of inconvenience, expense, or lack of medical care. Many Indians develop their attitudes toward illness and its treatment in this kind of atmosphere.

The Historical Background

In the space available, there is only room for a hurried sketch of the history of disease experience and medical care in Native Americans. We shall try to present traditional views of this history as well, since what informs people's behavior is how they perceive the world, not necessarily what official records may be.

Traditions have it that there were no significant diseases among Native American people before the Europeans came. Certainly smallpox, cholera, gonorrhea, mumps, and measles were brought directly by Europeans, and Africans brought malaria, hookworm, and yellow fever. The questions of the homeland of syphilis and tuberculosis are still being debated. Certainly the effects of these diseases were devastating in all areas of North America. Tribes were decimated by disease, the ability and will to resist white encroachment were sapped, farms were abandoned, and the subsistence base as well as the social and spiritual life of the people was distorted. Most of this devastation happened during the first 200 years after the arrival of Europeans, but the effects stay on. Ethnohistorians believe that it was during this period that Native American religion took on its preoccupation with disease and healing, a concern we shall examine more closely in subsequent paragraphs. Outside, the purview of this chapter is the influence on migration, political forms, warfare, and reaction to white colonization.

Early medical encounters between Indians and whites found Europeans learning from Indians. The lack of any qualified medial personnel in many of the colonies and the notion that God provides the cures for the afflictions

He sends in the areas where they occur, along with the general dependence on Native American knowledge for survival, drove colonists to rely on Indian doctors and native herbs, and there was some rough reciprocity. At the same time that Euroamerican physicians and druggists tried to gain prestige and credibility for their products by claiming that they had learned their secrets from an "Indian medicine man," Indians living close to white settlements were coming to depend on white medicine, with contradictory results. European medicine was not much more advanced than Native American medicine, and Europeans were almost as terrified and helpless in the face of smallpox as Indians in the seventeenth and eighteenth centuries. With the improvement of European medicine, the expansion of white settlements and the expansion of Christian missionization, Native American medicine and its practitioners became targets of concerted attack.

Missionaries provided some form of medical care, and later treaties with tribes carried provisions for the delivery of medical care by resident physicians. In 1832, Congress appropriated money for vaccination against smallpox, and this campaign slowly gained momentum through the century. West of the Mississippi, the War Department was charged with the responsibility of providing medical care through the post physician, and although responsibility was transferred to the Bureau of Indian Affairs in 1849, post physicians continued to deliver medical care in many areas until the turn of the century.

The Native American population continued to decline, from the estimated 9 or 10 million in 1492 to 250,000 in 1900, and Indians continued to be plagued by tuberculosis, pneumonia, trachoma, and other communicable diseases and malnutrition in the first half of this century. Hospitals were substandard, personnel was inadequate, and finances were inadequate. Indians looked to their treaties and expected the United States to live up to their promises to repay Native American people with medical care in partial payment for land lost; the United States was not living up to its part of the bargain.

After fact-finding commission reports in 1928, 1935, 1948, and 1954, responsibility for delivery of medical care to Native Americans was transferred to the Public Health Service, where it remains today. Since then the budget has grown from $34.5 million to $200 million, and staff has grown from 2,900 to 7,400. Hospitals have been improved and the incidence of communicable disease has declined dramatically, but medical personnel are still overworked and Indians are still suspicious and insecure about care, largely because of the lack of control of these institutions by Indians themselves. Recent legislation has provided opportunities for more control of programs by tribes, but implementation will take time. Besides, there are less than fifty Indian physicians, and only a handful of these and other Indian health professionals are involved in the design or implementation of these programs.

In short, experience with epidemics and with Euroamerican medicine in the past has left Native Americans with a religion that is concerned with disease and healing, with the feeling that "whiteman medicine" should cure "whiteman diseases," and that Euroamerican medical care is only part payment, stipulated in treaties, for land taken from Indians.

The Moral Basis of Native American Medicine

Native Americans are not unique in ascribing a moral component to disease theories. We can remember the obstacles placed in the progress of research in the control of venereal disease by those who believed that it was interference in God's plan to punish those who transgressed His laws concerning sexual behavior. But the moral component of traditional Native American medical systems, embedded in religious systems of control and cosmological explanation, is relatively explicit, coherent, and integrated. Christian influence has reinforced this feeling, at the same time tending to diffuse its systematic nature.

Ultimately, Native American medicoreligious systems proclaimed visions of a universe in balance—humans and natural forces, humans and the supernatural, and humans among themselves. Humans had the responsibility to maintain this balance by observing rules for correct behavior toward animals, plants, natural forces and their effects, and other humans, living and spiritual. These rules ranged from ancient contracts between humans and animals, for instance the giving of fresh water to freshly killed sea mammals (Eskimo); observing particular incest rules, menstrual isolation, or personal or group food avoidances (almost universal); and avoidance of lightning-struck objects (Navajo). The consequences of infraction of these rules may be interpreted in terms of the withdrawal of support by spiritual helpers or ancestral spirits, as the consequences of a mechanical breakdown comparable with the consequences of failure to lubricate an engine, or as punishment by spiritual forces on the behalf of an offended human. In the last case, interpersonal disputes as well as arrogance, stinginess, or conspicuous display may be instigating causes. The degree of "guilt" ascribed to the victim, or the amount of "punishment" ascribed to the illness, may vary from one tradition to another, but the explanation still follows the form (1) a person is sick because he or she did something wrong, or (2) a person is sick because somebody else has felt wronged, and (3) the sickness is a symptom of a local imbalance in the universe. (It must be noted here that illness is only one kind of misfortune brought about by wrongful actions. Loss of skills, bad luck, marital trouble, drinking problems, and court trouble all are possible effects of the distortion of the cosmos that comes from the failure to observe the rules that maintain balance. Naturally, we are only concerned here with illness, but the larger category should be kept in mind. Conversely, such discomforts as colds, headaches, digestive disturbances, and other mild acute conditions are not important enough to theorize about in this scheme.)

Not all infractions are known to the victim—indeed, not all the rules are known—and part of traditional treatment includes the search for infractions. This is the occasion for gossip and speculation on the part of the victim's associates, as well as reflection by the victim. The authority in these matters is the shaman, diagnostician, or other traditional healer, and this function gives him or her great influence and responsibility in traditional society. In societies that have been influenced by Christianity, illness may be ascribed to infractions of people's perception of the Christian moral code, yet brought about by the action of spirits as punishing agents. Traditional or Christian-influenced rituals may be parts of the healing process, but in most traditional cases, confession of the infraction is necessary to release the victim from danger.

> A 14-year-old Indian youth was brought to the emergency room following what appeared like a grand mal seizure. Thorough neurological examination demonstrated no organic cause for the seizures. History revealed that this boy had just heard in church that incestuous activities with sisters as well as mothers was forbidden. As he walked through an open field on the way back from church, he thought he heard a sound behind him. He looked back over his left shoulder, feeling an overwhelming sense of oppression. Believing that severe infractions morally would be punished by a "ghost," he was certain that this spectre was upon him and he fell into the seizure state. Since he had had sexual relations with his 16-year-old sister for two years, he felt he needed considerable expiation for his guilt. The result was a conversion reaction, which yielded to individual psychotherapy and concomitant counseling with his family [Schechter and Roberge, 1976].

This case illustrates the way in which spiritual forces enter into the interpretation of infractions of cosmic and moral rules and the way in which the consequences of these infractions can be somatized. Although the tribe is not specified in the report, any Northern or Midwestern tribe could contribute such a syndrome.

Cases such as this may have a certain reality that can be translated into Western psychiatric theory, and therapists may respond to them according to their interest and approach (see, for example, Jilek, 1977; Pattison, 1973). The moral content of nonpsychiatric conditions will be more obscure, and response to them by patient, family, and practitioner will not be as predictable. Some nodal points along a hypothetical continuum of mixtures of Indian and Western responses are as follows:

1. The condition is a minor disability itself and can be taken care of by empirical Euroamerican methods, but is one of a series of misfortunes, that

indicates a spiritual etiology: An elderly Lakota woman has recurring joint pains, she breaks her ribs in a fall off the roof of her house, and on top of this her sons are in trouble with the law. Her ribs are treated at the Public Health Service hospital; she endures her joint pains and takes her son's troubles repeatedly to shamans. She discovers that she has failed in her obligations to perform rituals appropriate to one who has dreamed of thunder, and the troubles will cease when she resumes her practice (Author's field notes, 1966).

2. The condition is a warning: A small child dies of pneumonia, and relatives of the parents state to each other and indirectly to the parents that this is a warning that they are leading dissolute lives, straying from Indian ways, and not paying enough attention to their children and their family. The father cuts off his finger at the funeral, and the parents start going to church again and try to reorder their lives. The topic is discussed by the spirits and shamans at various shamanic performances (Author's field notes, 1966).

3. The disease is caused by supernatural means, the symptoms can be ameliorated by empirical methods, Euroamerican or Indian, but the cause must be met by the Indian way: A Navajo singer says:

> They tell me . . . [tuberculosis] is inflicted by a person coughing in your face. . . . Right away I disagree with it. . . . We know of how a man gets to be afflicted with tuberculosis. One is the ceremony about the Wind Chant. If something goes wrong with that, it is tuberculosis, and if lightning strikes you, tuberculosis is the result . . . [Adair and Deuschle, 1970].

4. The condition is a member of a class of Indian sicknesses that must be treated in an Indian way, as opposed to a class of non-Indian diseases that must be treated by non-Indian practitioners. Pima and Papago Indians recognize the following two classes of sickness: "Wandering" sickness is characterized by its infectiousness originating from contact with foreigners (these "wandering" sicknesses come, change, and go; examples are measles, flu, and chickenpox); and "staying" sicknesses have always existed and always will (they never leave the Pima and Papago to afflict other people, nor do they pass by contagion from one person to another). These are diseases an individual gets by transgressing injunctions associated with certain animals, such as rabbits, horned toads, or caterpillars; plants (peyote, jimson weed); natural forces (lightning, wind); ceremonies; or concepts (enemy, saint, whore). In these cases, the shaman diagnoses the disease by symptoms and patient's history, performs sucking and massaging therapy, and appeals to the appropriate spirits. In refractory cases, the shaman refers the patient to a singer who will perform appropriate ceremonies. Lack of success with Euroamerican medicine may be one of the diagnostic signs of staying sickness (Bahr et al., 1972).

In short, while minor discomforts are generally treated empirically, multiple minor discomforts, chronic diseases, and those of obscure expression call for an explanation that goes beyond Euroamerican theories of etiology and treatment. The most common component of extrascientific explanatory systems is related, directly or indirectly, to ideas about spiritual, natural, or social balance. Measures that a patient or his or her family believe must be taken to deal with this aspect of the illness may hinder the physician's treatment regime, they may be neutral, or they may complement or reinforce the physician's efforts. However, each case must be considered on its own merits, because of cultural variations and individual variations in apprehension of tradition.

The mechanism by which disease and misfortune come about as a result of moral infraction is related to the concept of "power," which will be discussed in the next section.

The Idea of Power

Power, as the vital force of the universe, enters into health behavior in four ways: (1) the power of spiritual forces and objects to cause disease, (2) the power of medicine to counteract disease, (3) the power of an individual to manipulate spirit power to heal, and (4) the power of an individual to manipulate spirit power to cause disease and misfortune. All these are local aspects of the same pervasive vital force that activates living beings and imbues entities such as boulders, whirlwinds, rock crystals, and mountains with their characteristic personalities.

The details vary from tribe to tribe and tradition to tradition, but a synthetic statement would include the belief that power was concentrated at the creation of the world and has been diffused through all the beings; that humans, being created last, received the smallest portion; that individual humans can acquire power by entering into a relationship with an appropriate spiritual entity; that power is neither good nor evil; and that either the availability of power or the ability of humans to acquire it has declined since conquest by Europeans.

I have said enough about the power of spiritual forces to cause disease in the previous section. Here I shall discuss the relations of power to healing and healers.

In all Native American traditions concerning power, it is ultimately derived from a spiritual source. Skill and technology may accomplish some goals and may suffice their owners for a limited time and in ordinary situations, but there will come a time when the lack of power will result in failure. For example, among the Lakota, many people know ordinary herbal medicines for simple cuts, headaches, gastric upsets, toothaches, and general well-being. They have learned these usually from their relatives, and sprinkle tobacco where they gather them and protect them from the vitiating effects of menstruating women. However, at this level, the medicine works only pragmatically; its power must be called into action by one who has been given this ability in vision. The same herbal remedy that will work only in simple cases for a layperson will accomplish much more in the hands of a person who has power himself or herself to call on the power of the herb, as well as the power of spirit helpers who augment it. These individuals may be herbalists, who have received their power in a vision, or they may belong to one of a number of classes of shamans, who have relations with numbers of spirits. Just as herbalists may specialize in the administration of a few herbs for specified classes of conditions, so shamans specialize in the treatment of certain classes of diseases. Shamans, however, also claim power to find lost objects, affect luck, an aid in hunting.

All Lakota men traditionally are expected to receive some instruction and some power from visions, but shamans also usually inherit extra potential for power and make many vision quests throughout their lives. In addition, the time when they must start preparing for their vocation is announced by a serious illness, which only another shaman can cure. This episode initiates a period of apprenticeship and seeking of power visions. In this sense, power is somewhat equivalent to knowledge, and the supplicant, in addition to demonstrating his pitiable condition, asks for power "so that my people may live." Although power is knowledge, in the Lakota view, and is sought and given for socially useful ends, there is still a danger that the individual who controls it may abuse his or her relationship with his or her spirit helpers and thus lose control of the power, or the spirits may react to this abuse by withdrawing their support and allowing misfortune to happen or actively bring down misfortune on the miscreant or his or her associates. In addition, if a client neglects to sponsor a thanksgiving sing following a healing sing, bad luck may visit the client or his or her family.

Lakota individuals must gain their own power by direct experience with tutelary spirits, who provide them with knowledge, obligations, songs, designs, and objects that serve as collectors and repositories of power. Other tribes in the same area allow individuals to purchase power from people who have gained it in direct experience. In the Plains, Northwest, and Canada, the gaining and control of power are an individual matter, and constraints on its socially acceptable use depend on the individual's responsibility. There is always the danger that the shaman may use his or her power for evil, and individuals in some tribes have been known to use their powers for their own aggrandizement without any healing or socially useful practice at all. Technically, these are called sorcerers or witches. Nevertheless, their power ultimately comes from the same source. In the Southwest, socially useful power is controlled by priestly societies, and individuals who use power outside these societies are ipso facto witches. Referring to the previous section, even sorcerers may participate in the moral system, since they enter into interpersonal conflict resulting from failure to meet traditional obligations, either in actuality or in threat. In addition, since people do not want to be accused of sorcery, they avoid exhibiting the stereotypic traits of sorcerers—hostility, covetousness, sexual deviance, noncooperativeness, and lack of amiability.

The idea of power as the basis for the vitality of all beings and theories about the acquisition and control of power are basic to Native American cultures and pervade all aspects of social and religious life, in addition to contributing to individual ideology and self-image. Nevertheless, in spite of assertions about the superiority of Indian power, there is a widespread belief that spiritual power has diminished drastically since conquest by Europeans. It is unclear whether, in the world views discussed here, the source of power has weakened or the ability of humans to tap this source has diminished, but the result is the same. Shamans and sorcerers are less powerful than they used to be, and less dramatic miracles are performed.

Individual power depends on the power of the group. The power of the group is manifested in the amount of self-determination the group exercises, as well as the degree of cohesion in the participation in and support of traditional rituals and political life. As the tribe loses its ability to make decisions for itself, and as social and religious life becomes more fractioned, the ability of individuals to gain power, not only to heal, but to maintain good fortune (including health) in their daily life, has diminished. In addition, the introduction of diseases and conditions that indigenous healing systems had no power to control also has vitiated the strength of indigenous power.

"Whiteman diseases" and Euroamerican medicine introduce another source of tension in relation to ideas about power. While most Native Americans recognize, in varying degrees, a class of diseases that can only be treated by traditional methods, they also are only too aware of the fact that Euroamerican medicine has the technology as well as the responsibility to treat a large class of easily recognizable diseases. However, Euroamericans do not have access or, in some views, have only limited access to the source of power. Thus whites are only clever, but do not have the spiritual power without which one has only partial validation. As stated by a Kiowa Apache:

> Well, the white man, they have to go to a school to learn there. That's where they learn how to doctor, but Indian doctors have to learn in the hard way. They have to go way out somewhere by themselves. That way they learn to doctor. Something always tell them; they just brave enough to go out there like that. Something will show them how to doctor [Bross, 1971].

Not only do whites have no power, but, according to Ute thinking:

> The white is regarded as an interloper. It is not clear to Indians just what whites would do with power if they were able to acquire it. Who would turn to whites for advice, or for a cure, or for help in assuaging the wrath of a malevolent spirit? Orations at [sun] dances stress Indian integrity, the acquisition of power for Indian ends, and the need to respect and observe the practices of the "old people." Thus the focus is on Indian life, not white. It is a conscious, explicit, verbalized focus [Jorgensen, 1972].

In summary, the power to stay healthy, to heal, and to make ill is obtained and maintained by relations with the spirit world. Technology and skill are only partly responsible for success and depend on spiritual power for their social validation. Native Americans have seen their access to power decline as the fruits of Euroamericans' technology and cleverness increase. In this way, dissonance is induced and increased in Indian's views of the healing process.

Etiquette and the Healing Encounter

Moral components in an individual's disease theory influence the way he or she reacts to symptoms; ideas about power influence the way he or she will perceive the physician and his or her technology. Behavior in healing situations will be influenced by the patient's ideas about etiquette—that is, the way people are supposed to behave toward one another—and these are a function of ideas about the nature of man and woman, and of relations between people, as well as ideas about the way these relationships are to be expressed. Again, dissonance enters into contacts between Native Americans and Euroamericans because of differences in etiquette.

We may begin this discussion by a metaphorical description of the differences between Native American and European conceptions of the nature of humans, their relations to the universe, and their mission in life.

In this metaphor, Indians see the universe as a field of energy, with many small vortices here and there. These vortices are humans, animals, plants, and other natural entities. Being energy vortices, they have no boundary; thus they are all intangibly connected to each other by their mutual participation in the energy field; they all have a mutual responsibility to maintain this field; there is no hierarchy; and one vortex cannot manipulate another vortex, because there is no discrete boundary to push against.

In contrast to this view, Europeans conceive of humans as distinct atoms in the universe, with discrete boundaries at the skin. They are charged with the mission of subduing and controlling the rest of the world and thus consider themselves superior to the rest of the world, the highest in the *scala naturae*. Humans are also taught that it is not only possible to manipulate other humans, it is necessary to do this and at the same time resist manipulation by others.

While this metaphor may not be explicitly articulated by any Native American, it accounts for behavioral statements about Native American etiquette and the perception of unhappy experiences resulting from differences in etiquette.

Native American etiquette is guided generally by four principles: egalitarianism, self-determination, personalistic relations, and amiable social relations. Since behavior generated by the last principle is the source of most confusion, I shall spend more time with it, but all these principles are interrelated.

The first law of etiquette is egalitarianism. The ideal person "treats everyone equal the same." Strangers and kinsmen alike are to be met respectfully, without fawning or condescension. Although there is some variation in details, most traditional etiquette requires soft handshakes and averted eyes as signs of respect. Again, respect does not imply hierarchical relationships. Each person who gives respect expects the same.

The principle of self-determination not only results in the stereotypical parents who allow the child to choose his or her medical treatment, but also under this principle, each person has the right and responsibility to choose his or her course of action, without interference from others. This means that direct requests or demands are violations of self-determination, and one avoids them. At the same time, a person learns to be sensitive to the needs of others, so direct requests do not have to be made. A person who is not acting right, not fulfilling his or her obligations, who is impolite, greedy, or otherwise antisocial, is never told directly of his or her failings. The usual response is avoidance.

In contrast to the fractionation of roles characteristic of large-scale industrial society, the small-scale nature of Native American society has required multiple role relationships among its members. This has engendered a need in Native Americans to relate to people as whole persons, even when they are strangers in a bureaucratic setting. A nurse or an occupational therapist met years before can be described so vividly that the listener could recognize the person on the street, and the encounter is remembered in the same way. By the same token, Indians hope to be treated the same.

In spite of unmet expectations and conflict, the expression of hostility was, and is, repressed and looked down upon, as disruptive to society, symptoms of loss of control, and cause of illness (as described in the section on moral components of disease theory). The following kinds of behavior that are considered normal in Euroamerican culture are considered hostile in Native American culture: loud talking, fast talking, interrupting, arguing, making a direct request (including direct questions), refusal of a request, joking between strangers or between persons not in an appropriate relationship, and direct criticism. The proper response to these kinds of behavior is withdrawal. Thus a patient who has suffered one of these affronts will not make his or her dissatisfaction explicit, but will just not show up again.

These are traditional ideas, and as more Native Americans become familiar with strategies for coping with Euroamerican institutions, their results may not be so evident to outsiders and the use of third-party brokers or interpreters will decline. Further, Native Americans know that since whites do not have the relationship to spiritual power that Indians have, they also do not have the control that comes from the knowledge of spiritual and natural law; therefore they do not expect honest or courteous treatment. Most encounters with whites confirm this expectation.

Implications for Practice

It can be seen from the foregoing that there is no neat formula for "handling Indians" in medical settings. Indeed, any approach to Native Americans that is based on this idea is doomed from the outset. One could make a generalization that a successful approach would be based on the assumption that the patient is capable of making decisions based on evidence provided and the moral and cognitive framework that he or she brings to the situation. It is the job of the physician to provide evidence so the patient can make necessary decisions, with a minimum of intrusion into the patient's privacy. This may not sound unique to Native Americans, but we have seen how these feelings are maintained within a systematic world view in Native Americans. We also have seen that these attitudes are compounded from traditional views of the supernatural and expectations of Euroamericans and their ways.

1. Procedures must be explained carefully. A baby brought to the Indian Health Service Hospital dehydrated from diarrhea was treated with IV glucose, in the only position available, the temporal vain. Grandmother happened to see the infant and accused the IHS doctors of "sticking needles in baby's head." The resulting confusion was never satisfactorily resolved, but might have been averted by earlier explanation of procedures.

2. Scolding does not help. As part of a long series of attempts to convince a family to bring an adolescent tubercular relative in for treatment, one agent said that if they did not bring the young man in, "You might as well take a gun and shoot him." The family interpreted this as a direct threat and refused to talk to any representatives of the Indian Health

Service or the Bureau of Indian Affairs. The family accepted "whiteman" treatment only after advice from the spirits in a shamanic meeting.

3. Delay in seeking medical care may be for a good reason in the patient's view. Many conditions present as serious problems that could have been simple had they been brought for treatment earlier. The first response of the physician may understandably be anger, and he or she may communicate this anger to the patient without first discerning the reasons for delay or recognizing the validity of the reasons to the patient. Fear of "whiteman" medicine, a high value on self-healing and endurance, or "toughing it out," lack of money, or ignorance of procedure may act in combination to prevent early treatment. It does no good to try to find out the reasons if the patient does not volunteer, neither is this the time for direct teaching of the necessity for early treatment.

4. Respect for the patient includes respect for his or her privacy. Besides the suspicion of questions into aspects of life that are not justified as germane to diagnosis and treatment, Indians are usually threatened by unwarranted attacks on the privacy of their bodies—usually interpreted as modesty. As noted earlier, these threats and suspicions are more often met by withdrawal than by direct resistance.

In summary, the side variation in traditions and acculturation experience precludes any explicit schedule for dealing with Native American patients. Without knowing, the physician communicates his or her respect, or lack of it, for the Indian patient and his or her culture. Respect for Native American culture implies respect for the patient and family. This is expressed in honesty, sensitivity to individual needs and to subtle and indirect requests, and acceptance of a need for self-determination by individuals—a tall order.

Bibliographic Note

Most of the ideas in this chapter are derived from personal fieldwork with Lakotas in Pine Ridge, South Dakota and with Native Americans in the San Francisco Bay Area (Kemnitzer 1969, 1973, 1976, 1978). The moral basis of disease theory is best laid out in Hallowell (1963) and Reichard (1950), and power is best discussed in the contributions by Fogelson and Adams (1977) and Walker (1970). A good introduction to Native American religion, popularly written and well documented, is Underhill (1965). Most general books about Native American medicine are romantic, inaccurate, and misleading. Vogel's history (1970) concerns mostly pragmatic treatments and deals only lightly with theory and ideology. Good tribal studies include Adair and Dueschle (1970), on the introduction of a health program in a

Navajo area; Bross (1971), on Kiowa Apache body concept (unfortunately *not* body image—this badly needed topic has not been studied); Jones (1972), on a Comanche medicine women; Bahr et al. (1974), on Piman medical theory; Mooney and Olbrechts (1932), a translation of a Cherokee medical formulary with explanations; and Jilek (1974), on mental health. Fuchs and Bashshur (1975) report on socioeconomic factors in the use of traditional medicine by Native Americans in the San Francisco Bay Area.

Medical problems are best discussed in Bean and Wood (1969), based on Wood (1970), Wallace (1973), papers reprinted by AMS Press listed in the bibliography, and annual statistical reports issued by the Indian Health Service. Political and legal aspects are introduced by Kane and Kane (1972) and Sclar (1972), but the rapidly changing situation is best covered in *Wassaja,* a monthly newspaper published by the American Indian Historical Society in San Francisco.

References

Adair, J., and Deuschle, K. *The People's Health. Medicine and Anthropology in a Navajo Community.* New York: Appleton-Century Crofts, 1970.

Bahr, D.M., Gregorio, J., Lopez, D.I., and Alvarez, A. Piman Shamanism and Staying Sickness (ka:cim mumkidag). Tucson: Univ. of Arizona Press, 1974.

Bean, L.J., and Wood, C. The crisis in Indian health. A California example *Indian Historian* 2(3):29–33, 1969.

Bross, M.G. The Kiowa Apache body concept in relation to health. *Papers in Anthropology* 12(2): 1–80, 1971.

Diagnosis and Treatment of Prevalent Diseases of North American Indian Populations, Vol. 1. New York: AMS Press, 1974.

Diagnosis and Treatment of Prevalent Diseases of North American Indian Populations, Vol. 2. New York: AMS Press, 1975.

Fogelson, R.D., and Adams, R.N., eds. *The Anthropology of Power. Ethnographic Studies from Asia, Oceania, and the New World.* New York: Academic, 1977.

Fuchs, M., and Bashshur, R. Use of traditional Indian medicine among urban Native Americans. *Medical Care* 13(11): 915–927, 1975.

Hallowell, A.I. Ojibwa world view and disease. In *Man's Image in Medicine and Anthropology.* (ed.), I Gladston. New York: International Universities Press, 1963, pp. 258–315.

Jilek, W.G. *Salish Indian Mental Health and Culture Change.* Toronto: Holt, Rinehart and Winston, 1974.

Jones, D.E. *Sanapia, Comanche Medicine Woman.* New York: Holt, Rinehart and Winston, 1972.

Jorgenson, R.L., and Kane, R.A. *The Sun Dance Religion. Power for the Powerless.* Chicago: Univ. of Chicago Press, 1972.

Kane, R.L., and Kane, R.A. *Federal Health Care (With Reservations!).* New York: Springer, 1972.

Kemnitzer, L.S. Whiteman medicine, Indian medicine and Indian identity on Pine Ridge Reservation. *Pine Ridge Research Bulletin No. 10,* 1969, pp. 26–33.

Kemnitzer, L.S. Adjustment and value conflict in urbanizing Dakota Indians measured by Q-sort technique. *American Anthropologist* 75: 687–707, 1973.

Kemnitzer, L.S. Structure, content, and cultural meaning of yuwipi: A modern Lakota healing ritual. *American Ethnologist* 3: 261–280, 1976.

Mooney, J., and Olbrechts, F.M. The Swimmer Manuscript. Cherokee Sacred Formulas and Medicinal Prescriptions. *U.S. Bureau of American Ethnology Bulletin 99,* 1932.

Moore, W.M., Silverberg, M.M., and Read, M.S., eds. *Nutrition, Growth and Development of North American Indian Children.* DHEW Pub. No. (NIH) 72-76. Washington: USGPO, 1972.

Pattison, E.M. Exorcism and psychotherapy: A case of collaboration. In *Religious Systems and Psychotherapy.* ed. R.H. Cox. Springfield, Ill.: Thomas, 1973, pp. 284–295.

Reichard, G. *Navaho Religion.* New York: Pantheon, 1950.

Rimoin, D.L. Ethnic variability in glucose tolerance and insulin secretion. *Archives of Internal Medicine* 124(6): 695–700, 1969.

Schechter, M.D., and Roberge, L. Sexual exploitation. In *Child Abuse and Neglect: The Family and the Community,* ed. R.E. Helfer and C.H. Kempe. Cambridge, Mass.: Ballinger, 1976, pp. 127–142.

Schultz, J.L. *White Medicine, Indian Lives.* Fort Collins: Colorado State University, Department of Anthropology, 1976.

Sclar, H. Participation by off reservation Indians in programs of the Bureau of Indian Affairs and the Indian Health Service. *Montana Law Review* 33: 191, 1972.

Underhill, R. *Red Man's Religion.* Chicago: Univ. of Chicago Press, 1965.

U.S. Public Health Service, Indian Health Service. *Indian Health Trends and Services.* Washington: USGPO, 1976.

Vogel, V.J. *American Indian Medicine.* Norman: Univ. of Oklahoma Press, 1970.

Walker, D.E., Jr., ed. Systems of North American witchcraft and sorcery. *University of Idaho Anthropological Monographs 1,* 1970.

Wallace, H. The health of American Indian children: A survey of current problems and needs. *Clinical Pediatrics* 12: 83–87, 1973.

Whiting, B. Paiute Sorcery. *Viking Fund Publications in Anthropology* 15, 1950.

Wood, C.S. A multiphasic health screening of three Southern California Indian reservations. *Social Science and Medicine* 4: 579–587, 1970.

25 Health-Care Issues for Asian Americans

Reiko Homma True

Introduction

The American health-care system is under attack now as never before because of its high cost and often questionable quality of care. The issues related to service delivery to the poor and racial minorities, in particular, has attracted considerable attention among consumer advocates and legislators. According to the 1971 white paper issued by the Department of Health, Education and Welfare (HEW), the poor and the racial minorities have been found to be consistently underserved in their medical care as compared with the middle- and upper-income white groups. Recent legislative initiatives, such as Public Law 93-64, Health Resources Development Act of 1975, concerned with health-care delivery are placing an increasing demand on health-care providers to become better acquainted with and more responsive to the needs of these underserved minorities.

In the past, health-service delivery has been based on the assumption that America is a "melting pot," where people with different ethnic backgrounds are expected to be quickly assimilated into the mainstream Anglo culture. As a result of this assumption, there has been little emphasis on the development of strategies for health-service delivery for ethnic minorities. Recent studies have indicated, however, that significant differences are found among ethnic groups in their styles of coping with illnesses and that greater effort is needed to develop flexible alternatives for effective service delivery (Suchman, 1964).

In this respect, no group's health-care needs are more misunderstood than Asian Americans. This is true because of the marked differences between the traditional Asian health-care practices and those of Western medicine. This chapter attempts to highlight the special needs and issues related to the medical treatment of Asian Americans in order that health practitioners can respond with increased understanding and sensitivity.

Background

There are over 1.5 million Asian Americans in the United States, representing a diverse group of ethnic and cultural backgrounds. The term *Asian American* is becoming increasingly popular as a replacement for the term

Oriental, referring to as many as 16 different ethnic groups, for example, Chinese, Japanese, Korean, Indonesian, Guamanian, Samoan, Filipino (Although the spelling for the word *Pilipino* has been previously identified as *Philippino* or as *Filipino,* the pronunciation is believed to be more closely related to *Pilipino;* for this reason, the community people are now using the *Pilipino* as the preferred spelling), and Vietnamese. The term *Asian American* is misleading in that it gives the impression that a homogeneous group of people exist who share a common background and a predictable way of responding.

The immigration of Asians into the United States was spearheaded by the Chinese in the early nineteenth century. They were attracted by the news of the gold rush and the demand for cheap labor in railroad and other construction projects. During the next 150 years or so, successive groups of Asians have entered the country, settling primarily in the West Coast states of California, Washington, and in Hawaii (American Historical Association, 1974; Crane, 1970; Kitano, 1969; Nee and Nee, 1973; Morales, 1974). In 1965, the immigration law was liberalized to permit more Asians to immigrate. Since then, there has been a rapid growth of the Chinese, Koreans, and Pilipino communities. Most recently, in 1975, with the fall of the Saigon government and with political upset in other Southeastern Asian countries, an additional 150,000 Asian refugees were admitted (HEW Task Force, 1976).

It should be remembered that the term *Asian American* refers to various different groups of people with a diversity of history, religion, language, and culture. In addition, these various communities are also characterized by the experience of differential patterns of immigration and reception in this country. For these reasons, each community must be understood individually as a distinct and separate entity. However, because of the extensive nature of these differences and limitations in the available space here, it will not be possible for this chapter to delve into them all. Instead, the focus will be on the commonalities among these communities.

Although there are some common issues shared by most Asian American communities, there is difficulty created by the popular myth about Asian Americans. While there have been mostly negative stereotypes in the past about Asian Americans, they are now increasingly seen as being intelligent, law abiding, quiet, loyal, hardworking, and successful. Unfortunately, this picture has led to a prevailing belief that Asian Americans do not suffer the disadvantages associated with other minority groups.

However, in spite of the evidence of affluence and achievement among some, a substantial number of Asian Americans suffer from ghetto existence, characterized by below-subsistence-level income, unemployment or underemployment, substandard housing, inadequate health services, and insufficient social services. These problems are particularly prevalent among the elderly and the foreign-born immigrant groups (USDHEW, 1974; U.S. Commission on Civil rights, 1975). These are important considerations to be kept in mind as factors affecting the health needs and care of the Asian Americans.

Health-Care Issues

Compared with other ethnic groups, the utilization rate of health-care services by Asian Americans in this country has been very low (Wong, 1975; Oriental Service Center, 1970; Li, 1972). Although low utilization is often equated with, or considered related to, low morbidity rate or absence of needs, studies have shown that there are other factors involved in creating such a pattern (Eaton and Weil, 1955; Selltiz et al., 1959). Examples of these contributing factors may be physical and psychological barriers to service utilization, lack of information or availability or alternative resources, and lack of financial resources.

In the case of Asian Americans, previously cited studies also have indicated that there is a great need for health services and that existing services are not accessible to Asian Americans. Theses studies go on to suggest that services are not accessible because of language barriers, cost, transportation problems, and fear and/or distrust of Western medical practices.

Within the Asian American communities, the groups experiencing the greatest difficulties are the elderly and the immigrants. There is a myth about the traditional Asian value placed in the care and respect of the elderly. Actually many of the elderly Asians in this country, who came as immigrants, live alone, under poverty-level existence, and suffer serious illnesses. They lack the ability to seek adequate medical care (White House Conference on Aging, 1972; Kalish and Moriwaki, 1973). They are either separated from their families or their families do not have the resources to help them.

Although generalized needs for services have been reported for nearly all groups of Asian Americans, information concerning more specific types of health needs are limited to a few of the more well-known groups, that is, Chinese, Japanese, and Pilipinos. As an illustration to highlight the diversity among various Asian Americans, Weaver (1976) discussed the contrast between long-established, fairly stable populations, such as the Japanese, and those experiencing rapid growth in recent years, such as Pilipinos. He notes that while some consider the Japanese Americans to have more favorable mortality rate than Anglos (Gordon, 1957, 1967; Kitano, 1971), there are no substantiating data for such assumptions. Weaver (1976) cites a number of existing pathologies that plague Japanese Americans more frequently than other groups, such as a greater occurence of cancer of the esophagus, stomach, and liver, and psychosomatic illnesses. He also notes that changes in diet and lifestyle may account for the increasing incidence of the following pathologies: cancer of colon, rectum, and breast; cardiovascular and renal diseases; and Hodgkin's disease.

However, the Pilipino community, which is the fastest growing Asian community with the largest number of new immigrants, is experiencing a great deal of stress because of the lack of social and economic resources within itself. Some of the unique health problems experienced by the Pilipino in the United States seem to be related to a combination of genetic predisposition, psychosocial stresses, and changing lifestyles. Major health problems include high rates of hyperuricemia, particularly among adult males; cardiovascular and renal diseases among women; diabetes mellitus; and industrial diseases. Ailments occurring among Pilipino farm workers and factory workers include arthritis, pesticide poisoning, and bronchial conditions (Weaver, 1976).

Although there is very little published information on the health status of Korean Americans, the situation is quite similar to that of the Pilipinos in that the community is undergoing rapid expansion from the influx of immigrants. While the resources in the community have always been limited, there is an increasing number of problems related to health, and the gap between needs and resources continue to widen.

However, when considering the health-care issues for Chinese Americans, one needs to bear in mind that some very complex issues exist that reflect the diverse nature of the community. There are some who are established and affluent and others who are fourth- and fifth-generation Americans who experience only marginal difficulties in dealing with the health-care institutions of this country. However, there are others who are immigrants, whose language capability in English is limited and whose resources are limited. Among the latter, there is a greater gap between existing resources and health-care needs.

According to the health surveys conducted in various parts of the Chinatowns in the United States, the following were identified as high-need issues: significantly high incidence of tuberculosis, infant mortality and poor neonatal care, and problems related to the elderly (Huang and Grachow, 1974; Hessler et al., 1975; Wong, 1975; Chan and Chang, 1975). Since these surveys focused on residents of Chinatown, where there is a greater concentration of immigrants with marginal resources, they fail to provide an overall perspective on the needs of the native-born Chinese Americans and others who live outside of the Chinatown area. However, the findings are nevertheless instructive, since they identify the needs of the most vulnerable population in the community. Other studies also have identified the tendency among Chinese toward psychosomatic symptoms (Tseng, 1975) and the changing patterns of cancer incidence (King and Haenszel, 1973; Fraumeni and Mason, 1974).

In terms of their approach to health-care practices, the surveys conducted in Boston and New York (Hessler et al., 1975; Chan and Chang, 1975) seem to indicate that the residents have varying degrees of preference toward traditional Chinese and Western medical practices, with a substantial number of them having a dual orientation. They found that these preferences were related to their sociocultural backgrounds. For example, immigrants, particularly elderly immigrants or women with limited education, were more inclined to rely on the traditional Chinese practices.

Another finding of note is that those who rely on traditional practices often try to self-treat themselves until the condition becomes so exacerbated that they are no longer able to manage. For this reason, many of the patients who come to the attention of the Western practitioners are in much worse condition and require a greater degree of care than would have been needed initially. In addition, since the various traditional medications may bring about unexpected side effects which the Western practitioner may be unfamiliar with, it becomes more difficult to sort out the true nature of the illnesses.

Some Comments on Traditional Approaches to Health Care

Although Western medical practice was introduced to Asian countries in the eighteenth and nineteenth centuries and quickly became an established institution, it has never completely replaced the old healing practices in Asia (Wong and Lien-Teh, 1932; Huard and Wong, 1968; Palos, 1972; Quinn, 1972; Bowers, 1970; Mckenzie and Chrisman, 1977). This tradition has been carried over to the United States and is still persisting among the more traditional. Since healing practices in nearly all Asian countries were strongly influenced by the Chinese medical concepts and technologies, a brief overview of the traditional Chinese healing practice will be discussed here.

As in most other cultures, the earliest form of healing in China was based on superstitious and mystical folk beliefs that illnesses were caused by demons and evil spirits. It was believed that evil spirits had to be driven away through magical rituals, charms, and incantations. Although such beliefs were gradually replaced by healers with a more uniform and systematically developed belief system, these superstitious beliefs still have a considerable following among the folk and peasant cultures from which many of the immigrant populations have originated.

During the early stages of the development of Chinese medicine, the medical profession was closely intertwined with the priesthood. This historical relationship is reflected in the Chinese ideograph character, referring to the term *i* ("doctor"), which is a composite of characters referring to priest and wine. For this reason, the medical profession has incorporated various religious beliefs of Taoism, Buddhism, and Confucianism and the use of the medicinal herbs by priests.

The period between 1100 B.C. and 900 A.D. is referred to as the "golden period of Chinese medicine," during which time the two basic doctrines were perfected. The nature and etiology of the diseases are explained in the doctrine of the five organs of spleen, liver, heart, lungs, and kidneys.

The illnesses were believed to be caused by disturbances in any of the combination of the Yin-Yang forces and elements. The healing methods used to deal with these disturbances included acupuncture, moxa treatment, massage, herbs, meditation, and breathing and other exercises. Among these methods, the least understood is probably the moxa treatment. It is a form of healing practice developed in China which involves applying heat to acupuncture points through the use of combustibel cones of powdered leaves.

Although most U.S.-born Asian Americans are not strongly influenced by these traditional practices, many elderly and immigrants still believe in the efficacy of these treatments. There is a following observation on the moxa treatment among Japanese Americans who were placed in a concentration camp during the War:

> A piece of punk is burned on the skin "to stimulate the nerves" in selected spots, the malfunctioning of which nerves being responsible for specific illness. Another group had a pseudo-neurological theory behind its curing technique, which consisted in sticking gold needles in the patient to stimulate his nerves. On a non-institutional basis, one, of course, often observes such masochistic behavior in individual neurotics; here evidently a group neurosis is elaborately tailormade to fit the characteristic anxieties of the people [LeBarr, 1945].

Now that the Western medical community has been introduced to acupuncture, Yoga, and other alternative Asian health practices, it is hoped that such a negative perception no longer exists among our practitioners.

Some Suggestions for Treatment Approaches

While there is a substantial number of Asian Americans who are thoroughly accustomed to dealing with Western practitioners thereby needing little special attention, there are many others who have considerable difficulty communicating their needs for medical assistance. With the growing number of Asian immigrants here in this country, such difficulty is likely to continue, if not increase. In order to break down the barriers that exist, the practitioner should be open and sensitive to the individual and cultural differences of the various Asian American patients. In situations where patients are maintaining dual approaches to medical care, the practitioner should not be openly critical of them or make frontal attacks on such practices.

In terms of the more obvious problems that exist in the Asian American community, such as the language barrier, lack of financial resources, lack of health-care information, and physical and psychological barriers to services, changes will need to be made at social and institutional levels. For example, attention should be given to some type of change in the following areas:

1. Training and hiring of more bilingual, bicultural health-care personnel, including professional and paraprofessional workers, to remove the communication barriers.
2. Location of health-care facilities so that they are easily accessible to minimize the transportation problems.
3. Making low-cost services available to those with limited funds.
4. Outreach services appropriate to the cultural and family organization of the Asian population.
5. Bilingual health-education programs through use of pamphlets and media presentations to inform the residents about the existing resources, the need to seek early professional care, and so forth.

At the same time, there is also a need to deal with the more subtle attitudinal barriers to health care. The role played by health-care practitioners is critical in this respect. In order to improve the process of effective communication, interviewing, diagnostic assessment, and treatment, the following factors should also be considered:

1. *Stoicism and maintenance of face.* One of the most deeply rooted cultural values among Asian Americans is the value placed on stoicism, that is, ability to control the expression of pain and suffering and to endure and persevere. Closely related to this is the concept of shame and pride and the belief that one's inability to control self-expression will lead to loss of face and a sense of shame. The concept of shame is frequently referred to in several Asian languages as *haji* (Japanese), *mentzu* (Chinese), *chaemyun* (Korean), and *hiya* (Tagalog). When applied to the clinical situation, it will be useful to bear in mind that many Asians will try very hard to minimize their pain and discomfort. It may be that when the patient states that he or she is feeling a little bit of pain, it may actually mean that there is a considerable amount of pain. An effective approach for a practitioner in such a situation would be to maintain an actively empathic and supportive posture and become more directly inquisitive about physical pain than with Anglos.

2. *Reserve.* Closely related to stoicism, another trait stressed in the Asian culture is what is known as *enryo* (Japanese), *Him Huy* (Chinese), or

Pakikisama (Tagalog). It is akin to the Western concept of reserve and is related to the need not to create burdens or demands on the other person. Asians are taught to be as reserved and unobtrusive as possible, which appears at times to Westerners as passivity. In clinical settings, this may influence the patient not to create any inconvenience for the physician, to the point of not asking for clarification when there are questions or when the patient disagrees with the physician. In order to maintain a clear line of communication, it may be necessary to go beyond asking questions. There is the need to be sensitive to indications of various cues, including nonverbal ones, as well as to allow sufficient time for explanation and discussion.

3. *Modesty and Asian women.* When dealing with Asian people, particularly with those who were born and raised in Asia, another issue to be kept in mind is the impact of the cultural emphasis placed on modesty, particularly for women. It is generally a very stressful situation for Asian American women to be examined by physicians who are males and non-Asian. This will often exacerbate the already existing communication difficulties. A Western male physician could include a woman assistant in the examining room to be of support for the Asian woman. Also, the physician should be as supportive as possible, such as providing explanations concerning the examining procedures and the purpose for such steps (see chapter 14).

4. *Fear of laboratory procedures, surgery, and other medical procedures.* While blood drawing, x-rays, and surgery are important aspects of Western medical practice, there is considerable cultural fear of such procedures among some of the less-educated foreign-born patients (Chan and Chang, 1975). Although such fears can be allayed eventually through careful explanation of the needs and the benefit to be derived, it also would be helpful to include someone representing the patient's potential support system in this purpose. Such person could be one of the respected family members, community workers, or ministers. In addition, there also should be an effort to organize bilingual community education programs to increase the understanding and appreciation of the Western medical practices.

5. *Fear of hospitals and hospitalization.* While hospitalizations are frequently used for nonfatal illnesses in United States, in Asian countries, hospitalization is instituted in cases involving serious illnesses that are often terminal. For this reason, a physician's decision to hospitalize an Asian patient may create more anxieties than it does for American patients. The kind of anxieties experienced by men and women in this regard are somewhat different. Because of the need to maintain the masculine facade of strength, Asian men may feel unable to admit their fears. However, women may be more concerned about what will happen to their families in their absence.

For whatever reasons, Asian patients will tend to be reluctant to talk about their anxieties and concerns. For this reason, it would be helpful to carefully explain the need for hospitalization, allaying unnecessary anxieties whenever possible. It also will be helpful for the physician to be sensitive to the complications that may develop out of the need for hospitalization, for example, need for a family caretaker, and to help arrange for social workers or others to make necessary arrangements.

6. *Special problems of pregnancy and childbirth.* Many of the Asian immigrants are from backgrounds where medical care is sought only during the periods of medical crisis and where the concept of preventive medicine is unfamiliar. For example, it is not unusual for a pregnant immigrant woman to come in contact with a clinic for the first time when she is already 6 or 7 months pregnant. It is believed that this poor prenatal care is responsible in large part for the high early infant mortality rate among Asians. A great deal of painstaking effort is needed to educate Asian Americans regarding sound health-care practices.

Summary

At a time when inadequate health-care treatment of the poor and the ethnic minorities is attracting public attention, the problem of service delivery to Asian Americans is probably least understood. Asian Americans are often thought of as one homogeneous group, when in reality there is a tremendous diversity. The fact that their traditional health-care practices are different historically and culturally from the Western practices contributes to this misunderstanding.

Studies have indicated that the utilization of health-care services by Asian Americans in the United States is very low despite documented need for such services. In addition to the obvious barriers to services, such as language difficulties, transportation problems, and high costs, there are other more subtle psychological and cultural barriers exacerbating this problem. Physicians and other health-care providers need to be sensitive to the impact of Asian cultural values, such as stoicism, reserve and modesty. Health providers also need to recognize the fears and anxieties some Asian patients have about hospitalization and treatment delivery by non-Asian practitioners. There is much need for greater understanding and a supportive attitude among existing care providers.

References

American Historical Association. *Pacific Historical Review: The Asian Americans* 153: 4, 1974.
Bowers, J. *Western Medical Pioneers in Feudal Japan.* Baltimore: Johns Hopkins Press, 1970.
Chan, C., and Chang, J.K. The role of Chinese medicine in New York

City's Chinatown. *American Journal of Chinese Medicine* 4(1): 31–45, 1975.

Crane, P.S. *Korean Patterns.* Seoul: Hollyn, 1970.

Eaton, J., and Weil, R.J. *Culture and Mental Disorders.* Glencoe, Ill.: Free Press, 1955.

Fraumeni, J.F., and Mason, T.J. Cancer mortality among Chinese Americans, 1950–69. *Journal of the National Cancer Institute* 52(3): 659–665, 1974.

Gordon, T. Mortality experience among the Japanese in the U.S., Hawaii, and Japan. *Public Health Reports* 72: 543–553, 1957.

————. Further mortality experience among Japanese Americans. *Public Health Reports* 82: 973–984, 1967.

Hessler, R.M., Nolan, M.F., Ogbru, B., and New, P.K. Intraethnic diversity: Health care of the Chinese Americans. *Human Organization* 34(3): 253–262, 1975.

HEW Refugee Task Force. *Reports to the Congress.* Washington: USGPO, 1976.

Huang, C., and Grachow, F. *The Dilemma of Health Services in Chinatown, New York City.* New York City Department of Health, 1974.

Huard, P., and Wong, M. *Chinese Medicine.* New York: McGraw-Hill, 1968.

Jacobs, P., and Landau, S. *To Serve the Devil,* Vol. II; *Colonials and Sojourners.* New York: Random House, 1971.

Kalish, R.A., and Moriwaki, S. The world of the elderly Asian Americans. *Journal of Social Issues* 29: 187–193, 1973.

King, H., and Haenszel, W. Cancer mortality among foreign and native born Chinese in the U.S. *Journal of Chronic Disease* 26: 623–646, 1973.

Kitano, H. *Japanese Americans: The Evaluation of a Subculture.* Englewood Cliffs, N.J.: Prentice-Hall, 1969.

Kitano, H., and Sue, S., eds. Asian Americans: The model minorities. *Journal of Social Issues* 29(2): 1973.

LeBarr, W. Some observations on character structure in the Orient. *Psychiatry* 8: 349–351, 1945.

Leslie, C., ed. *Asian Medical System: A Comparative Study.* Berkeley, Calif.: University of California Press, 1977.

Li, F.P. Chinese community health task force study. *American Journal of Public Health* 62(4): 536–539, 1972.

Mckenzie, J., and Chrisman, N. Healing herbs, gods, and magic: Folk health beliefs among Filipino Americans. *Nursing Outlook* 25(5): 326–328, 1977.

Morales, R.F. *Makibaka: The Pilipino American Struggle.* Los Angeles: Mountainview Publishers, 1974.

Nee, V.G., and Nee, B.C. *Longtime Californ': A Documentary Study of an American Chinatown.* New York: Random House, 1973.

Oriental Service Center. *Health Surveys.* Los Angeles, April 1970.

Palos, S. *The Chinese Art of Healing.* New York: Bantam Books, 1972.

Quinn, J.R., ed. *Medicine and Public Health in the People's Republic of China.* National Institute of Health. DHEW Pub. No. (NIH) 72-67. Washington: USGPO, 1972.

Selltiz, C., Jahoda, M., Deutch, M., and Cook, S. *Research Methods in Social Relations.* New York: Holt, Rinehart, and Winston, 1959.

Suchman, E.A. Socio-medical variations among ethnic groups. *American Journal of Sociology* 70: 319–331, 1964.

Tseng, W.S. The nature of somatic complaints among psychiatric patients: The Chinese case. *Comprehensive Psychiatry* 16(3): 237–245, 1975.

U.S. Commission on Civil Rights. *Asian Americans and Pacific Peoples: A Case of Mistaken Identity.* Washington: USGPO, 1975.

U.S. Department of Health, Education and Welfare (DHEW). *Towards a Comprehensive Health Policy for the 1970's. A White Paper.* Washington: USGPO, 1971.

U.S. Department of Health, Education and Welfare (DHEW). *A Study of Selected Socio-economic Characteristics of Ethnic Minorities.* Vol. II: *Asian Americans.* DHEW Pub. No. (OS) 75-121. Washington: USGPO, 1974.

Weaver, J.L. *National Health Policy and the Underserved: Ethnic Minorities, Women, and the Elderly.* St. Louis: Mosby, 1976.

White House Conference on Aging. *The Asian American Elderly.* Washington: USGPO, 1972.

Wong, K., and Lien-Teh, W. *History of Chinese Medicine.* Tientsin, China: Tientsin Press, 1932.

Wong, M. A Survey Report on Medical Care in Oakland's Asian Community. Oakland, Calif.: Asian Health Services, 1975.

Part V
Delivery of Health-Care Services: Patients and Families

The great Samuel Johnson was seldom at a loss for words, but on one occasion he said, "What can a sick man say, but that he is sick?" This book is full of accounts of various psychological considerations in health care, written by those on the caregiver's side of the medical interaction. There is not a great literature written by the sick, but Virginia Woolf, in expressing her ideas about that dearth, also described some of the phenomenology of illness in quite as powerful a way as Susan Sontag did in the quotation we gave in the introduction to this book. In her essay "On Being Ill" (from *The Moment and Other Essays*), Woolf wrote:

> Considering how common illness is, how tremendous the spiritual change that it brings, how astonishing, when the lights of health go down, the undiscovered countries that are then disclosed, what wastes and deserts of the soul a slight attack of influenza brings to view, what precipices and lawns sprinkled with bright flowers a rise of temperature reveals, what ancient and obdurate oaks are uprooted in us by the act of sickness, how we go down into the pit of death and feel the waters of annihilation close above our heads and wake thinking to find ourselves in the presence of the angels and the harpers when we have a tooth out and come to the surface in the dentist's arm-chair and confuse his "rinse the mouth—rinse the mouth" with the greeting of the Deity stooping from the floor of heaven, to welcome us—when we think of this, as we are so frequently forced to think of it, it becomes strange indeed that illness has not taken its place with love and battle and jealousy among the prime themes of literature.

In this section, we address three issues: the first-person description of the impact of illness on a patient, the problems with objectification of patients in the supposed service of more efficient medicine, and the impact of illness on family members. All are areas that are frequently neglected when considering the psychological aspects of diseases. The authors all write from extremely personal perspectives: Winkler and Birrer (chapters 26 and 27) as patients, Marcia and Al Ross (chapter 28) as parents of a terminally ill child. Perhaps more than any other chapters, these will impress on the reader the extraordinary nature of the psychology of illness and are hence a fitting way in which to conclude this book. All shades of emotion, from despondency to relief, appear; we have not wanted the authors to underplay the impact of circumstances.

26 The Doctor-Patient Relationship in the Mastectomy Experience

Win Ann Winkler

The doctor-patient relationship in specialized medicine has created a false nostalgia for "the good old days," the horse-and-buggy doctor, the "bedside manner," and other turn-of-the-century practices that probably were responsible for the average lifespan of 40 years in an adult and an exceptionally high infant and child fever mortality rate.

While one of the side effects of medical progress has been the doctor-on-the-golf-course jokes, the general consensus has been that the neuter-sex doctor simply does not give a damn about the neuter-sex patient. However, the doctor-patient relationship never reached "criminal" proportions until the early feminists got into the act. Then, of course, it was allegedly the *male* doctor perpetrating his phallic imperialism against the *female* patient in female-related disorders only. There are no cases on record of a male dentist working out his hostilities against women by suggesting root-canal procedures, nor has any doctor been accused of removing gall bladders for the sake of mutilation in either male or female patients. If any dermatologist ever attempted to cure dandruff in a male patient by performing a prostatectomy, it was never recorded in feminist literature.

Although it was never made clear by the orthodox feminocracy whether the desire to mutilate human beings was the only motivation for every medical practitioner from Hippocrates to St. Luke to Marcus Welby, certainly any male practitioner who chose to specialize in female-related disorders could never have had any other motivation. Women gynecologists, obstetricians, and breast surgeons have received the same treatment from the women's movement as low-income men—they simply do not exist.

With all due respect to antimale epithets coined by the women's movement in the general area of obstetrics and gynecology, it is specifically the area of breast cancer, and mastectomy in particular, that has come to epitomize the victimization and mutilation of women by men. There are actually two schools of thought on the nature of this crime: (1) if the medical profession were not male dominated, breast cancer could never have come into being in the first place, and (2) mastectomies are not necessary.

In any area of specialized medicine, the term *doctor-patient relationship* becomes a misnomer. Once an illness progresses past the flu shot from the rapidly disappearing family practitioner, the patient is dealing with the medical bureaucracy—laboratories, receptionists, x-ray technicians, secretaries, nurses, bookkeepers, answering services and answering machines, busy signals—all of whose prime function seems to be to protect the specialist from the most serious threat to his or her effective practice of medicine, namely, any sort of human interaction with a patient.

In addition to the severity of the illness, or the suspected illness, the patient's desperation increases with the inability to contact the doctor. This desperation reaches panic proportions when the patient's social network— spouse, lover, friends, and family—can react only with a level of anxiety that is greater than the patient's.

The patient who suspects breast cancer is handicapped by her social network to the degree that the patient who suspects cardiac disorder is not. The suspected breast cancer patient's friends will tell her not to be silly, not to worry, that there is nothing wrong with her, while the man with chest pains will be encouraged to see his doctor at once. As the patient's social network becomes increasingly paralyzed in the area of comfort and emotional support, hyperdependency will increase on the doctor initially, not so much for competent treatment, but for a denial that the suspected illness may indeed become a reality. While a woman with abdominal pain may seek the advice of a doctor fully prepared to undergo an appendectomy, if required, the woman with a lump who consults a breast surgeon is not quite that willing to undergo a mastectomy, if required.

Thus, in the case of breast cancer, the doctor-patient relationship is handicapped by two overwhelming factors: (1) the lack of support and encouragement for the patient by sociocultural factors, and (2) the patient's reluctance to go ahead with the only life-saving procedure currently available.

A double fantasy is set up by both doctor and patient. The doctor fantasizes about a cooperative patient who will have her emotional needs met by friends and family, and the patient fantasizes about a doctor who will (1) tell her that the tumor is benign or (2) if a mastectomy is required, turn his back on his entire practice in order to fulfill her emotional as well as physical needs following surgery.

In addition, the patient is handicapped because a mastectomy is the only experience in which a woman will be completely bereft of the "female support group." In virtually every female physical experience from the onset of menarche through pregnancy, contraception, abortion, childbirth, breast feeding, hysterectomy, or menopause, a woman has a "female support group" that is not necessarily limited to family and friends. Two pregnant women who have never met before may strike up a conversation concerning morning sickness, swollen legs, and method of delivery, although they do not know each other's names. Two women who are total strangers may discuss hysterectomies on the supermarket checkout line. This peer-group support is, to my knowledge, unique among women. This same lack of peer support has been noted and remarked upon among men. It is not common for two executives on a plane to close their attaché cases and discuss their respective problems with premature ejaculation or their sense of inadequacy at their wives' failure to achieve orgasm.

Breast cancer is the exception to the rule of the female support group. It is also the only female disorder that will evoke a reaction of "My God, how disgusting!" from other women. Except for the younger, outspoken group of patients who are decidedly in the minority, mastectomy is still regarded as a private shame whose most serious implications involve the possibility of someone "finding out." The woman who may have discussed contraception freely with comparative strangers will not acknowledge the nod of greeting on a bus from the saleswoman who fitted her with a prosthesis. The younger woman who may well reach out to her peer group for support and encouragement will receive one of two reactions: misguided attempts at reassurance that she could not possibly have had cancer (and besides, if she did, no man would think twice about it), or the solemn pronouncement from the feminists to the effect that if male surgeons had their penises cut off, mastectomies would no longer be performed. For the friends of the mastectomy patient, breast cancer falls into virtually the same category as child abuse; no one wants to acknowledge that it exists, but if it does, certainly not among anyone they know. Husbands and lovers are no more eager to acknowledge the possibility of a mastectomy than are a woman's friends and family.

As the patient's rocks of emotional support progressively turn into paper maché, hyperdependency on the surgeon reaches unmanageable proportions for both surgeon and patient. The patient's dependency on the surgeon and hatred for him or her increase proportionately. The surgeon, as a survival mechanism, has learned to hide behind the medical bureaucracy and clinical rhetoric. This is where the second major unmentionable of the feminist orthodoxy comes into play. No one is ever permitted to acknowledge the snide insolence of female members of the medical profession in contrast to the sympathetic understanding of the male doctor. This is where the patient is in for her second major shock, even before the mastectomy, or even if the tumor turns out to be benign. Her possible need for a mastectomy will make her the target of venom and viciousness from female members of the "helping" profession. Her ambivalence and guilt increase with her resentment at what she knows are her friends' and family's attempts at supportiveness. The doctor, during all this, seems to become more elusive and evasive the more he or she is needed.

In all areas of specialized medicine, the higher the doctors' credentials and reputations, the higher their caseloads, the more frequently they are called away from their office practices for hospital emergencies, the lower their availability for personal interaction with each patient. The patient, on her part, has the choice of a highly qualified practitioner who will never remember her name or a hand-holding charmer who last performed a mastectomy 20 years ago. Sometimes she can get a combination of the two. If she has never undergone surgery before, this could be the patient's first experience with the medical bureaucracy, which can be far more traumatic than a diagnosis of cancer. From the moment a mammography is ordered until months, and often years, following the mastectomy, the patient's cries for human understanding are met by recorded phone messages, terse cliches, syrupy runarounds, glib evasiveness, and ad lib bitchiness. She very quickly learns that her need for human interaction in a time of crisis will only earn her the label of, to lapse into the nonmedical vernacular, "pain in the ass."

Patronizing, putdown, and *belittling* are the favorite adjectives used to describe the male doctor's attitudes toward female patients. The mastectomy patient rarely has enough time with her surgeon for him to display any classic male chauvinist characteristics. She has to wait until she gets into the hospital for any serious colonialism to take place. It is not only mastectomy patients who are promptly placed in the category of "good girl" or "bad girl," it is any woman who enters a major teaching hospital for any suspected illness or treatment. Moreover, if the woman is 40 or over, it is simply assumed that all she needs to allay her anxieties is a good healthy dose of daytime television soap operas. She is first-named by the nurses and social workers, who are convinced that their professional status cannot tolerate anything less than "Ms." She is supposed to be grateful for basket-weaving activity prescribed for her, even if she is a renowned interior designer. She may regard organized religion the way she regards daytime television, but that will not stop a zealous hospital clergyman from giving her "consolation" on his appointed rounds.

The "good girl' patient will keep her hospital gown open and her mouth shut. The "bad girl" patient may try to express shock, anger, annoyance, and demand an explanation of what has happened to her, what her prognosis is, and generally manifest other forms of survival instinct—blasphemy where hospital procedure is concerned. She will quickly be spoon-fed by the time-honored mastectomy clichés—"Think how lucky you are; be grateful you didn't lose an arm or an eye"; "It sure is a beautiful scar"; "Certainly you're not going to worry about a little thing like a breast."

The surgeon, by this time, has lost whatever minimal interest he may ever have had with the patient, who, by now, has been transformed from a human being into an open wound. If the patient is in a major teaching hospital, which the medical gospel tells us is the best place to be, her mastectomy also will become an interesting object lesson for the entire kindergarten class of the medical school with which the hospital is affiliated. Her visitors will either shift their gaze while shifting from foot to foot, making bad jokes about hospital food, or telling her honestly that they do not know what to say.

If the surgeon is merely indifferent to the patient's emotional needs, she can consider herself lucky. Some of the world's leading surgical oncologists are known by their reassuring classical statements, which run the gamut from "What are you so concerned about a breast for? After all, you're forty-three" to "Now you can join the men's club, ha ha!" (if the latter patient is lucky enough to be a bilateral).

In the midst of all this, depending on her surgeon's orientation, the patient may be force-fed by a visit from a Reach to Recovery volunteer. Reach to Recovery is a branch of the American Cancer Society, and its volunteers, recovered mastectomy patients, earn their "Brownie points" by greeting patients with "Don't worry, your husband will continue to love you," which does not always go over too well with the woman who is either going through a divorce or is in a living-together arrangement. But the really *beau geste* of Reach to Recovery is the standard training-manual practice of taking the patient's two hands, placing them on the volunteer's breast and prosthesis respectively and asking, "Tell me, Darling, which one is real?" There are quite a few recovered mastectomy patients who swear that recovering from Reach to Recovery was more difficult than recovering from the mastectomy.

In all fairness, it should be stated that, like invitations to join the Shriners, the visit from the Reach to Recovery volunteer is considered a blessing from heaven by women of a particular sociocultural orientation. There are many surgeons who become as livid at the words *Reach to Recovery* as some beneficiaries of this experience do, and unfortunately, some of their patients who could benefit from this 1950s *Jello* magazine philosophy are denied the experience. No surgeon, to my knowledge, has ever regarded Reach to Recovery the way they have regarded penicillin; that is, it may be contraindicated for some patients. The concept also has been set forth that the Reach volunteer saves the surgeon an unsavory job, namely, that of dealing with the psychoemotional aspects of the mastectomy. It also should be stated in fairness that the arm exercises designed by Reach to Recovery are, in many instances, the only form of physical therapy the patient receives after surgery, which is not saying that much for hospital policy.

However, for the woman whose breast(s) meant more to her than a contribution to the national economy by the purchase of brassieres, the standard Reach reassurance of "Once you get fitted with your prosthesis, you won't even know which breast was removed" is about as supportive as the promise of a large doll to a woman whose child has just died.

It is only when the patient is out of the hospital that the full realization of the loss of a breast (or two) and the diagnosis of cancer becomes a reality.

She is in for a few more shocks, such as the polite leprosy treatment, the very real job and insurance discrimination, possible inability of her husband to cope with the situation, and comments from her children to the effect of "I don't want my friends to know that my mother is a freak." By the time these experiences have been digested, the occasion arises which the Reach to Recovery volunteer has assured the patient will become the rite of passage or reentry into the world of total womanhood: the prosthesis fitting. One patient describes it as follows:

> The worst ordeal was being fitted for a prosthesis. . . . After traveling 30 miles to find one [prosthesis shop], I went through two hours of tedious fittings, excuses, apologies and still returned home without a prosthesis of any kind. . . . When I was about three months post-op the garment shop owner telephoned that she was prepared to fit me. After extensive adjustments I came home happy. But by the end of the sixth month my body shape had shifted considerably. . . . [1]

Other women also report the prosthesis fitting as second only to the Reach to Recovery experience on the trauma scale.

Theories are not lacking regarding the emotional adjustment of the mastectomy patient. The Playboy philosophy is often blamed for women's feelings of inadequacy following a mastectomy. Are we supposed to assume that Russian women have fewer problems in adjustment?

Like widowhood, the mastectomy experience presents different problems for different women. Can the 72-year-old postmastectomy patient be compared with the 27-year-old woman who discovered a lump while she was breast feeding? Can the 55-year-old financially secure woman be compared to the 55-year-old clerical worker who finds herself unemployable following surgery? How about the woman whose mastectomy triggered off a divorce? The 42-year-old mother of three teenage daughters will react very differently from the 42-year-old childless single woman. Assuming the disease was brought under control by the mastectomy alone, is the loss of one or both breasts more severe for the woman who had a full and satisfying sex life prior to surgery than it is for the woman who had problems with "sexual dysfunction"?

Along with the mythical supportive surgeon, the equally mythical supportive husband or lover is supposed to smooth over the trauma of a mastectomy. In other words, he is asked to play a supportive role when he needs support himself. This emotional paralysis on the part of husbands can only increase the patient's dependency on the doctor, who is now expected to assure her of her womanliness as well.

After the mastectomy patient leaves the hospital, the mass media is probably her worst enemy. While prior to her suspicion that a mastectomy might be necessary, she pointedly ignored any media coverage of the subject, following the surgery, her repression turns into an obsession. She will devour anything in print on the subject of breast cancer, and the college-educated woman will suddenly find herself snatching copies of the *Star* and *National Enquirer* with their regularly headlined stories of cures for cancer, breast cancer in particular. The women's service magazines as well as the feminist service magazines will reinforce her fantasy that the mastectomy was unnecessary. General interest magazines will not spare her either. The following is excerpted from a *Newsweek* article entitled "Too Much Surgery?"

> Since the late nineteenth century, most surgeons have opted for radical mastectomy, a disfiguring operation. . . . "I would say at this point that there is little or no justification for doing radicals," notes study director Dr. Bernard Fisher of the University of Pittsburgh.[2]

The truth of the matter is, however, that the patient who has had a modified radical is not spared the trauma of the loss of a breast. The woman who had a radical will be told that she did not need a radical; the woman who had a modified will be told that her breast need not have been removed.

Where is the mastectomy patient's surgeon during all this? Hopefully, reading the *AMA Journal* rather than the *Ladies Home Journal.* What is happening to the doctor-patient relationship? The doctor has been deified in the patient's emotions and vandalized in her intellect. Often, the patient is ashamed to voice her anxieties about the mastectomy and fears accusing him or her of removing the breast unnecessarily. Simultaneously, her friends tell her that she has been taken for a fool; she was at best an inno-cent victim, at worse, a gullible idiot.

Added to this is the very real postoperative discomfort and, possibly, radiation and/or chemotherapy—and this is when the doctor(s) cannot be reached. The patient is completely at the mercy of the medical bureaucracy; she has learned to become apologetic if she asks for an appointment to speak to the doctor on the phone. This is also where the absence of the female support group is felt most intensively. She has no one to tell her that the numbness under the arm, which seems to go on indefinitely, is part of the healing process. She is convinced that every ache and pain, from head to toe, is a sign of the dreaded "recurrence," which she fears will only be laughed off if articulated. In the hospital, she was never prepared for the posthospital experience, either physically or psychoemotionally. She may have received a list of "don'ts" regarding care of the affected arm, but she has been programmed to suppress any anxieties by both her social network and the medical bureaucracy. Her doctor will hide behind the mask of the clinical vernacular in relation to the scar, but will answer all other com-plaints with a terse "It's normal."

The denial mechanism that is operative in virtually every cancer patient becomes intensified in the mastectomy patient in direct proportion to the success of the surgery. Thus, the expression "I didn't need this mastectomy; the doctor made a mistake; I couldn't possbily have had cancer" is heard far more frequently among women who are 10 and 20 years postoperative than among recent patients.

As far as premastectomy preparation is concerned, the doctor is damned if he or she does and damned if he or she does not. While the bitter "My doctor told me I wouldn't need a mastectomy" can be heard from most patients, the women whose tumors proved to be benign will complain with equal bitterness, "My doctor put me through all this worry and aggravation for nothing." In each case, the doctor probably said, "Although everything looks all right, we have got to do a biopsy to make sure."

The one-step procedure, specifically, the patient signing for a biopsy and mastectomy should it be necessary, has come under particular attack by feminists, who have argued and, to a degree, won their battle for the two-step procedure; that is, have the patient sign only for a biopsy, and should a malignancy be found, she should then "shop around" for a doctor who will offer her something other than a mastectomy, or if she does opt for a mastectomy, she will be prepared for it. Women who have gone through the two-step procedure have reported that the week or two wait from diagnosis until surgery was the most harrowing aspect of the experience. Except for a few underground "hotlines" from other mastectomy women, there is no preparation for the mastectomy experience. Patients who have asked their doctors' nurses or attempted to call the hospital have usually been told "Bring your Blue Cross card and a toothbrush." Reach to Recovery, on principle, will not give out any information to the premastectomy patient other than "If you should need a mastectomy, a volunteer will visit you."

Contrary to popular belief, the woman whose biopsy did not necessitate a mastectomy is not dancing with joy, nor does she regard her surgeon as a hero. She knows she will have to receive annual checkups, semiannual if she is high risk. In addition, her breasts have made the transition from private source of sensuality (hopefully) to be shared only with someone whom she has chosen to public property of the medical bureaucracy.

Paradoxically, one of the most heartbreaking disappointments occurs in the woman whose lesion was discovered in the earliest stages and whose prognosis is the most hopeful—specifically, the carcinoma in situ which was not detected during the biopsy. This is the woman who goes home to the congratulations of her friends only to be told, when she returns to the doctor to have her bandages removed, that there is something called the paraffin section, which showed a malignancy. Although this is a rare occurrence, the patient is once again in conflict. While her medical outlook is excellent and surgery can be kept minimal, this is also the occasion where her well-meaning friends will bombard her with epithets against her surgeon, the hospital, and the entire medical profession.

In addition to the woman who was diagnosed and underwent a mastectomy within a relatively short period of time, there is also the woman who went to a series of doctors over a period of months and even years before she was diagnosed. This is the woman who received everything from a "Don't worry; it's nothing" from her doctor(s) to vitamin injections to a lumpectomy, only to be told by the surgeon who diagnosed her that had she gotten competent medical care earlier, her chances would have been better.

Like the words *car accident,* the words *breast cancer* are indicative of a wide variety of extent. Carcinoma in situ is not the same thing as nodal involvement with metastasis, just as a dented fender is not the same thing as an overturned automobile. A modified radical that did not require additional treatment cannot be compared with an extended radical requiring radiation and chemotherapy. Physical and emotional recovery for the same extent of surgery is not going to be the same for women in different age, socioeconomic, and psychoemotional brackets. Different women have different coping mechanisms and different relationships to their breasts prior to the surgery.

By all rules of logic, it would seem that the younger, physically active woman whose surgery was minimal would make a far better emotional adjustment to the mastectomy than the older woman whose surgery was more extensive and required additional treatment. In reality, it is the older woman with strong family stability who will make the better adjustment than the younger woman especially the unmarried. This is what most breast specialists cannot understand. They feel that most of the emotional complaints come from the women who are the "luckiest."

The younger woman, who may feel that she is repulsive to men as a result of the surgery, will now expect validation of her sexual desirability from her doctor, who, she assumes, has seen enough mastectomies to take them in stride. The doctor is now expected to become a fountain of emotional strength and support for validity of the patient's sexuality in addition to a guarantee of her perfect health.

The psychoemotional pressures on both doctor and patient are enormous. Charges of emotional indifference or downright callousness on the part of doctors are, in many cases, justified. However, it must be stated in all fairness that even patients of "available" doctors, including women surgeons, have reported that even though their doctors could not have been more wonderful and understanding, they still have difficulty in adjusting to the mastectomy. The doctor, on his or her part, feels that he or she is hated for performing the very procedure that saved the patient's life. In addition, he or she often feels that his or her professional opinion is regarded as being somewhat lower than a gossip columnist's. He or she also may be regarded as more of a sex object than a competent practitioner.

It may be fashionable and, certainly, convenient to point the finger of accusation at the "clinical distance" of the doctor in diagnosing the patient's psychoemotional problems, but it is neither constructive nor realistic. Postmastectomy depression (PMD) has simply been denied by the medical bureaucracy or, if acknowledged, treated by band-aid syrupy clichés by those who cannot face their own anxieties in relation to cancer.

The medical profession cannot continue to deny or gloss over the psychoemotional problems of the mastectomy patient. Surgeons will have to come to the realization that mastectomy patients have problems that are beyond the control or area of expertise of most surgeons. The problem has best been summed up in the words of a nurse who underwent a mastectomy:

> Sometimes I wish I could wear a placard saying, "Forget that I once had breast cancer. Please treat me as you did before—as a whole person." . . . How I hate the platitudes—like "Well, you *look* good"—used so often to answer my complaints. Yet, how many times have I, as a registered nurse, used this phrase with cancer patients to avoid a deeper conversation? I had hoped that I was making these patients feel better. But I lacked the knowledge and understanding that only a patient has. I realize now that I didn't fool my patients any more than I am fooled by evasive reassurances from people caring for me.[3]

Fortunately, we are on the threshold of the emergence of the psychoemotional aspects of breast cancer from the closet, which is a good thing, considering it took approximately 5,000 years for this to occur. Psychiatrists, psychologists, and social workers are focusing on the problems of the mastectomy patient. Mutual support groups are being formed by individuals and medical and community organizations, and these are expanding the female peer group to include problems related to mastectomy. Exercise as well as "rap" groups are being formed, and virtually every responsible organization requests physician approval before accepting a new member.

One of the prime objectives of these groups is to reinforce the doctor-patient relationship, encouraging the patient to discuss specific details with her doctor rather than her hairdresser. Women are encouraged to express their ambivalence toward their surgeons, especially their resentment that none of them was Marcus Welby, M.D. (fortunately). The patient learns that her anxieties are stages to be worked through, not lifelong deadlocks. Most important, she learns that having sought competent medical care classifies her as a responsible, dignified woman, not the brainless little fool that the popular press makes her out to be.

Probably the most supportive service a surgeon could offer mastectomy patients is a thorough knowledge of all community practitioners and organizations that offer emotional support to such patients, from psychiatrists in private practices to YWCA-sponsored ENCORE (postmastectomy swim, exercise, and discussion group) programs to dance and exercise teachers who have special classes for postmastectomy women or who accommodate them into regular classes.

When a patient expresses anxieties about the mastectomy, she should be told that her concerns are healthy, not neurotic. She also should be encouraged to take advantage of whatever services are available to her in coping with her adjustment.

When the doctor trades in his or her guilt, inadequacy, and impatience at not being able to meet the patient's emotional needs for encouragement to seek the help of those who can benefit her in this area, both doctor and patient will be able to hold their heads a little higher.

Notes

1. Sadie L. Kennerly, R.N., "What I've Learned About Mastectomy," *American Journal of Nursing* 77(9), September 1977.

2. *Newsweek,* April 10, 1978, pp. 66–67.

3. Sadie L. Kennerly, R.N., "What I've Learned About Mastectomy," *American Journal of Nursing* 77(9), September 1977.

27 Psychological Aspects of Neurological Diseases: A Patient's Efforts to Disprove Being Labeled Crazy or Hysterical

Cynthia Birrer

It was nearly the end of 1973 before I was willing to admit, even to myself, that I was not well. But the day dawned when the physical and psychological changes that had so insidiously been permeating my consciousness for some time could no longer be ignored. I felt that I knew exactly *what* was happening, from the physical point of view. The sequence of events and my experience of them were quite specific and easy to detail, even though the web of underlying circumstances was so insubstantial that I pushed it far back into the recesses of my mind. Psychologically, too, I was aware of what was going on, but I had not even the suspicion of an idea as to why. I had read nothing that could throw a glimmer of light on the apparent metamorphosis I was undergoing—obvious not only to myself, but to those who knew me well.

The emotional debilitation I felt was echoed by the real fatigue of my body. I was generally fatigued, waking tired in the morning, going to bed in a state of exhaustion. But there also was fatigue that was induced by specific activities: walking, driving back and forth, climbing stairs in particular—all this sort of thing tired me. The tiredness was exacerbated by some odd difficulties with my right leg. After walking even short distances, I often found that I literally could not take another step with it. There was no pain, but if I pushed myself beyond this limit, the leg dragged badly. Fortunately, it soon recovered with rest, but its annoying quirk considerably limited how much I was able to do each day. The knee was a problem, too. There was consistent, though not unbearable pain in it, and it had the frequent and disconcerting habit of giving way, almost as if in response to pressure on the sole of the foot. I kept tripping over my own feet, and sometimes I fell, twice in the street. I did not know how I came to be there, I was not conscious of the knee reneging or of stumbling, but there I was, sitting on my bottom in the middle of the sidewalk. Walls and doors on my right acted like a magnet; I bumped into them, over and over again, as well as into low tables and the sharp corners of desks, always leading with the right side, so that upper arm, thigh, and shin were seldom completely free of bruises.

The leg also was troublesome on waking. I learned to open my eyes, keep still, and move on only very slowly. Nevertheless, as soon as I rolled onto my right side or stretched the leg toward the bottom of the bed, spasms would convulse the calf, and the toes would ache with a violent cramp that forced them downward. The spasms were intensely painful and seldom abated within 15 to 20 minutes. When I was at home, my husband, Bill, often had to help me with massage or hot water bottles. I cannot remember a single morning during 1974 when the spasms did not occur, although once I was up and about there was no recurrence. I did have severe cramps on the odd occasion when I woke during the night and moved my legs around. I also learned to avoid sitting too far back in a chair or crossing my legs at the knees or below, since doing this had the tendency either to put my right foot to sleep or to set off sharp bouts of pins and needles, sometimes in both feet.

I had my first bout of double vision in January 1974. I was in a book shop studying the shelves when the objects in front of me began to peel apart. It was the first in a long series of attacks, and although their frequency varied from once in 8 to 10 days to only once or twice in 3 weeks, their form did not. They were always preceded by a short period during which I felt very ill. Then there was a "V-ing" sensation; that is, the split would yield two images of the same object at the top, but only a single image at the base. The separation would become complete within a few seconds, resulting in two distinct images at some distance from each other on the horizontal plane; subjectively, I had the impression that if I moved forward I could pass between them. They retained their clarity, their color, and their dimensionality for approximately 15 minutes, when they would become misty and muted and appear to exist on a flat surface; I was looking at a canvas that was distinctly concave at the center. This impression would last a short while before the images fused again. At that point I would move unsteadily, falling sideways easily and banging into everything while I concentrated on positioning my feet. Within about half an hour my head would seem numb. One of two things then followed: either I got a headache in my eyes, which ached on rotation and if I pressed on the closed lids with my fingers (there was some pain), or else I experienced pain over the top of my head, an even, deadened effect with no throb. In both cases I had then to sleep for a long period. Since the attacks never occurred after 11 A.M., this meant until the next morning. Sometimes I woke for dinner, but more often I did not feel like eating, although I was never nauseous. Sleep was imperative: I simply canceled the lectures scheduled for the day and left the campus.

That was my long-distance double vision, but there also were difficulties at closer range when reading or writing, particularly in artificial light. This was a huge problem to me until treatment of the disease began in

December 1975: the rising and falling of oncoming headlights drove me wild, the "flicker" mechanism of the EEG, like the candle, could induce great agitation, and sitting for any length of time in a brightly lit auditorium was well-nigh impossible. Doing book work induced patchy vision; the center portion of the print would lose its inky gloss, become grayish, and within seconds bleach out entirely. Some print would be visible on the periphery, more at the top and bottom than on the sides. However, when the middle came back into focus, the remainder would patch out. This alternation would persist for variable lengths of time. When it was short-lived, I was generally left with a mild headache and blurring in the right eye. I tried to clear this by slitting the eye, tugging gently at the outside corner. When it was of longer duration, my right hand would begin to tremble. If I was writing at the time, the trembling could travel up the arm into the right shoulder and then, somehow, affect the left arm very slightly. The upper limbs felt extremely weak, and the right-hand tremble and arm shake usually continued until I went to bed, feeling thoroughly squeamish. I retched once or twice, a horrid, tearing experience.

I contemplated the situation and finally decided to go to an ophthalmologist. It was as good a place to start as any—and surely the one where the least harm could be done. I made an appointment for October 22, 1974, with Gerald Davids (names of physicians and others mentioned in this chapter have been changed to protect their anonymity), whom I knew slightly through my work at the university. He suspected myasthenia gravis and referred me to a neurologist.

"A neurologist, like who?"

"Bruce Green."

"But is he any good? You're talking about my nervous system—I want the *best*."

"He is."

"All right. But I'd like to make a few inquiries first."

I did. I solicited the opinions of several doctors and they unanimously acclaimed Green's neurological expertise.

Seated opposite Dr. Green on 20 December I began my litany. There were several factors I wanted to stress. First of all, the excessive fatigue that had dogged me for the past year.

"Are you tired, or are you weak? There is a difference."

Yes, there was. My lower limbs were fatigued; the upper limbs seemed weak. I gave him examples of what I meant. "And there's pain, too, particularly in my knee."

"Well, then, that is not myasthenia. Myasthenia is painless."

I didn't know about that, but certainly what I had was not painless. I told him about my sight, trying to make a clear-cut distinction between double and patchy vision. He listened to it all carefully and hardly interrupted. He asked about the incidence of illness in my past, but put no specific questions.

"Come on, let's have a look at you."

Afterwards, I walked up to his desk, struggling with the buckle of my belt. He continued writing for a few seconds and then came around and sat next to me.

"Sit down. Do you know any anatomy?"

"A little."

He sketched the lower portion of the brain and the cervical spine. He added what he called a "horn" protruding from the cerebellum—the more usual term is *tonsil*. He crooked the index finger of his right hand. "This is known as an Arnold-Chiari malformation." He explained that this is a lesion of the hindbrain, characterized by the downward displacement of the cerebellum and medulla through the foramen magnum into the cervical spinal canal. "That's your problem; you have a Chiari."

I looked at him. He was very alert, the archtype of invincible certainty, and he issued his pronouncement with the unwavering ring of unassailable confidence.

And so, on 20 December 1974, Bruce Green decided, after a conscientious medical examination lasting approximately three-quarters of an hour, that I had a congenital anomaly of the hindbrain and that this was responsible for fatigue and pain in my right leg, made walking a grave effort, and instigated attacks of double and patchy vision; it was also responsible for weakness and trembling in the right and, less frequently, the left arm and trunk, as well as the almost total loss of sensitivity over my entire body.

On 28 January I was admitted to a hospital for a myelogram. I expected an ordeal, but was pleasantly surprised.

At about 5 P.M. that evening a very bad bout of leg spasms and cramps in the toes began, probably triggered by the Iophendylate. I gripped the head rail with both hands and felt the sweat beading on my face. I hung on for 20 minutes before I rang for the nurse. Fifteen minutes later she came in.

"Green's here now, I'll get him." She returned with a syringe.

"What's that?"

"A muscle relaxant."

"I want Green, not drugs, thank you."

"No, look, let me give you this. It will help that leg."

"Not until Green has seen my leg, thanks."

"It's nothing to worry about, just a reaction to the myelogram."

"Yeah, maybe. But I go through this every morning of my life, dye or no dye. It's slightly more severe now, but it's identical in every other way. I want Green to see it."

He came in and watched in silence as the leg convulsed. "You know those horns I told you about?" He crooked that index finger. "You've got one."

I could not mistake the triumphant look on his face. Se he *was* right. If I had not *been* on my back, I would have *fallen* on it, and I told him so. He looked like the proverbial Cheshire cat, although the grin was confined to his eyes.

"So that *is* what my problem is?"

When Green came in the next morning to discharge me, I asked what happens to a Chiari.

"In my experience, it throws up symptoms. The equivocal ones are the difficult ones."

I did not like it one bit. A lesion so capricious that its very existence seemed uncertain, with all-embracing consequences, sounded more like an alchemist's conundrum than a serious medical explanation of the queer quotidian events of the past year. Nor was it a happy augury.

"You can go home now."

"Not so fast. What are you going to do about my leg?"

"I can't do anything about it. It's a Chiari leg."

"You mean, it's a live-with-it leg?"

"Yes."

We stared at each other for a long moment. "There must be *something* you can do about spasms."

He looked wary. "Try Benadryl, two tablespoons in the evening. See me in a fortnight."

In their discussion of diseases of diagnostic procedures, Hess and McDonald (1969) note that some authors felt that in adequate dosages, antihistamines, especially intravenous diphenhydramine hydrochloride (Benadryl), can prevent or ameliorate allergic reactions. In higher dosages, diphenhydramine may protect against the nonallergic, unpredictable, dose-independent shock reaction that "probably is due to drug idiosyncracy." But, they add, "the literature does not generally support this hopeful attitude." And neither do I. (Hess and McDonald, 1969).

On 18 February a brain scan was taken. It was negative. When I saw Green again on 3 March the only new development was four ordinary faints. Twice I had fallen straight forward, eyes closed, onto the dinner table, and twice I had passed out briefly at the university.

"Forward faints are quite characteristic of a Chiari," Green said, mimicking the action of falling forward with his right hand.

"What about the fits?"

"There's something funny on the EEG."

"Funny?"

"Well, there's something in the temporal area. The institute wants to repeat the EEG in 6 weeks. I think you should. Meanwhile, I'll try you on an anticonvulsant.

A week later I reported by phone that my right leg was no longer convulsing, but that it had become spastic instead; nor was there any decrease in the number of fits.

"Step up the anticonvulsants to three a day."

Within 2 weeks of starting the drug I found that the spasm in my right leg had disappeared completely. I was overjoyed; I could thrash around in bed to my heart's content without any hint of a convulsion. But although the spasms in the leg were gone, the pain had not. The spasm on the left side of the trunk also did not recur, nor did the faints; the severity of the fits had lessened, although their frequency was unaffected.

Green had the results of the second EEG when I saw him on April 8. The picture had not changed, and another reading in 6 weeks was advised. I told him bitterly that I now had a lot of pain in the right leg and that walking was not easy.

"Patients with a Chiari often get pains down the legs." He ran both hands down one of his own.

"It's only the right leg. Are you quite sure about that wretched Chiari?"

"It's there all right."

"I just don't know. I'm getting so damned fatigued again, it's difficult to get around."

"I think it's neurasthenia."

"Do you mean a *neurotic* fatigue?

"Yes."

"Psychosomatic?"

"Yes."

I hooted. "My friend, in this case, neurasthenia, if you define it like that, is as mythical as you claim myasthenia to be."

"I don't know, you've had problems."

I looked at him sharply. What on earth was he referring to? He noticed my stupefaction.

"I mean, you have *got* problems."

"Yes, and I suppose they must be creating some anxiety—it would be extraordinary if they were not. But there's a great deal more to it than that."

Since humans are thinking beings, psychological phenomena are involved in any disease, even if only in the form of anxiety or despair. But labeling a patient neurasthenic or neurotic because these factors undeniably play a part in pathology seems to me to be a very queer ploy indeed. Way out, in fact. Actually, among doctors, Green is the worst psychologist I have come across in my various experiences as a patient. And in this particular instance he was doubly out of order because it was one of his own breed, the great French neurologist Pierre Janet, who first showed that it is quite worthless to define the neuroses in terms of the intervention of psychologic phenomena.

I walked into Green's room again on 7 July. He had the report of the fourth EEG of 25 June in his hand. He passed it to me over the desk. There had been a marked deterioration.

"What am I going to do with you?"

"I don't know; but I do know that things are going downhill—fast." I went over it all in detail. He watched me quietly. "Some things seems to be so wrong, and yet others are still going well—my writing for example."

There was a marked silence. "I am quite prepared to accept that an EEG is only a piece of paper until I hear the kinds of things you're saying. Then I get cold feet. I must do an angiogram." In this procedure, a dye is injected into the left carotid artery in the neck to facilitate x-raying the arterial system in the head.

I hesitated. There was something on my mind, but I could not bring myself to say it. "You think an angiogram is necessary?"

"The EEG report indicates that it is, and so does your story. Frankly, I'm chicken. Go and get undressed.

As usual, I sat on the couch. He stared at me and gave an involuntary start. "I have never seen your ptosis like that. It is awful."

"Yes. Sometimes I have the greatest difficulty in keeping the eye open at all."

Green always took pains with his examinations, but this time he was back-checking. Everthing was much as before—no double vision, same extent of insensitivity to pin pricks—until he started on the reflexes. There was no response from either ankle. He tapped the knee, eliciting a series of rapid and exaggerated contractions. He tried again, with the same result, and then again.

'Shit." That was my sentiment, too. Seconds later I felt the oncoming rush of a head explosion. The upper portion of the right arm and shoulder began to convulse violently. I twisted onto my right, lifting my left side off the couch. I leant heavily on the upper right arm. The shoulder shuddered and writhed. I leaned harder, feeling the panic rising. I also felt a bit sick. Green's astounded eyes were glued to my arm.

"It's your *shoulder*," he exclaimed, unable to refrain from stating the obvious.

"I get . . ." I tried to force out a sentence, but I could only make the harsh, rasping sound that was characteristic of these attacks and that always prevented me from calling for help. I made another effort.

"Don't talk while it's happening."

I let the avalanche take its course. My head exploded twice before the disturbance subsided. I asked for a drink of water. Green was grave, brooding.

"I don't know what that is." He was almost inaudible.

He helped my off the couch. We stood facing each other. "I must do the angiogram." He ran his finger down my neck. "I expect it to be negative," he said firmly. But he was shaken, and it was not at all clear that he really did.

I went to his desk and sat down. He turned to his phone. "Now, about that angiogram. . . ."

"No, no angiogram."

There was no doubt that further neurological investigation was clearly indicated. But an angiogram is used to detect abnormal vascularity, for example, in an aneurysm, or the displacement of the cerebral arteries by a tumor. I could not see that my problems were necessarily being caused by either. Eventually, I supposed, the possibility of both had to be excluded, but right now I thought Green ought to review the whole case with a colleague, just to make sure he was not barking up the wrong tree, diagnostically speaking. There *are* other things besides aneurysms and brain tumors that can affect the nervous system in strange ways. I could not shake off the vague feeling that something was being overlooked.

Green fingered the receiver. "You don't have to have it if you don't want it." His forehead furrowed. "But you *must*. What are you going to do if that happens in a lecture?"

"It has. What are you going to do if the angiogram shows nothing?"

"I am going to push pills."

"Drug therapy?"

"Drug therapy," he affirmed, nodding his head.

I nodded too, wordlessly. I had to leave it to him.

The psychologically most stressful period during the progressive capitulation of my body to disease started toward the end of March 1975. I had begun to feel desperately ill. The experience was not entirely novel; the bouts of double vision and fits had always been heralded by an acute physical unease, but now this was magnified a thousandfold. Green wanted to know exactly what I meant when I said I felt ill, and I was rendered helpless and frustrated by his probings, floundering in an inchoate welter.

"Headache?"

"No."

"Nausea?"

"No."

"Pain?"

"No."

"Well, what then?"

"Peculiar, just peculiar."

From the look on his face, he obviously thought me so too. But it was impossible to put the sensation into words. When I tried, they echoed as hollowly as the strained and stilted vocabulary the English language offers to lovers, and I could not rescue the rhetoric from its shackles as a Michener might do, falling back on some graphic and picturesque argot.

Over 20 years I have developed a good sense of the functioning of my own body. Among other things, I am aware of when I begin to ovulate, even though my cycle is irregular, and it is easy to describe the process in such terms as heaviness, or fullness, or distension, or whatever the immediate experience is. But in this situation, there were no really appropriate linguistic labels. Somewhere, deep inside, I was undergoing destruction by some form of physiological pollution, much as the mind might disintegrate under the impact of the subtle and insidious persuasion of various methods of torture. There was a strong feeling of dissolution, of decomposition, a loss of the definition of internal boundaries, a gradual but resolute slaking of tissue rendering the body anomalous, and it was as if the cumulative effects were being swept through every vessel by the blood, suffocating vitality. It was a rapacious invasion of the vital principle that destroyed its power to quicken; it would not be repulsed, and it made me feel very sick indeed.

After the worst attack I suffered during the period of head explosions, I stood staring out my bedroom window at the cascading grace of the weeping willow, sweeping and sinuous in the afternoon balm against the white garden wall. I no longer felt ill, by in my heart of hearts I knew that all the king's horses and all the king's men were not going to be able to put together the pieces inside me again. I understood then, in an idiosyncratic way, the incorporeal predator that had been my constant companion for at least the preceding 21 months. It was my first real grasp of the Kafkaesque dimensions of my condition, and while I never dwelt on it, it prepared me for the unvarnished truth when I was forced to face it. It also enabled me to take the first steps toward my own emotional rehabilitation. What I had lost on the swings, I gained on the roundabouts.

Friday, 1 August 1975 is branded into my memory, deeply, clearly. I did not know it then, but it marked the beginning of a time, not yet ended, that has given me poignant personal insight into some of the infinite and subtle connotations of physical pain. The limp was pronounced. Toward midday there were marked twinges low in the back. They spread, like tentacles, into the right of the rump. A strip across the lower third of both buttocks, from far left to far right, seemed chafed, and I became increasingly uncomfortable, constantly shifting my position from one side of the chair to the other. At about 2 P.M. the toes and ankle and heel of the right foot began to ache in a numb sort of way. Later, I came to call this my weeping pain; there were times when I could get no relief from it during all my waking hours; I wanted to weep, wretchedly, miserably, and once I did. The knee seared; my screaming pain, which screams, could never vanquish. The lower spine flared spasmodically and sometimes, though not often, the agony swept upward, above the waist; my gasping pain, electric charges briefly but intensely felt.

These sensations, sometimes experienced alone, but more generally in concert, were to consume all my energy in the weeks to come, so that while I obediently ate whatever was put in front of me and kept it down, my weight plunged in the first 30 days from 52 to 47 kilos, from 47 to 43. A further 3 kilos slipped away rather more slowly.

But on that Friday I had no inkling of what lay ahead. I stood up—and screamed. From the lower vertebrae of the spinal cord to the tip of the big toe of my right foot, I was on fire. The area from the sole of my foot, now host to a thousand sharp, penetrating pins, to just above the knee was the most badly affected by the scorch. Of the thigh only the inner surface burned. Much later, when the burn (but not the pain) became symmetrical, affecting each leg in exactly the same way, I became consciously bowlegged, to prevent any irritating contact between the thighs. There also seemed to be a great deal of activity in the right calf and knee, although there was only mild local pain in the latter. A thong ran up the back of the calf, binding ankle to knee. Sometimes, when this was flexible, I walked fairly easily, until it contracted and stiffened, preventing further activity—and, thank God, driving sensitivity into numbness. But on that day its effect was crippling and I could barely make it over the 10 meters from the desk in my study to my bed.

One day melted into the next. The pain tore into the flesh, stripping a little from the bones each day; it dulled the wits, so that the daily newspapers became a serious intellectual challenge; it weakened the will, although it never quite crushed it. I wanted to be up, away from that austere room with its white stucco plaster and wooden rockers. But the pain resisted everything; there was no elixir, no relief to be found in any pill.

I grew drawn and pale, hair stringy and unusually greasy from the eternal twisting and turning against green striped pillows that became damp and hot and creased. I supposed ruefully that this was how Jill thought I should look when I saw Green. "Whenever you see him, you look as though you've had a holiday," she said furiously, staring at my freshly washed hair as I slipped into the front seat of her car one day. Bill had also once, before a dinner date, glanced at me, sparkling outwardly and shrunken inwardly, and remarked that it was difficult to believe that I was ill. But I do not see a doctor unless I have a tale to tell. Do I have to look like a hag in order to be believed?

The pain scourged my body, sapped my mind. That was bad enough. But with equal ferocity it flayed those who cared. Bill also had to live through those excruciating night hours when I could barely move my limbs at all, when I could not tolerate the merest pressure of a sheet, or of night wear, or of bed socks, against the skin of back and limb and upper instep; when all he saw was me shrouded in misery, and he could do nothing, nothing but bring another glass of water and another pain killer. He became irascible, tenser, thinner. My parents too saw most of it, keeping steadfastly cheerful as they fetched and carried, but inwardly fuming, fretting, breaking their hearts a little more each day. My friends saw a great deal of it, keeping in constant contact by telephone, arriving gay and leaving gray.

On 26 September I kept an appointment with Green that I had made with great difficulty more than a month and a half previously. Drugged, in great pain, weak from bed rest and rapid loss of weight, I remember very little. He dug his thumb into the flesh beneath my big right toe. I yelped.

"Ah-*ha*! What *you* need is a good orthopod. This pain can be fixed easily, with a metatarsal bar in your shoe. We'll get onto that."

The leg was in spasm. Green thought that it was due to whatever Iophendylate remained in the spine from the myelogram he had done on 28 January. Arrangements were made to remove it the following day. About the addition to my foot gear I said nothing. I knew from experience I would not be seeing an orthopedic surgeon, not on Green's initiative anyway.

Green said that as far as he was concerned, there was no sign of prolapsis in the lumbar region on the x-rays Dr. Peters had taken on the instructions of my family doctor. The next day, 27 September, the myelogram was rescreened to confirm this.

"There is nothing there. I told you so," said he, sanctimoniously, setting my teeth on edge. I was trapped face downward on the x-ray table, with Pethidine dripping slowly, blessedly, into a vein on the back of my left hand. Apart from the fact that this particular situation enforced inactivity, I scarcely had the strength to swat a fly. But my inclination was to hit him. Hard. And it had nothing to do with being crazy, either.

Earlier, Green had been quite prepared to confine me to bed for the customary 14 days for a pain that *may* have resulted from a prolapsed disc. On the other hand, it may not have had anything to do with a disc; after all, no one had ever claimed that there was more than a hint of prolapsis. He had checked neither plates nor patient to assess for himself what the cause of the pain might be. And yet, as the neurologist in charge of the case, no one knew better than he that for the preceding 18 months I had been victim to one strange symptom after another. Even if he did think I was a raving nut (which I was beginning to suspect he did), he had not actually said so. Had he done so, I would, of course, have sought help elsewhere. As far as I was concerned, therefore, he was obligated to search unremittingly for some medical basis for my pathology where this appeared to exceed the limits of the early diagnosis he had fixed his mind on, as it was surely beginning to do. I did not see then, and I do not see now, how he could possibly have formed an accurate assessment of, let alone pass judgment on, my psychological state. He knew next to nothing about me as a person, and he apparently understood even less about the infinite complexities of psychological growth, its resilience, its fathomless potential. To allow his psychological prevarications to bedevil his medical commitment was impudent at best, heinous at worst. If the Iophendylate was causing the burn, or if it was responsible for the pain in the leg, I might have been spared weeks of agony.

The dye came out on Saturday, 27 September, and the pain eased for 24 hours. I left a message of appreciation at Green's home; at least he had ensured that what is often an unpleasant procedure had been painless. I also said that I thought it had made a difference. By 6 P.M. on Sunday I knew I was mistaken. Dr. Rice, my family doctor, phoned Green, who was surprised. Surprised. Period.

The conduct of my case during the days following grew more curious and more curious; there was a second opinion, then a third, followed by a flight to Cape Town for a fourth. This began promptly at 1 P.M. on 10 December 1975.

As Dr. Bell moved from the top of my head to the soles of my feet, he probed things I had been conscious of for the previous 2 to 2½ years, but which had not been considered by the other doctors. He wanted to know what my thought processes "felt" like. It took me some time before I found the word *compressed,* and that was not very apt. Having a "head explosion" is one thing, readily identifiable and amenable to description. I experienced the angiogram, which was negative, as a series of head explosions, attenuated by the effects of the anesthetic, which cannot be held completely at bay. But the experience of being crowded out of your own body, squeezed aside, by your own thoughts turned in upon themselves is not something that I really felt I wanted to talk about—or could, for that matter.

In the short period since the diagnosis of my condition I have given some thought to the psychology of the disease. Apart from the erosion of emotional life, the thinking process, which I believe generally remains intact throughout, plays some peculiar tricks, and there are times when mental activities proceed at a rate that is thoroughly exhausting. They are so lucid and vivid, they constitute very real noise. But the din does not *displace* words, thoughts; it *is* the ideas that chase each other around, eventually crashing tumultuously into an unseen barrier, piling up, high, high, high, one on top of the other, pressing down hard when they reach their bony limits: thoughts demanding to be expressed. They spill over into the motor system, but the tongue refuses to convey them and the legs cannot run from them. The mind does not lack clarity, nor is it tormented by formless images; it is not beset by vague fears. But the coherence beats hopelessly against the massive force of inertia. It seems to me that this tragic dilemma, more than anything else, holds the seed of the final act of self-destruction, for as the disease progresses, it must become virtually synonymous with the abolition of the spirit that powers the intention to act, while leaving the ability to form the intent inviolate. It is one of the more diabolical twists of fate. My safety valve is writing, since my right arm is only slightly affected; the hand cannot exceed a certain rate and the mind is bridled by it, providing some degree of volitional control over thinking.

Bell's examination was very similar to those conducted by the other doctors. In addition, he examined the skin on the forehead for evidence of more profuse sweating on one side than on the other. He found this on the right, and I gathered that he was satisfied that the constricted pupil there was Horner's syndrome. Later in the examination he attempted to elicit abdominal reflexes. These were present. His face, tautening as he worked over the legs and hips for more than 10 minutes, relaxed. "Good, good," he muttered.

While I dressed, he moved into an adjoining room with the x-rays. He came back 12 minutes later. He did not agree that there was a Chiari. "Whatever you call it, it is not causing your problems." By now, those sounds were familiar. We both sat down and I waited while he wrote up his findings. When he looked up, Bill asked him if he had reached any conclusion. He raised both hands a few inches above the desk, placed the tips of his fingers together and leaned forward. I don't think he enjoyed the next few minutes very much.

"The burning you are experiencing in your lower back and legs is due to a condition known as arachnoiditis. It is a rare and dreaded reaction to a myelogram. It makes one wonder whether myelograms ought to be done, particularly when a patient is as severely affected as you are." Arachnoiditis is the inflammation, or scarring, of one of the three meninges, or coverings of the spinal cord. "You ought to have hydrocortisone in the spine—three shots should be enough. But even so, it will be a few months before it subsides. Without it, the painful burn will continue indefinitely. If you were my patient, you would have the first shot today."

Bell glanced downward, and leaned back. "The more critical question, however, concerns the nature of the problems that caused you to have the myelogram in the first place."

I thought the wrinkling at the corner of his eyes increased, just a little. There was no need for either of us to speak. He leaned forward again, fingertips now pressed tightly together.

"Mrs. Birrer, you have consulted other specialists, and my opinion carries no more weight, but no less, than theirs. This is an exceedingly complex clinical picture. However, it is my opinion that you have multiple sclerosis."

I looked at him. Maybe he was wrong.

He looked at me. "Maybe I'm wrong. When you get back to Johannesburg, I want you to see Dr. Evans. He has taken a special interest in this disease for a number of years. He can confirm the diagnosis. Maybe he can also help you."

Between the fateful day and 18 December, when the diagnosis was unequivocally confirmed, I experienced one episode after another. On admission to a Johannesburg clinic on 29 December 1975, I was partially paralysed, half blind, generally disabled by a multitude of minor dysfunctions, and in excruciating pain. The following day, treatment to arrest the progress of an incurable disease began.

Part of this chapter is to advise health-care professionals on how to avoid the gross errors of omission and comission, many of them not recorded in these pages, that were made in my case. A consideration of the side effects, or aftereffects of the technological imperative that holds dominion over the medical profession today is beyond the scope of this chapter. However, a few points can be made regarding the doctor-patient relationship, which is the source of so many difficulties.

It is a truism that the majority of sick people do not find it easy to relate to their physicians. Doctors, we so often say or hear others say, act as though they are God. Dr. Donald Hayes (1978) agreed at a conference in Houston, Texas that many doctors do indeed seem to glory in this role, but he went on to point out that the fault for their having assumed it is only partially theirs. "If you want your doctor to come down off that pedestal," he aptly remarked, "*you* have to get up off your knees and quit worshipping him. It works both ways."

Yes, it does. Hayes suggested that the demystification of the medical mystique would probably answer the largest single area of need in professional and patient, or client, relationships that we presently face. He outlined different modes whereby a professional relates to a sick person, beginning with the one most frequently represented on television and exemplified in the Green-Birrer relationship: the engineering approach. The engineer who is a structural master, works on the patient who is a body. Now, there are circumstances where this is appropriate—in the case of traumatic injury following an accident, for example. But in a situation that requires decision making about the outcome of the illness, then, Hayes insists, he would wish to have a say in the matter, as would most people.

Hayes therefore holds out as the ideal a relationship that he calls "colleaguial." Here the physician and client address the problem mutually as colleagues, both equally concerned about it. The physician brings to the situation a fund of knowledge and experience which the individual does not have, while the patient brings a fund of emotional, physical, and financial investment which the doctor does not have. Together they broach the problem as colleagues.

If such a relationship were a reality, which it is not, it would represent a large step toward alleviating timidity, fear, confusion, inarticulateness, and ignorance among the sick; it would also mean an end to doctors who will not explain, teach, listen, inspire, guide, or care. It would herald the beginning of a truly helping participation between doctor and client, with multitudes of lives enriched and, perhaps, meaningfully extended.

Dr. I.M. Cooper (1976), in his book *Living with Chronic Neurologic Disease,* appears to offer such a relationship to those who seek his help. "Very often, following a consultation with someone who has been ill for a long time, I ask the patient to think over all the things we have spoken of during our visit together. Then, when the patient has had a few days to contemplate whatever diagnosis or opinion I have offered, as well as any treatment I may have suggested, it is extremely helpful to both of us for the patient to write or dictate a letter to me questioning matters that are still not understood, expressing frankly any fears or doubts about the therapy I have recommended and stating anything not previously mentioned that now seems important. "This communication influences me, and I believe should influence all doctors, in the ultimate decision for or against some elective surgical procedure, or prolonged hospitalization, or further extensive examinations" (Cooper, 1976).

Turning now to what sufferers can do for themselves, both directly and indirectly, with the support of their doctor, Dr. Cooper (1976) also offers a questionnaire which, he says, is invaluable in learning as much as possible about a sick person and his or her problems. If you suspect that a client has multiple sclerosis—and public education concerning this disease being conducted through the media, local chapters of the National Mutiple Sclerosis Society, and books by sufferers may have alerted both of you to this possibility—ask him or her to answer this questionnaire thoughtfully, it may help the patient define more clearly the specific symptoms and disabilities that affect daily life.

The question of self-care in health has come to the fore recently for many reasons, economic and political among them. When doctors talk about self-treatment, they usually mean self-medication. However, this is a very narrow perspective that should be widened to cover health maintenance, which includes disease prevention and care of the self in illness (Birrer, 1980). Improving people's methods of self-treatment requires that they be educated about what to treat, when to treat, how long to treat, and with what.

The task of "patient" education is particularly difficult when the illness requires complex changes in lifestyle. I have argued (Birrer, 1980) that this has a definite etiologic link with multiple sclerosis, which appears to be a syndrome rather than a disease. If so, the significance of the requisite changes to the suffered as a symbol of social apartness is so profound that it would be difficult for someone who has not been similarly affected to appreciate their effects. This failure on the part of the nonafflicted, *including members of the medical profession as well as paramedics,* to appreciate the dimensions of chronic disease has led to the establishment and proliferation of self-help groups.

Some doctors do accept that these groups have a valuable educative function, in respect of themselves, their clients, and the general public. Sufferers, particularly, can learn much from the experience of others about their disease and about ways in which life can be made as normal as possible. Conversely, neither medial training nor much medical knowledge is concerned with the psychosocial aspects of chronic disease—a problem such as sex for the disabled is barely comprehended.

Williamson and Danaher (1978) point out that this does not necessarily mean that doctors are uninterested in such issues, merely that they have no specific training to enable them to be particularly sensitive to them. For this reason, *self-help groups are developing the special function of informing the medical profession itself of the combined experience of people suffering from specific diseases.* Particularly in multiple sclerosis, which remains as great a mystery now as it was when Charcot identified it over 100 years ago, doctors need to rely less on research than on what sufferers say about their experiences if they are to offer genuine care to the sick. Self-help groups in the fields of chronic disease and disability are undoubtedly one of the most significant advances in Western medical care in the past decade. As the etiologic complexity of the diseases from which modern human beings suffer increases exponentially, I think that self-help groups have a function equal to that of the laboratory in finding solutions, or at least the means of returning sufferers to an appropriate level of health. Doctors need to recognize this function of the self-help group, to promote its development and to cooperate fully with it.

At this point in time, the most important means of reducing the suffering of the multiple sclerotic are the links that could be established between the relevant self-help groups and the medical profession. Supporting the person through the often extraordinary experience of multiple sclerosis requires exquisite tact in balancing encouragement with coercion and its consequent reinforcement of dependency. Self-care in multiple sclerosis demands an interdependence between doctor and client. Unless this can be achieved, primarily through educative liaison between the profession and self-help groups, faith in the value and efficacy of medicine will plummet even further.

References

Birrer, C. *The Medical Cop-Out.* Cape Town, Human and Rousseau, 1976.
Birrer, C. *Multiple Sclerosis: A Personal View.* Springfield, Ill.: Thomas, 1980.

Cooper, I.S. *Living with Chronic Neurologic Disease*. New York, Norton, 1976.

Hayes, D. *The Doctor/Patient Relationship: Colleaguial or Engineering?* Holistic Health Association, Houston, Texas, April 1978.

Hess, R.J., and McDonald, H.B. Diseases of diagnostic procedures. In *The Diseases of Medical Progress: A Study of Iatrogenic disease,* ed. R.H. Moser, 3rd ed. Springfield, Ill.: Thomas, 1969.

Williamson, J.D., and Danaher, K. *Self-Care in Health*. London, Croom Helm, 1978.

28

Commentary: The Parents' Experience of Health Care for the Terminally Ill Child

Marcia Ross
and *Alvin P. Ross*

Our son is gone. Bruce Nolan Ross is dead. This is a chronicle, of sorts, of our participation in his struggle and our need—his need—for that participation in the last months of his life, his coping with death, his dying with dignity—at home. This is a story of love, a journal of the love of a mother and a father and a son for one another, a love that grew and was nourished and came into full bloom as our son lay dying of leukemia.

Leukemia! Acute myelogeneous leukemia. There is nothing soft or delicate or gentle about the words or the process. Indeed, all the words, the nomenclature associated with the diagnosis, treatment, and medical care are hard and harsh: Chemotherapy. Bone marrow. Oncology. Metastasize. Cancer. Kill the cells. Fungi. Terminal. Hard words, hard feelings, harder times. The hardest of all to endure is the pain. Physical pain, spiritual pain, and emotional pain. Pain hurts, and no one wants to be hurt. Yet, we the parents had to fight for and demand the right, our God-given right, to become involved in the health-care system. We who could best balance the equation by offering tenderness and love and a sharing of the pain had to force our way into the treatment process.

Now that the ordeal is over and Bruce is at peace, it is time to reflect on what could have and should have been done to add a softening to the hard times endured by all concerned.

Yes, this is a critique of the medical profession and its many components: physicians, psychologists, nurses, and medical technicians. A lesson learned through experience during the 8 months of fighting for life and learning to accept death. There were a few individuals along the way who were capable of expressing a tolerance and an understanding of needs beyond the technology of medicine. However, our frame of reference convinces us that most doctors (even oncologists and psychiatrists) and nurses are not trained to deal with the terminal patient. They are even less capable of dealing with the parents and families of the terminally ill. They are adept at quoting statistics and admitting that some medical protocols are experimental and that "there is always hope."

They, the health-care practitioners, are not capable of dealing with the need to bring comfort, caring, and love into the lives of those who have little time to live. They are not able to bring dignity to death. They are systematic, mechanical, and materialistic in their approach to the patient and the patient's family. Generally, the whole care "package" that Bruce—and we—endured was without feeling for emotions, attitudes, or mind factors.

If we were to design an equation to be symbolic of the ratio of care and caring involved in our experience, we would put deficiency on one side and efficiency on the other side, and we would discover that the only way we could balance the equation and overcome the weight of deficiencies would be by adding feelings to the efficiency side of the equation. That's the word: *feelings.* It is so easy to say to someone who is devastated by the news of a terminal illness, "Don't cry," and offer them a tissue to wipe away the flood of tears. It makes a world of difference to say to that same distraught parent, "Go ahead and let it out," while comforting them with an arm around the shoulder. Someone must educate physicians to put away their handkerchiefs and offer their arms, a piece of themselves, the warmth of the body and the soul.

It is our conviction that single-minded efficiency, professionalism, skill, and competency allopathically can be combined and integrated with feelings and human connectiveness to aid in the alleviation of stress and ease the acceptance of losing a child. From day one, we observed that the stern and sober professionals involved with our case had seemingly abdicated from the world of shared emotions.

The psychodynamics of the family were not pursued beyond our being told that we were invited to ask questions. What questions? We did not know what to ask other than the still persistent, Why? Why Bruce? Why us?

Communication with the family must be encouraged, since the family can be critically important as the child's life ends. Parental involvement can be healing for the entire family.

For the patient's sake it is important that the health-care practitioners open the doors to the mystique and let us, the parents and family-at-large, in. Instead of acknowledging us as a viable part of a support system capable of contributing considerable love and sharing in the care of the child, we were cast aside. It was very disturbing to be treated as if we already knew all possible was being done and thus were expected to observe in a nonparticipatory manner the mechanics of the health-care delivery system. It was even more irritating to be regarded as intellectual midgets incapable of comprehension, leaving us to make assumptions and presumptions about the techniques being utilized for our loved one. These irritations only added to our stress, anxiety and hurt and reduced our ability to cope with this unnatural situation.

Our son, although under the sentence of death, was still a living being responsive to external stimuli and able to perceive our distress to such an extent that his anxiety increased. His ability to maintain confidence in the treatment and the hospital staff was reduced. He responded to our feelings, for we were his only link to the world of wellness.

We can understand that physicians, by virtue of their training and in order to maintain a balance in their own lives, do not allow themselves to become emotionally involved with their patient's. Why though should they expect us, the family, to share that separateness with them? Why sever the human connection just because death is imminent? We did not expect the doctors to give the intimacy needed by us or our son, although such action would have been highly therapeutic. Neither could we understand their inability to grasp our need to reach our son intimately. It was almost as if they viewed his body as a machine, beyond repair and continued productivity, but worth experimentation so as to prevent other machines on the line from breaking down. The message we received from their aloof mechanical composure implied that "since it can't be fixed, just accept its obsolescence and learn to exist without it."

We refused to receive that message. We were sure that we could be a vital part of a support system. We believed, and we now know, without equivocation, that our support improved the quality of our son's last months of life and improved the quality of his dying. We fought and overcame the obstacles placed before us by the system, a system striving so hard for goals of competence and skill achievement that it reduces interpersonal relationships to irrelevance. We encouraged family communication and we took responsibility for connecting with our son at every plateau along the way in his dramatic struggle for life and his acceptance of death. We balanced the equation by adding sensitivity, intimacy, and caring that the professionals preclude (in order, we suppose, to maintain their own sanity) from treatment of the terminally ill. Our Bruce was treated as an object by the professionals and a person, a subject, by us. Thus a holism, an equilibrium, was created. We are convinced that our membership on the support team extended his lifespan by many weeks beyond that predicted by the technologically oriented professionals. Sometimes knowingly and often without conscious awareness, we dealt with the psychological factors involved.

It is our hope that by expressing and sharing our feelings and our experience, a more humanistic approach to the care of the terminally ill, and an understanding of their right to die with dignity, will evolve. As a consequence, the environment surrounding youthful victims of catastrophic disease will be improved.

We encourage all concerned with the health care of the terminally ill to recognize that in the essence of dying must be the sense of living. Our son died at home, in our bed, getting love and life out of every remaining minute. He was free of needles and tubes and poking and probing and out from under the care of impersonal strangers. Some call it dignity. We called it love.

This, then, was our story:

Week One

Our son complains of lethargy, excessive sweating at night, and loss of appetite. It appears that he is fighting a virus or flu.

Week Two

The malaise increases. Fever is present, and vomiting anything ingested increases weakness. We sense something more than flu or a viral infection and urge him to see a doctor.

Week Three

Day One

A most competent diagnostician realizes that this ailment is very serious. An office blood test, quickly analyzed, has Bruce hospitalized at noon with a white blood count (WBC) exceeding 50,000. At 2:00 P.M., the doctor suggests we call in a hematologist. Perceptive Marcia asks, "Do you suspect Leukemia?" and the doctor answers, "I don't suspect it. I am diagnosing it as leukemia and signing off the case in favor of the specialists he needs." By 6:00 P.M. the hematologists have completed their testing and have confirmed the diagnosis. Arrangements are made to transfer Bruce to the oncology section of a major teaching hospital in Los Angeles. The WBC is climbing by the hour and now is approaching 150,000.

It is near midnight of the first day of hospitalization, and many tests later, Bruce is in "protective isolation" and on chemotherapy complete with IV tubes and cooling blanket and the incessant hum of life-sustaining equipment. The WBC is over 200,000. All that can be done is in process, and we are invited, for the first time, to sit down with the medical team and are told the gravity of the situation.

We know now that we are in a life or death day-to-day struggle. Numb with shock, devastated beyond description, and barely able to concentrate on the words, we find ourselves overwhelmed with medical jargon and then the inevitable invitation to ask questions. What questions?

How? Sorry, says the doctor, we just don't know enough about the disease yet. *Why?* Sorry, says the doctor, we don't know. *What* are the chances? Statistics. *What* will you do? Chemotherapy, bone-marrow examinations to determine the type of leukemia and enable a proper protocol to be put into operation. *Protocol?* That is the treatment procedure. *Then what?* We wait and we hope.

Day Two

The diagnosis is acute myelogenous leukemia (AML), and more-serious and less-hopeful statistics are quoted to us. More doctors probe and poke and confer. Residents come and go. Additional IVs are set up, and patient stabilization seems to be the immediate goal. Now we know, by questioning, that what is going on is the introduction of extremely powerful poisons into Bruce's system to kill the leukemic cells in the hope that after the intense course of chemotherapy and the destruction of the abnormal cells the body will manufacture normal cells.

Days Three, Four, and Five

We wait and watch and suffer. We robe and disrobe in sterile gowns and masks and gloves as we go in and out of his room. And still no one has really offered to orient us, to educate us. We hunger for information so we become knowledgable about AML on our own. We read, we listen, we observe, we question. How much easier it would have been to introduce us by way of a brief seminar, an orientation course, to the aspects of the disease, the treatment, the consequences of chemotherapy. Yet no one was prepared to prepare us, patient or family, for the horrors we were to face.

It was at this stage of the process, as the initial shock was wearing off and the awareness of the inevitable was encroaching on us, that we asserted ourselves into the treatment process. No, we did not attempt to insert our thoughts relative to the medical treatment, but we did impose our attitudinal values and our feelings and sensitivity into the psychological void created by the lack of personal attention on the part of the medical team members.

After all, we the family know the emotional needs of the patient during times of good health and normal living conditions. Why not then accept the fact that as adaptable, reasoning people, we could best gauge those needs during a time of crisis and allow—no, encourage—us to join the team as supporting ancillary components in the battle? Why cast the parents aside? Why not use the family to fill the breach developed by the physicians who need to stay detached and uninvolved in protection of their own psychological well-being?

From day one, the various members of the medical team and the staff nurses persisted in sending us home. "Get some rest" and "Don't let your-self get run down" were commonly and frequently repeated to us. And the ever familiar, "Bruce shouldn't become so reliant upon your presence." Why not? To quote an old simile, "Home is where the heart is," and cer-tainly our hearts and our total beings were there in that room with him. Reliance! It was his reliance upon us that allowed the connections between us to grow to such an extent that he could later give us the support we needed as the end came near. The ultimate in reciprocation.

Please understand that we are not condemning the health-care profes-sionals for their impersonal posture. We are fully aware that they could not act differently. They did not know how. They did not know how to react subjectively. They had not been trained in feelings. Consequently, they reached to our emotional problems by throwing all sorts of medical and sci-entific terms at us. We were bombarded with the rhetoric and vernacular of the oncology section and sent into even deeper states of frustration by our lack of familiarity with their jargon. So often, as we sat staring into space, doctors and nurses tried to reach us and bring us back to the here and now by their invitation to "ask questions." We did not know what questions to ask. We did not know what it was all about, so how could we frame ques-tions?

The total situation of terminal illness was foreign to us. It was made more difficult by the strange and unfamiliar terminology and the glossing over, ever so lightly, of the expectations of the extent of the pain and levels of consciousness we should expect Bruce to exhibit. Naturally, we became even more anxious and did not know what to expect. For example, when we were given details about chemotherapy, we were warned that there would be *some* hair loss and *some* nausea. No one prepared us for the transforma-tion we were about to witness. Facts. Bare limited facts. No feelings, no soul.

The professionals were so mechanical in their overall approach that no one took the time to develop a personal history of Bruce's lifestyle. Or ours either, for that matter. No personal rapport was achieved. There was a total lack of awareness of our beliefs, our lifestyles, our culture, thus precluding their use of our personal capabilities and/or techniques familiar to us which could appreciably ease the pain and discomfort of the patient. We were all, including Bruce, experienced in meditation and in self-hypnosis. Yet with-out a knowledge of this, how could the professionals encourage us to utilize these tools to alleviate the stress buildup? Bruce was proficient at achieving deep states of meditation, but was laughed at for using such a tool to alter his state of consciousness in attempting to achieve a reduction of stress and pain and overcome excessive nausea. Why make light of something that just might help? Especially with the admission that they had so much to learn about the disease. And yet, they did scoff and ridicule.

We experienced a refusal by the members of the healing profession to accept that healing could occur any other way than through the puncturing of the body with a needle. We attempted to acculturate the physicians and nurses into our way of thinking. We did not, Bruce did not, attempt to play down the need for drugs and chemicals and traditional medical treatment. We did want to complement that process with other methods that might produce a synergism in the approach to healing. No attempt was made, by us, to exclude or override the knowledge and skills of the doctors. Yet all our attempts were frowned upon and, for the most part, ridiculed.

We persisted and we finally wore the staff down. Their fear of family interference, of violation of their mystique, of our mingling in their sacred fraternal-like order was an immense barrier to overcome. The prevailing question is, why did we have to use so much of our limited energy fighting a system that itself should have been receptive to any help, from any quarter, to make the patient more comfortable.

Admittedly, it has to work two ways. The family must let the professionals do their thing. But the professionals should become familiar with the family support team available to them and educate that team component fully, in lay language, concerning the medical protocols being used as well as detailing all the possible consequences. In this way, an extended support system is created to service the patient with equal portions of bitter pills and soothing love. If this is to work effectively, then the professionals must be receptive to the emotional needs of the family. Then, and only then, are the channels of communication open between the two elements vitally concerned with the patient's well-being.

In our own situation, we experienced such reluctance to understand our need, as parents, to be there with Bruce and to watch and touch and stroke him that an atmosphere of opposition existed. Two forces, with like goals, pushing against each other when we should have joined hands and worked in harmony. Even the staff psychiatrist failed to recognize our needs. He virtually told us to stay away and leave the healing to professionals. He stated that our constantly being around was detrimental to the functioning of the staff. The one professional trained in the therapy of the psyche was so indoctrinated with traditional medical practices that he could not realize the value of feelings and of caring in the medical process. Someone must redefine *care* for the health-care professionals!

The whole element of personal interaction and shared feelings becomes even more important to all concerned after the revelation, by the physicians, that, "we have done all that we can do," and now it is just a question of time. The rhetoric of that moment is the classic, "Now we have to wait and see." Their conception of wait and see is to wait somewhere else and see by virtue of an occasional, once-a-day, 5- to 10-minute visit. Were we to follow the advice of those professionals, including the psychiatric staff, at this point in time, Bruce would have been not only a terminal patient, but also a prisoner in a state of solitary confinement called "protective isolation."

Weeks Four through Ten

Bruce has been through three courses of chemotherapy with over 70 blood transfusions. Dad has been on the pherisis unit 7 times for transfusions of white blood cells. Bruce has undergone a metamorphosis from a 150-pound curly headed and bearded youth to a 104-pound skeleton-like creature infested with sores and fungus. The pain never diminishes, but steadily increases.

Death is constantly nearby and occasionally so close as to be frequently imminent. And during this period when touching and intimacy are so important to ease the fear and alleviate uncertainty, we have to fight for information and cope with the hospital's impersonal systems. More important, Bruce drifting in and out of lucidity is seeing only eyes, beneath sterile caps and over masks, feeling only gloved hands, and encountering doctors who stand back from the bed, some with their hands clasped beneath sterile gowns, exhibiting an inability to touch, to stroke, to be one with him. They act as if he is contagious. They seem to forget that it is they who he has to be protected from.

And it goes on. The daily admonishment to "stay away." Leave him to us, for we know what is best.

Week Eleven

The wait-and-see period. Chemotherapy is over. Weak and unable to take anything orally, he now has IVs in both arms. Semiconscious, for the most part, he fights to live. Veins are constantly collapsing. Sores and fungi are prevenlant and the ever-present IVACS are beeping in the quiet.

This period, it seems to us, is the critical period for closeness, for personal interaction between healer and healee. The occasional taking of vital signs and the visits by phlebotomists and IV nurses are not enough to maintain calm in the patient. Yet now the physicians became even more remote from us all. And still the reluctance to accept our constant attendance as if by our very presence we would invade their privacy and encroach upon their territory. A prime example of professional indifference to a patient's feeling occurred at this time. The toxic chemicals of the chemotherapy had done their job. The leukemic cells were dead and gone. Each day a blood sample was taken to determine the quality of the blood being reconstituted by the body. In spite of his and our obvious anxiousness over the reports, which could tell the difference between remission or failure, no effort was made to understand that anxiety and ease it by prompt communication.

Many times we had to fight our way through staff bureaucracy to obtain the results of testing. Add to that the confusion of a mentally weary patient in accepting that a negative report was a good report.

We discovered that instead of being elated when told that the test was negative, Bruce was dejected and slipped into a deeper state of depression. In his frame of reference, negative meant bad. No one bothered to tell him that a negative report meant that there were *no* leukemic cells in the blood and that that was a good thing. Marcia realized his confusion and, with a great deal of difficulty and motherly patience, tried to enlighten Bruce. In his weakened state, with an inability to concentrate and under the influence of heavy doses of morphine, he just could not accept Marcia's explanation. We had to corral a resident, from the oncology staff, whose eyes were familiar to Bruce to affirm her explanation and substantiate that the negative reports were good reports.

Had we not been there at his side in constant attendance, he might well have given up his courageous struggle at this time, out of pure futility, thinking that nothing had worked. Along these same lines, no one took the time to explain to Bruce, or to us, how long it might be before a conclusive remission could be established. It was solely because of the family support team's awareness of the patient's state of mind that he was able to emotionally survive that week-long "wait and see" period.

In our opinion, it is necessary to reacquaint the physician with the use of everyday vocabulary. He or she has been in an environment dominated by medical jargon for so long and in the narrowness of the tunnel of medical technology begun in his or her training and lengthened, but not broadened, in practice that he or she is unaware of the communication gaps created by the terminology. It is also important that we overcome the mystique of the medical profession perpetuated by the physician with the concept of keeping everything confidential. They do not share the records with the family, and they do not share thoughts with the family.

We acknowledge and agree that not everything has to be shared and/or interpreted for the patient and the parents. Certainly, however, test results should not be classified as "top secret" to such an extent that only a select member of the fraternal order has the authority to divulge the results at the cost of needless hours of anxious waiting by the patient. There is no reason that a floor nurse, or intern, cannot impart good or bad news to a waiting patient or immediate family member as soon as the results are available. Instead, additional stress is created as we wait for the primary physician, the doctor in charge, to disseminate the information when he or she makes the rounds.

This sort of elitist "rites of spring" ritual we had to become acclimated to is unquestionably unnecessary and definitely most harmful to the state of mind of all concerned, especially the patient.

It became apparent to us that a hierarchical structure existed among the health-care group. The physicians of record were at the top level, and staff doctors were at the next level down. Resident physicians and nurses were in constant competition for the next two levels in the system. Those on the lowest levels, although in possession of critical, quite possibly mind-stabilizing, information, would not impart such data to us. The fear of reprisal by the power bloc of the upper echelons was so strong as to remove any human feelings from the subordinates. The emphasis was on adhering to and monitoring rules and regulations and jockeying for position in the chain of command—to hell with human feelings. All of them, regardless of their position on the ladder of hierarchy, had to cope with the hospital administration. On more than one occasion we had to combat the dehumanized bureaucracy by expressions of anger and hostility and make almost violent threats to support an instantaneous decision of a nurse or resident precluded, by the system, from taking prompt action to relieve an immediate crisis.

During this period of our son's hospitalization, the oncology unit of the institution was always full. Among some 30 patients, there were several other youthful AML victims. Not only was nothing done to build community among the families and create a network of mutual support, which would have been beneficial to all concerned, quite to the contrary, we were admonished by the staff, including the psychological team, not to get close to other sets of parents. We were all advised that such would be detrimental to ourselves and the patients and so were repeatedly warned, yes, warned, not to communicate with each other. The hospital staff felt that interaction between families might lead to confusion and possibly interference with the medical teams as we discovered that different protocols were in operation. No concern for human feelings, just the ever-present concern that someone might learn something that might, could, maybe, would interfere with the staff's performance.

Most of the other parents were less forceful than we were. They had not acquired the knowledge about leukemia that we had been able to assimilate through self-study and observation. Easily influenced by the God-like awesome aura of the medical professionals, they paid heed to the command and withdrew. They also bowed to the authoritarian advice to "stay away, since there is nothing you can do here" and unquestionably suffered emotionally as a consequence of such adherence. There was a total disregard for us, the parents and the immediate families, and for our emotional needs as the survivors-to-be. How much it could have helped us all to comingle, share, and establish by virtue of our common problem a network wherein we could contribute to each other and be with each other dispelling the loneliness that accompanies such deep emotional pain. The best mode of therapy we parents, as a collective, could have been directed to would have been involvement with each other. To share the burden of grief. To realize that we alone were not singled out to endure this punishment.

It is true that our culture has a built-in stigma concerning death and we are programmed from an early age to fear our own mortality. However, at a time when a child is pronounced terminally ill, we, the parents, thirst for and need to be involved with the act of their dying, just as we were involved with their conception and birth. The institutions of our social structure do not prepare us for this exigency, and the health professionals and their institutions do even less to enable us to cope. Instead of encouraging dialogues and conversations about death and making that final act an accepted part of the conditions of living, it is feared and allowed to become a sort of cancer itself by virtue of the way it is hidden beneath the surface.

The hospital's conception of providing for the family of the terminally ill was to provide a waiting room. In our experience, that room was often offlimits to us, since the staff frequently locked us out of the waiting room so that it could be used for meetings and shift-change reports. No one cared that parents suffering exhaustion and anxiety and trying to overcome the feelings of devastation, of being violated, were sitting on corridor floors. We should not have been there in the first place. Had they not told us to go home and stay away?

Week Twelve

Remission! Now it is just a question of gaining strength and learning to walk again. Isolation is over, and the door is open. Eyes become people, and Bruce smiles for the first time in weeks. He hungers to identify the nurses and doctors, the residents and technicians who he has known only as eyes peering over a mask.

Yet, not even now is physical contact with the patient made unless it is necessary for examination purposes. The exception is our private-duty nurses, who hug and stroke and do a lot of hand holding with Bruce. And, of course, we are in constant touching contact with him. The physicians, including the staff psychiatrist, are still walking in with their hands in their pockets. They have a hands-off syndrome. They are classic examples of disdain. We are convinced that a required course in medical school must be one called "touch aversion." Physical contact between the bearer and the recipient of news can ease bad news and enhance good news. Touching a shoulder or stroking a head or chest while talking to a bed-ridden patient can do so much to raise their spirits, to let them, through that momentary connection, feel wellness instead of sickness. It can increase the patient's self-confidence as well as confidence in the healer and thereby reduce fear. Why the reluctance to touch?

Very often we observed a physician enter the room and stand back away from the bed in such a posture as to impart to the patient an aura of contagion and negative vibrations. This was more prevalent and more adverse in the "protective isolation" situation. However, even now with the door open, they still maintained that distant, aloof attitude. During the previous weeks of "protective isolation," the patient saw only eyes above a mask and beneath a cap. He had no idea of who he was dealing with or what people looked like. In spite of the protective clothing, the doctors refrained from touching, stroking, feeling—little touches that impart a message of warmth and caring and compassion were totally absent.

When you smile at people, they tend to smile back. When you frown or sulk, people tend to avoid your look. The same is true of touching. It is reciprocal. Yet it is almost as if the professionals are afraid to touch for fear that such a display of emotion would negate the mystery and topple them from their perch of authority and knowledge.

In our experience, it was almost a competitive situation between nurses, residents, staff physicians, and the primary physician that constrained the latter, as well as most resident and staff doctors, from becoming humanistically supportive of the parents. The competition was so keen as to preempt the development of community in an environment where communal thought could have been a tremendous asset to all.

It is obvious that the trained health-care professionals were not educated in the realization that the terminal patient and the family, in any catastrophic disease situation, need preparation for what is in store for them and what they will have to cope with. We recognize and applaud their technical competencies. We also are painfully aware of their limitations. It is a question of deficiency in their education. A deficiency that can and should be corrected so that they can properly orient the patient and the family and utilize this heretofore invisible support team as an adjunct to their technology.

We are inclined to think that medical training dehumanizes individuals. Most graduates come out as good, or adequate, or outstanding technicians, but somewhat less than humane and feeling beings. Even the psychological teams that we dealt with were not programmed for holistic thought. Their primary function seems to be to minimize the problems between the patient and the family and between either or both of those and the hospital administration. They are more concerned with reducing friction between patient and/or parents and the staff than in dealing with the emotional needs of the child or the parents. They, of all concerned in the total health-care delivery system, should be aware that the emotional needs of the parents directly affect the child and vice versa. They lack awareness of the need to develop a rational state of mind and thereby create a balance among all the individuals involved in the totality of the situation.

In order to help someone, to ease the physical and emotional pain, you must make contact. There must be a bridge to allow that connection. A relationship is a bridge connecting two people. It is built of trust, openness, respect, and care. It can be the strongest bridge ever known—it can support and comfort and sustain life, and it can, when need be, ease the path of dying. We do not ask, nor do we expect, the medical practitioners to build such bridges. We dare them to cross over bridges the parents are willing to build. We defy them to cross and to allow themselves to experience caring and understanding and maybe even love.

During our hospital experience, great numbers of people worked with, on, or around Bruce. Possibly 40 or 50, even 60, different individuals saw him and us with some regularity. Yet of all, only a very few, possibly 4 or 5 individuals, crossed the bridge and made a connection. And each of these was a private-duty nurse, hired by us to complement the staff and maximize attention to Bruce. They were proof to us that bridges can be crossed. Some of the private-duty nurses were pure technicians operating right out of a manual of standard operating procedure in spite of their experience with terminal patients. Others, just as proficient in the technology, allowed themselves to become involved. They touched and were touched. They dared to become emotionally involved with our son and with us. They provided listening ears and warm hands. They were not afraid to cross over, bridging the deep chasm between technology and feelings.

Weeks Thirteen through Twenty-Five

At home: Bruce is gaining in strength and spirit. We are continuing a maintenance chemotherapy by injections (at home) and visiting the doctor's office once a week for blood tests and so forth. In spite of the reemergence of body hair, his weight gain, and his ability to go out among people and trees and even ride his bike on his own, we all recognize that the odds are thousands to one that he will remain in remission. We hope, and sometimes we tend to forget that death is still very close to us. We allow ourselves to speculate that Bruce will be the *one* in the thousands-to-one odds. The one to have a lasting remission. We dare to dream. Yet always we know to savor these moments, these days, and take them one at a time, for reversal is a strong possibility.

Week Twenty-Six

And then it occurs. It is here! Remission is reversed. The dirty words, the hard words—*leukemic cells*—came back to burst the dream. Decision time is at hand. We are advised that there are two medical alternatives, and both require immediate hospitalization. Both are drastic, and both are bleak in outlook. One is to undergo more courses of chemotherapy, as in the past, only more intense and with the chance that it will not work. The other is to resort to the highly experimental and rarely successful bone-marrow transplant procedure. In either case, the oncologists paint such a grim and pessimistic picture that Bruce rejects both alternatives and elects to stay at home.

It is, in his words, too dehumanizing to undergo such treatment with so dubious an outcome, and he would choose to die at home with the conscious awareness of death. He says he is ready to die if it is his time. He tells us, "I want to be able to consciously experience the act. It must afterall be a wonderful thing if God saves death for the last and final act".

He has become a very spiritual person in these last few weeks, and he seeks affirmation of his decision not only from us, but also from several religious leaders, of various denominations and order, whose opinion he respects.

Two days later, with our support, Bruce announces his firm decision not to undergo further hospitalization and experimentation. While the oncologists understand the nature of the decision, they find it an uncomfortable one to accept. Their composure is momentarily shattered. Then at our urging, they predict a time frame of 2 to 3 weeks before the expiration of life. The physicians strongly urge us to hospitalize Bruce. They state that even without chemotherapy or any other type of procedure to attempt to combat the rising leukemic cell count, the proper place for him to be is in a hospital where he could best be cared for in these last days. These healers, no strangers to death among their patients, cannot conceive of the comfort, love, and caring that would be (and was) achieved in the home environment. They cannot sense our ability to deal with each other. They think only in terms of physical needs and not of happiness or emotional peace. Every attempt is made to impress us with the relief from pain the hospital can offer Bruce and the relieving of personal discomfort we, his parents, can gain by absenting ourselves from the constant observation of his rapid wasting away.

In consideration of their obvious lack of knowledge of the needs of the family unit, we can understand their pleading. From their perspective, limited as it is, the arguments are valid. We counter with the facts that we are willing and feel we must be constantly together at this time and that we know we can bring registered nurses, as private-duty nurses, into the home to handle the administration of pain-killing drugs such as morphine when that becomes necessary. At this point in time, medical care, to relieve pain, is less important than the ability for us to be together in a warm and familiar home environment. In that constant togetherness, we can talk through the fears and the reality or the death we are about to experience. Unaccustomed to such feelings, the doctors virtually withdrew from any further contact other than that of dispensing the required perscriptions for morphine and other pain-killing drugs from that day forward. Once, and only once, during the ensuing 9 weeks did one of the oncologists make a house call to visit the patient. And that call was made at our urging to validate the need for increasing dosages of morphine. Even then, in spite of what the doctor saw and heard—color and music, personal paraphenalia and people, laughter and joking, the smells and sounds of life—he could only think to advise us to move Bruce to a hospital to spare us the shock that he imagined we would endure with the encroachment of the finality of death.

As survivors we look back and we know that the choice was right. We only regret that, for those like us who are equipped emotionally to handle dying at home, there is no professional help to ease the acknowledged burden. The child and the parents have the right to decide where they want to die, how they want to die, and who they want with them at the end. In making this choice, we went against the institutional prescriptions of the health-care profession, and the members of that group could not cope with this abrupt violation of their norms, their established customs. The obvious lack of traning in dealing with the terminal patient and our willingness to confront such a situtaion must have presented the physicians with a condition so foreign to them as to create a fear of the unknown negating their ability to become involved. The respected physician implies that we are wrong and he or she is right by virtue of his or her medical training and abundant experience in matters like this. He or she states that we are dealing from emotion and that he or she is dealing from knowledge—a paradox. At this point in time when knowledge had failed and the admission has been made that there is "nothing more that we can do with any certainty to reverse the condition," it is time for emotion to prevail and knowledge to take a back seat.

Weeks Twenty-Seven through Thirty-Six

Bruce outlives the prediction by almost 8 weeks. He was lucid, aware, happy, and fulfilled until the very last. He was free of needles and tubes and really enjoyed the environment of home and friends and family. His life was surrounded by familiar smells and sounds and furniture and people. He had the motivation and the will to stretch his life out to the fullest possible.

During this last period of his life, we shared with each other a togetherness that could not have been possible in any other setting but home. Hope took a back seat to the imminence of death, yet was never totally cast aside. Miracles could happen. Maybe, just maybe, something radical might occur and his body might fight off the foreign invaders and he could recover.

These last weeks were the fullest of our lives. They were full of pain and pleasure, laughter and tears, happiness and sorrow, and in the end the fullest and most complete love one person is capable of giving to another. Three days before he lapsed into the 18-hour coma that preceded death, Bruce asked, ''Why is it that we really don't feel what love is until it is too late?''

Annotated Bibliography of Selected Materials in Health Psychology

Linda J. (Tik) Menefee
and *Joseph Nieberding*

The purpose of the annotated bibliography is to provide a limited and select review of the literature in health psychology, primarily from the past ten years. No attempt was made to retrieve and annotate all relevant materials in health psychology. Attesting to the difficulty of such an attempt, Kahana (1972), assisted by the computerized MEDLARS retrieval system, surveyed those studies in medical psychology which considered both the patient's personality and his or her physical illness. He likens the results of the flood of printout from the computer to the final scene from Walt Disney's "The Sorcerer's Apprentice." Within the two- to four-year period reviewed, 5,000 references were found, of which half were determined to be relevant for his purposes. The large number of references that resulted from his search alludes to the diversity of topics and interest in psychological aspects of physical illnesses as well as the difficulty in arriving at precise definitions of health-psychology terms in order for the computerized retrieval system to categorize and organize information. This is further complicated by the diversity of terms currently in use (that is, medical psychology, health psychology, psychosomatic medicine, behavioral health, behavioral medicine, and so on). Hopefully, the current efforts to arrive at more precise and uniform terminology will simplify future attempts to search particular aspects of the literature in health psychology.

This bibliography is divided into five sections and the articles are arranged in chronological order within each section to give a perspective on the development of concepts and theory. The selected articles are by no means exhaustive. Rather, the intent is to provide a starting point for further reading and inquiry.

Reference

Kahana, R.J. 1972. Studies in medical psychology: A brief survey. *Psychiatry in Medicine* 3:1–22.

Theoretical Perspectives of Psychosomatic Medicine

Mechanic, D. 1962. The concept of illness behavior. *Journal of Chronic Diseases* 15:189–194.

> Illness behavior is defined by Mechanic as the ways in which a set of symptoms may be perceived, evaluated, and acted (or not acted) upon by others. Mechanic hypothesizes, and later shows through studies that illness behavior influences when and how an individual seeks treatment and the ways in which an individual responds to that treatment and cooperates in it. Several factors contributing to illness behavior are detailed.

Lipowski, Z.J. 1969. Psychosocial aspects of disease. *Annals of Internal Medicine* 71(6):1197–1206.

> Lipowski states that total medical management should include the social and psychological aspects of the patient's illness. Although most medical personnel agree with this philosophy, Lipowski feels that this is more lip service than actual practice. He then states that in order to evaluate how a patient responds pyschologically to a given illness or injury the following four aspects of the patient's life must be considered:
>
> 1. personality and relevant factors in the life history;
> 2. current social and economic situation;
> 3. characteristics of the nonhuman environment; and
> 4. the disease or injury process as it is perceived and evaluated by the patient.
>
> He goes on to explore more fully the determinants of the patient's psychological reaction, including the meaning of illness for the patient, and the behavioral components accompanying different reactions.

Lipowski, Z.J. 1970. Physical illness, the individual and the coping process. *Psychiatry in Medicine* 1:91–102.

> Lipowski discusses the ways in which people cope with the stresses and challenges of disease. Coping includes all of the cognitive and motor activities that patients use to preserve bodily and psychic integrity and to deal with the outcome of the illness or disability. He distinguishes coping styles from coping strategies and notes that these may be adaptive or maladaptive.
>
> The determinants of coping, within an individual, include intrapersonal factors, disease-related factors, and environmental factors. An individual's coping style is a relatively enduring quality. Cognitive (minimization and vigilant focusing) and behavioral (tackling, capitulating, avoiding)

styles may be combined in response to illness. The various coping strategies are more variable and changeable than the individual's style. Some of the major patterns of strategies are:

1. Illness as challenge.
2. Illness as enemy.
3. Illness as punishment.
4. Illness as weakness.
5. Illness as strategy.
6. Illness as irreparable loss or damage.
7. Illness as relief.
8. Illness as value.

Lipowski suggests that the specific meaning of a given illness significantly affects the coping strategy chosen.

Mechanic, D. 1972. Social psychologic factors affecting the presentation of bodily complaints. *The New England Journal of Medicine* 286(21): 1132–1139.

Mechanic begins by stating that patients frequently seek medical assistance for complaints for which physicians can find no physical basis. He cautions against assuming that all of these patients are hypochondriacal. Mechanic reviews how individuals learn about illness through socialization, including the learning of what symptoms are to be considered legitimate. He then classifies these patients into two categories: those who are aware of and willing to use psychological language and concepts and those who are not. He goes on to indicate that many patients with these complaints may be under stress or are expressing emotional distress and the physician should evaluate for this possibility.

Abram, H.S. 1972. Psychological dilemmas of medical progress. *Psychiatry in Medicine* 3:51–58.

Abram raises and discusses three questions relating to chronic hemodialysis and organ donors, as well as other new medical techniques that serve to prolong life in complex ways. First, he discusses the issue of who should receive such treatment, reviews available studies, and concludes that psychological screening does not seem to eliminate serious psychological problems. Second, he discusses organ donors and notes that serious consideration should be given to whether the individual is donating an organ for altruistic or neurotic reasons. He feels that careful psychological screening should be undertaken. Finally, Abram discusses the problems involved in prolonging life. He feels that the frequently rigid routines that must be followed by those patients can sometimes become a living death.

Lowy, F.H. 1975. Management of the persistent somatizer. *International Journal of Psychiatry in Medicine* 6(1/2):227–239.

Lowy defines the somatizer as a patient who complains of bodily symptoms that cannot be adequately explained on the basis of organic pathology. He states that somatizers are among the most unpopular patients seen by physicians and are frequently felt to represent only one symptom pattern. However, somatization may be representative of a number of psychological problems or syndromes. Especially among the lower classes somatization is used as an expression of emotional distress. Early life experience and particular personality characteristics have also been associated with somatization. Lowy feels that primary prevention is a logical final goal, but that there is currently an insufficient understanding of predisposing factors to make this feasible. Therefore, he recommends secondary prevention through early diagnosis and treatment. Recommendations for management by psychiatrists and primary physicians are made.

Spaulding, W.B. 1975. The psychosomatic approach in the practice of medicine. *International Journal of Psychiatry in Medicine* 6(1/2): 169–181.

Spaulding strongly recommends the use of a psychosomatic or holistic approach to medicine by all physicians. He notes that as many as 30 percent of patients seen by internists in private practice and 60 percent of patients in nonpsychiatric units of community hospitals have psychological concomitants that contribute to their physical distress. These factors may be causing the symptoms, may contribute to the symptoms, or may serve as background features. Spaulding recommends that physicians elicit histories of psychological disturbances and physical complaints concurrently. This history taking may be significant in treatment, as the patient may be more willing to recognize psychological factors if he or she perceives the physician to be considering them seriously. In difficult situations Spaulding states that he utilizes psychiatric consultation, sometimes in sessions conducted jointly by himself and a psychiatrist.

Reichsman, F. 1975. Teaching psychosomatic medicine to medical students, residents, and postgraduate fellows. *International Journal of Psychiatry in Medicine* 6(1/2):307–316.

Reichsman describes the psychosomatic teaching program at the Downstate Medical Center College of Medicine in Brooklyn, New York. The teaching objectives of the program include (1) teaching skills to accurately observe and take histories relevant to the psychological and social aspects of disease and injury; (2) assisting trainees in acquiring an understanding of body-mind relationships to health and illness; (3) helping trainees acquire reasoning skills; (4) producing change in attitudes and behavior; and (5) presenting as a model a physician with an interest and competence in both the psychosocial and physical-physiologic-biochemical areas of medicine. Reichsman works with medical students, interns and residents, psychiatric residents, and liaison fellows. He views as the greatest difficulties toward the development of psychosomatic medicine the attitudes of medical practitioners and the shortage of well-qualified teachers. Reichsman also recommends that with so much medical care being delivered within the community a move be made toward providing this training and service in nonhospital settings.

Lipsitt, D.R. 1975. Some problems in the teaching of psychosomatic medicine. *International Journal of Psychiatry in Medicine* 6(1/2): 317–329.

Lipsitt states that estimates of 20 to 80 percent of patients who present to a doctor with physical complaints have psychosocial problems of either primary or secondary import. He reviews the history of psychosomatic medicine and notes that its success is in some ways also its failure. Psychosomatic medicine became the study of only a few diseases. There has not been an agreement among physicians of the need to attend to the psychological and social needs of all patients. Lipsitt suggests that this lack is partially the result of the segregation of psychiatrists, by themselves and by general medicine practitioners, from concern with general medical needs. Thus, students do not have models of physicians who integrate the medical and psychosocial aspects of patients. Lipsitt also points out the Cartesian philosophy in medical education as a difficulty. Lipsitt feels that new ways of teaching medicine are necessary and that new criteria for selecting future physicians may be needed.

Rappaport, M. 1975. Medically oriented psychiatry: An approach to improving the quality of mental health care. *Psychosomatic Medicine* 26(12):811–815.

Rappaport argues for the use of the medical model by psychiatrists in order to ensure an integrated treatment plan. His use of the term "medical model" implies that at times a definitive diagnosis can be made, with effective treatment being initiated quickly and resulting in a satisfactory outcome achieved in a cost-effective manner. Rappaport points out that it is generally accepted that many patients who complain of medical problems to a physician also have concomitant psychosocial difficulties. However, there are many physical problems which first appear as psychosocial difficulties. He argues that the psychiatrist is in the unique position of being able to fully evaluate patients who come for psychotherapy, both medically and psychologically. Additionally, he feels that all nonmedical mental-health workers should be required to work under or in close association with psychiatrists in order to rule out these medical disorders. Finally, Rappaport presents a plan whereby a patient would fund increasing amounts of his psychotherapy as the therapy continues beyond the reduction of disabling psychological dysfunction into an emphasis upon human growth.

Lazerson, A.M. 1976-1977. The psychiatrist as teacher in primary care residency training: The first year. *International Journal of Psychiatry in Medicine* 7(2):165-178.

Lazerson reports on the first of a three-year multidisciplinary primary-care training program for internists and pediatricians at Boston City Hospital and the Boston University School of Medicine. The goals of the program are to train primary-care physicians for the inner city with a curriculum which emphasizes psychosocial aspects of medical practice while maintaining training in the traditional medical subjects. Some of the difficulties encountered include the overwhelming demands placed on the trainees, the tendency for senior medical personnel to have more interest in patients on the inpatient services, the tradition of faculty working alongside interns and residents in the outpatient clinic, and the rotating schedules of interns and residents. Additionally, it was initially difficult to demonstrate the importance of psychosocial factors within medicine to the trainees. The author worked through these difficulties by assigning each trainee to the outpatient clinic for a specific time period each week and by having the trainee follow each patient throughout the training period (three years). Lazerson did not begin by presenting lecture and literature material, but rather sat in with trainees for a short time period during an examination. He then discussed the patient with the trainee, pointing out relevant psychosocial factors. After the trainee was able to recognize the importance of psychosocial factors, curiosity led to perusal of relevant literature.

Cousins, N. 1976. Anatomy of an illness (as perceived by the patient). *The New England Journal of Medicine* 295(26):1458-1463.

Cousins reports on his experience as a patient with a life-threatening illness given little hope of recovery by the medical profession. Having read several books about the effect of the mind on the body, Cousins decided that the hospital environment was not a positive one. With the cooperation and agreement of his physician, Cousins decided to take an active role in his own recovery. He moved from the hospital into a hotel, obtained humorous books and films which he read and viewed frequently, and took massive doses of vitamin C. Cousins also set about maintaining a positive attitude and exercising his own will to live. After two weeks he had recovered enough to go to Puerto Rico for a vacation in the sunshine, and within several months was able to return to work. Although he does not claim total recovery, Cousins is doing relatively well. He attributes to his physician a major role in encouraging him to become a respected partner in conquering his illness. He also discusses relevant literature in the area of placebo effects and effects of positive attitudes.

Singer, M.T. 1977. Psychological dimensions in psychosomatic patients. *Psychotherapy and Psychosomatics* 28:13-27.

Singer reviews five major changes in the field of psychosomatic medicine over the past fifty years, including:

1. a broadened scope of study and a shift from studying psychological factors in chronic illness to studying psychological factors in all illness;
2. a shift from studying the patient's intrapsychic processes to a study of his or her interpersonal transactions;
3. use of the transactional and systems viewpoint to study the patient's style of communication with others relative to the illness;
4. the appearance of literature that deals with different psychotherapeutic methods in the treatment of all physically ill patients; and
5. an increase in staff at teaching hospitals and clinics, enabling them to offer more psychological and psychiatric services to the physically ill. This has led to the general public becoming more aware that its health may be influenced by attitudes and responses to changes and stresses in life.

Singer sees four important dimensions, when formulating designs for research and therapy, in evaluating psychosomatic patients. These are (1) the patient's cognitive style, (2) the ways in which the patient invests him- or herself in transactions, (3) the attitude a patient holds regarding changes in his or her life, and (4) concern for research which represents adequate sampling, including factors such as ethnicity, age, social class, and so on in matching the ill and healthy. Singer then briefly reports on current research that attempts to measure these dimensions with some critical review.

Wright, L. 1977. Conceptualizing and defining psychosomatic disorders. *American Psychologist* 32(8): 625–628.

Wright questions the usefulness of the concept of psychosomatic illness as physical problems caused by emotional stress. He presents the areas that he feels are within the area of psychosomatic medicine. Wright begins by discussing organic problems which do not result from stress but are created by difficulties of learning or development, citing children who develop abnormal breathing patterns and encopresis after tracheotomies as examples. Second, Wright discusses organic problems which are created as the result of personality problems and character development, such as self-mutilating behavior. Finally, Wright discusses psychological problems that are caused indirectly by organic disease when patients are placed in the position of dealing with the added burdens of illness and psychological problems that are caused directly by organic disease.

Karasu, T.B. 1979. Psychotherapy of the medically ill. *The American Journal of Psychiatry* 136(1):1–11.

Karasu reviews the literature on psychotherapy with the medically ill. His review indicates that most of this literature consists of case studies with comparative research or systematic evaluation. Karasu found that psychotherapy is successful with some patients, resulting in some physical or psychological improvement. However, clear conclusions are difficult to draw because of the nature of the reports. Karasu recommends that more systematic research is needed which would consider not only the individual psychotherapeutic techniques but also focus attention on the therapeutic process, longitudinal data, and specific variables in the patient and the therapy.

Health-Care Psychology

Kahana, R.J. 1972. Studies in medical psychology: A brief survey. *Psychiatry in Medicine* 3:1–22.

Kahana performed a MEDLARS search of the years 1968 through 1972 to review the available literature relating a person's personality to the nature of illnesses incurred. His search resulted in over 5,000 citations, of which 2,500 related to the topic and Kahana felt that approximately one-fourth of these were useful. This article specifically describes some 367 of these articles under the categories Systems of the Body, Age Related Studies, Special Problems, Medical and Surgical Treatments, and Relationships between Professionals and the Patient. Each article is briefly cited in relation to its specific subject area.

Kimball, C.P. 1975. Medical psychotherapy. *Psychotherapy and Psychosomatics* 25:193–200.

Kimball defines medical psychotherapy as the application of psychological concepts and methods to the individual and/or family experiencing catastrophic and/or chronic illness. He reviews basic techniques for establishing rapport and facilitating communication. Kimball feels that the medically involved patient should be viewed as going through a grieving process. He reviews Lindemann's process identified in his studies of survivors and relatives of victims of the Coconut Grove fire and applies those to medical psychotherapy. The stages of this process include denial, ventilation of affect, the defensive stage, and the restitutive stage.

Brumback, G.B. 1974. Symposium: Toward a psychology more responsive to the nation's health care crisis. Introduction. *Professional Psychology* 5(1):83–84.

This symposium contains articles by psychologists whom Brumback states have broken away from traditional psychology to think innovatively about ways to respond to the health-care crises. He feels that the solution to the discontent within psychology is in the branching into unusual roles. Brumback feels that health psychology may serve this purpose and emphasizes that the training of health psychologists should be responsive to the role preferences involved.

Taylor, C.W. 1974. New manpower selection and educational programs for more effective health care performances. *Professional Psychology* 5(1): 85–88.

Taylor describes a research project in which he was asked to develop criterion measures of physician performance. Results showed that neither performance in premedical and medical education nor scores on the Medical College Admissions Test predict later career performance well. Success was more accurately predicted by using a specially constructed and keyed biographical inventory. Taylor notes that this presents medical educators with some direct questions regarding selection of students. However, he cautions that individuals who are good physicians today may not have characteristics which will satisfactorily meet demands in the future. Taylor then briefly notes what has been done in the area of selecting and training nurses with regard to measuring performance or objectively selecting students. Taylor feels psychologists have a potentially important role in developing methods for selecting future medical personnel.

Ort, R.S. 1974. Effects of psychological factors on the delivery and utilization of health care services. *Professional Psychology* 5(1):91–94.

Ort reviews the psychological factors that influence a physician's performance. Physicians identified two factors leading to effective practice that include the physician's view of his or her professional responsibility, including concern for the patient, individual competence and motivation, and the exercise of impartial control, facilitated by objectivity. Ort also discusses the effect of poverty upon the development of maladaptive health behaviors.

Rizzo, J.R. 1974. Toward a system of health care delivery. *Professional Psychology* 5(1):94–95.

Rizzo discusses the need for the knowledge of organizational psychology to be used to improve the present nonsystematic methods of health-care delivery.

Mensh, I.N. 1974. Consulting in medical, educational, and training settings. *Professional Psychology* 5(2):129–132.

Mensh reviews the University of California at Los Angeles training procedure in consultation skills for psychologists and psychiatrists. The role of the consultant is seen as twofold: aiding the inquirer in focusing consultation needs and exploring and developing available options.

Asken, M.J. 1975. Medical psychology: Psychology's neglected child. *Professional Psychology* 6(2):155-160.

Asken reviews the gradual increase in medical knowledge among psychologists and presents a proposal for the establishment of a professional-degree program as evidence that psychology is now seriously attending its potential role within the health-care system. Asken notes that the development of medical psychology in most countries has been through the efforts of psychiatrists and he feels that psychology has much to offer with its scientific base and stricter methodologies. He also reviews various aspects of medicine in which the patient's personality is a major variable.

Drotar, D. 1976. Psychological consultation in a pediatric hospital. *Professional Psychology* 7:77-83.

Drotar reviews the establishment of a psychology consultation unit within a pediatric hospital. He describes the difficulties including the unfamiliarity of the hospital for a psychologist, the multitude of disciplines under different administrations, the transiency of training personnel, and the need for relatively quick solutions to patient problems. Additionally, both the social and the psychiatric services were developing consultation programs. Drotar began by responding to individual patient requests promptly, with detailed discussions and written reports following. He encouraged the use of ward meetings and consultation on rounds. The mental-health departments met together and found that by being less rigid regarding traditional professional lines they were able to work cooperatively and without duplication of services. As more psychologists were added to the staff, the consultation service was able to place more emphasis upon environmental changes and specific patient groups.

Ruphuy, R.S. 1977. Psychology and medicine: A new approach for community health development. *American Psychologist* 32(11):910-913.

Ruphuy describes a developing system of integrated services delivered by medical and psychological practitioners in Costa Rica. He notes that the specialized health-care systems of the developed countries are not practical for developing countries. Costa Rica has developed a program in which the professionals work within the rural communities, taking into account the people's social and economic situation. Psychological services are delivered by intermediate psychologists trained in psychodiagnostics and elementary psychotherapeutic techniques. Efforts are made to have the areas' inhabitants view their health care in a preventive way and to take steps themselves to improve their development.

Schwartz, G.E., and Weiss, S.M. 1978. Behavioral medicine revisited: An amended definition. *Journal of Behavioral Medicine* 1(3):249–250.

Schwartz and Weiss present the definition of behavioral medicine developed at the Yale Conference on Behavioral Medicine in 1978. Although the Yale Conference noted the integration of behavioral and biomedical factors, it was felt that the definition of behavioral medicine contributed to the traditional body/mind dualism. Thus, at the April 1978 meeting of the National Academy of Sciences the definition was altered to emphasize the interdisciplinary nature of behavioral medicine and to encourage the integration and application of behavioral and biomedical knowledge and techniques.

Asken, M.J. 1979. Medical psychology: Toward definition, clarification, and organization. *Professional Psychology* 10(1):66–73.

Asken states that greater interest is evidenced in the field of medical psychology by the number of journal articles appearing. However, he notes that the term has no standard definition and proposes one that subsumes four major areas: psychosomatics, somatopsychology, behavioral medicine, and health-care studies. He describes each of these and then proposes that a formal organization be created to promote the advancement of medical psychology.

Masur, F.T. 1979. An update on medical psychology and behavioral medicine. *Professional Psychology* 10(2):259–264.

Masur responds to Asken (1979) and his proposals for a definition of medical psychology and the creation of an organization to promote this area's interests. Masur questions Asken's use of the term "psychosomatics" on a historical basis, but is particularly concerned regarding his statement that medical psychology subsumes behavioral medicine. Masur points out that the new definition of behavioral medicine (Schwartz and Weiss, 1978) states that it is an interdisciplinary field. Therefore, no one field within it can subsume behavioral medicine. Mazur further notes that since the preparation of Asken's paper several organizations have been formed in the area of behavioral medicine, most particularly Division 38 of APA, the Division of Health Psychology. Finally, Masur notes recent books published or in preparation in the field of health psychology.

Budman, S.H.; Feldman, J.; and Bennett, M.J. 1979. Adult mental health services in a health maintenance organization. *American Journal of Psychiatry* 136: 392–395.

The authors describe the delivery of mental-health services at the Harvard Community Health Plan in Boston. This health-maintenance organization serves some 69,000 members. The authors begin by emphasizing that mental health is seen as an integral part of primary care and that social and psychological issues are addressed throughout the system by members of primary-health-care teams. Within the mental-health division emphasis is upon short-term services. Longer-term therapy is available for twenty sessions on a copayment plan and beyond that for fees comparable to private practitioners. About 15 percent of the plan's members have availed themselves of the mental-health division's services.

Pomerleau, O.F. 1979. Behavioral medicine: The contribution of the experimental analysis of behavior to medical care. *American Psychologist* 34(8):654–663.

Pomerleau reviews the involvement of psychology in medical care and the definitions of psychosomatics, medical psychology, and behavioral medicine. He notes that the two techniques that have shown the most promise in behavioral medicine are biofeedback and self-management. He reviews different areas in medicine where these have been used (for example, seizure control and obesity). Adherence by patients to the techniques has proved to be the most difficult problem in achieving success. Pomerleau emphasizes that psychologists must devote considerable energy to the understanding of behavior with health implications. Some cautions regarding the use of behavioral techniques are also mentioned.

Wright, L. 1979. Health care psychology: Prospects for the well-being of children. *American Psychologist* 34(10):1001–1006.

Wright reviews the history of pediatric psychology and notes that health-care psychology for children has predated its adult counterpart considerably. He sees the roles of the pediatric-health-care psychologist in many aspects of primary mental-health care. In the area of diagnosis, Wright notes the need for diagnosis in considerably less time than in traditional mental-health delivery. Psychologists can contribute substantially to more-descriptive and meaningful classification of medical-psychological problems. They also have a role in the prediction of the sequelae of physical illnesses. Finally, psychologists can contribute a major part in the treatment of medical-psychological problems. Wright describes several different treatment modalities.

Consultation/Liaison Psychiatry

Enelow, A.J., and Adler, L.M. 1964. Psychiatric skills and knowledge for the general practitioner. *Journal of the American Medical Association* 189:117–122.

This article presents a series of training courses, offered by the University of Southern California, that provide psychiatric information and training for general practitioners. The training was offered through case conferences at the Los Angeles County General Hospital, regional workshops, and two-day intensive case seminars. Three levels of courses were offered. The basic psychiatry course was designed to provide the physician with primary skills, especially careful observation and accurate description of patients and their behavior, and cognitive information regarding psychiatric symptoms. Intermediate-level courses were designed to provide skills through actual practice and observation. The advanced courses enabled the physicians to learn psychotherapy in a medical setting. Brief psychotherapy techniques to be used at irregular intervals were taught, as well as the proper use of psychoactive medication.

Two major research projects were conducted concurrent with the training program. One project studied the characteristics and the interests of the physicians enrolled in the program. Physicians enrolled in this training series were found to be more similar to psychiatrists than physicians who enrolled in general medical continuing-education courses. Their interest was greatest in the areas of office psychotherapy, practical management of less-severe psychiatric disturbances, and psychiatric diagnosis. They were not found to be particularly scholarly.

The second research project was designed to measure the effectiveness of psychiatric case conferences in producing learning. The major goal of the basic psychiatry course was to promote accurate observations of patients and their behavior during unstructured interviews. Participants were not found to make a higher proportion of psychiatric statements about patients following the course, but they were found to make a higher proportion of statements regarding the patient's appearance and behavior and were more in agreement with the instructor regarding statements with psychiatric content.

Information obtained from the research studies is used to modify and improve the courses.

Treusch, J.V., and Grotjahn, M. 1967. Psychiatric family consultations: A practical approach in family practice for the personal physician. *Annals of Internal Medicine* 66:295–300.

This article reports on the experience of a psychiatrist providing consultation within the office and practice of an internist. The advantages of this approach are reported to be:

1. The psychiatrist becomes a part of the continuing relationship between the patient and the physician.
2. The psychiatrist is able to step in with a brief comment or question and then step out without disturbing the ongoing relationship.
3. Consulations are arranged with ease and without the usual resistance by the patient toward being sent to a psychiatrist.
4. The patient gains a direct understanding of the relationship between medical problems and emotional problems.
5. An increased awareness of the significance of family interaction in psychiatric conditions which were likely to be presented in the internist's office was gained.
6. The flow of conversation and sense of relaxation was continued when the psychiatrist entered the interaction between the patient and/or family and the physician, thus allowing for more spontaneity and development of the theme of the consultation.
7. The internist remains as a witness to the consultation, thus providing the physician with more understanding and information than would be gained from a more traditional consultation.

This model of consultation results in a practical postgraduate course in psychiatry for the internist and in internal medicine for the psychiatrist. It increases the diagnostic skill of each and reinforces the understanding of the relationship between medical and emotional problems.

Lipowski, Z.J. 1967. Review of consultation psychiatry and psychosomatic medicine. I. General principles. *Psychosomatic Medicine* 29:153–171.

Lipowski reviews the scope and functions of consultation psychiatry within a general hospital setting. He defines the scope of consultation psychiatry as including those areas of clinical psychiatry that relate to all of the diagnostic, therapeutic, teaching, and research activities of psychiatrists in the nonpsychiatric parts of a general hospital and uses the terms "liaison" and "consultation" psychiatry interchangeably. Consultation psychiatry is generally concerned with the psychological aspects of illness and medical practice within the general hospital.

Information regarding the number of liaison services within North America is lacking. Lipowski feels that consultation staff members should function as a team and share experiences through weekly staff conferences. Additionally, each consultant should be a part of the medical team in the department to which he or she is assigned.

The consultant should be readily available to the medical team and thoroughly familiar with its members. The success of the consultant depends on the degree to which the consultant proves to be useful to the medical team. The consultant should be available when needed, communicate adequately with all concerned, and follow up with the team and/or patient as appropriate. He or she should not only be competent in the fields of psychodynamics and psychopathology, but also have a sound knowledge of general medicine and the specialty to which he or she is assigned. Additionally, the consultant should possess personal qualities that allow him or her to be an acceptable member of the team.

Consultation is the main focus of liaison psychiatry. This may be either client-centered consultation or consultee-centered consultation. In both, the consultant must consider the social milieu of the hospital in relation to the consultation question.

Consultation is viewed as a process with three primary elements: receipt of a request for consultation; gathering of information; and the communication of the consultant's findings, opinions, and advice. The main functions of consultation are diagnosing, advising in patient management, therapy, resolving conflict within the medical team, and teaching. It can be conceptualized as a branch of preventive psychiatry and as the practice and teaching of psychosomatic medicine.

Lipowski, Z.J. 1967. Review of consultation psychiatry and psychosomatic medicine. II. Clinical aspects. *Psychosomatic Medicine* 29:201–224.

Lipowski reviews the types of diagnostic and management problems presented to the consultation psychiatrist in the nonpsychiatric areas of a general hospital. Data regarding the prevalence of psychiatric illness among medical patients is reported to be limited and inconclusive. Generally it is felt that depression is the most common reason for referral to a psychiatric consultant. There is a significantly low number of referrals of psychosomatic patients.

The primary reasons for referral are: diagnostic uncertainty on the part of the physician and a need for advice regarding patient management. The patients referred can be grouped as presenting the following symptoms:

1. psychological presentation of organic disease;
2. psychological complications of organic disease;
3. psychological reactions to organic disease;
4. somatic presentation of psychiatric disorders; and
5. psychosomatic disorders.

Up to one half of all requests for consultation are for management problems. The most common problems are:

1. suicidal attempt or threat;
2. grossly disturbed behavior;
3. excessive emotional reactions;
4. refusal to cooperate;
5. delayed convalescence;
6. conflict between patient and personnel;
7. patient with psychiatric history;
8. psychiatric side effects of drugs;
9. selection and/or preparation of patients; and
10. disposition.

The consultant's role is widening and there is an increasing opportunity to show, through consultation, the important interaction between organic and psychogenic factors in health and illness.

Lipowski, Z.J. 1968. Review of consultation psychiatry and psychosomatic medicine. III. Theoretical issues. *Psychosomatic Medicine* 30:395–422.

Lipowski points out the difficulties and disenchantment within medicine and psychiatry with the concept of psychosomatic medicine. He states that the task of psychosomatic medicine is the attempt to integrate the biological, psychological, and social aspects of health and disease. It is seen as more than a set of techniques or an approach; it is a science whose purpose is to formulate hypotheses and to study the relationships between biological, psychological, and social phenomena as they pertain to individuals. It is an approach to the practice of medicine that considers all of these aspects and the consultant's activities should reflect this philosophy. Lipowski expands on these concepts by presenting relevant research and clinical activities of consultation psychiatry.

Schwab, J.J., and Brown, J. 1968. Uses and abuses of psychiatric consultation. *Journal of the American Medical Association* 205:65–68.

Schwab and Brown point out common problems in the use of psychiatric consultation and provide suggestions for proper consultation. They note that consultation should not be a measure of last-resort but should be part of a well-thought-through plan to understand and assist the patient. It may be used when discrepant views are held by the medical team. When making a referral the physician should summarize the results of the medical work-up and give the patient's current medical status. The physician should provide data regarding plans for treatment and indicate how he or she feels about the patient. Referral should be timely. Common abuses of the consultation process by the physician are:

1. the "either/or" question;
2. the social-distance problem;
3. ignoring the nurse's role;
4. inability to evaluate denial;
5. failure to refer the dying patient;
6. incomplete history;
7. inconsistent referral of patients with personality disorders; and
8. not diagnosing an organic brain syndrome.

The psychiatrist can also contribute to poor use of the consultation process. Response should be quick, usually within twenty-four hours. The consultant should become familiar with the patient's history. The response should be concise. It should answer the consultee's question as well as implicit concerns regarding the patient. Facts and data to support the psychiatrist's impression should be given and a plan for treatment and disposition must be presented. The consultant should discuss findings directly with the consultee and clarify who will implement the proposed plan.

Zabarenko, R.N.; Merenstein, J.; and Zabarenko, L. 1971. Teaching psychological medicine in the family practice office. *Journal of the American Medical Association* 218:392–396.

The authors describe an educational experiment in which a psychiatrist and an internist met weekly for one year in the latter's office. The proposal was to emphasize the teaching of disease concepts and to produce changes in the style of the internist's practice. No special selection of patients was done. Rather, the psychiatrist consulted regarding a general sampling of the physician's patient population.

The method consisted of the psychiatrist being present while the physician saw scheduled patients. The psychiatrist observed and then provided consultation to the physician in the corridor. Eventually, the psychiatrist made interventions in the patient's presence. As fewer new patients were seen, consultation occurred following the patient's visit.

The physician found the consultation useful because it allowed a focus upon the total patient without the patient being forced to agree to consciously accept the emotional bases of his or her medical complaints. Additionally, the physician learned to be aware of the clues to the patient's personality, defenses, and probable reactions to stress without the need to communicate this to the patient before the patient was able to accept the information. Rather, the physician was able to make note of this information and use it to plan future patient management.

The psychiatrist felt his role as an impartial observer allowed him to follow the process more readily and to note where it was impeded or deflected. Intervention was always to facilitate the process. Primary teaching principles were: (1) to observe the patient in totality; (2) to help the physician to learn that every patient behavior is an effort to communicate; (3) to pay special attention to the psychopathology of life eras as a guide to the totality of the patient and complaints; and (4) to teach quick recognition of major, but hidden, syndromes.

Two major points were made in summary. The physician who had previously attended teaching seminars finally integrated the concept of not forcing the patient to accept the lack of organic bases for his or her medical complaint. This suggested that insufficient emphasis and support had been given to the learner to integrate techniques of accurate observation with the proper timing within the summarization of clinical material. The psychiatrist noted that he was able to refresh his knowledge of general medicine and to consult on patients not usually brought to psychiatric attention.

Lipowski, Z.J. 1971. Consultation-liaison psychiatry in the general hospital. *Comprehensive Psychiatry* 12:461–465.

Lipowski points to the spread of consultation-liaison psychiatry in the United States, noting that 76 percent of all psychiatric training programs provide instruction in consultation and related skills. He notes that this reflects the current trend toward person-oriented, community, and preventive medicine. The role of the consultant is to act as an interpreter between the medical and psychiatric fields, bringing to his or her work a unified, holistic, or psychosomatic approach to patients. The consultant role is also to mediate between patients and members of the medical team.

Krakowski, A.J. 1972. Doctor-doctor relationship II: Conscious factors influencing the consultation process. *Psychosomatics* 15:158–164.

Krakowski studies the conscious and unconscious motivations that cause physicians to choose medicine as their careers and the relationship between those motivations and the physicians' feelings toward the consultation process. He found that his sample of fifty physicians chose medicine for various reasons. The following are their responses to the question, "Did you perhaps want to

		N
1.	serve others?"	40
2.	achieve independence?"	38
3.	enjoy social status and prestige?"	28
4.	feel omnipotent?"	7
5.	feel omniscient?"	9
6.	make lots of money?"	10

The attitude toward medicine is that twenty-one respondents feel it is a science, four feel it is primarily an art, and twenty-five view medicine as a combination of the two.

The majority of physicians reported that they request consultation to obtain better information about diagnosis and treatment. Professional qualities expected from the consultant are knowledge and competence, thoroughness, common sense, promptness, availability, and humility. Sixteen percent implied a refusal to accept consultation from someone in the same type of practice and specialty as their own. Twenty-two percent were inhibited for fear that the consultant might find something wrong with their management of the patient. The majority of respondents approved of psychiatry as a branch of medicine. However, 20 percent expressed doubts regarding psychiatry, its position as a branch of medicine, and the trustworthiness of its practitioners. Two-thirds of the sample felt uncertain with psychiatric patients either because of lack of knowledge or because of negative feelings. No clear trend was elicited regarding how to make psychiatric consultation more acceptable and useful.

Krakowski, A.J. 1974. Consultation psychiatry, present global status. A survey. *Psychotherapy and Psychosomatics* 23:78–86.

Krakowski reports on a global survey which he conducted to learn the status of psychiatric consultation services. Generally the supply of psychiatrists is inadequate and unevenly distributed throughout the world. The frequency of requests for service was uniformly low. The prime reason for requests was usually an emergency situation. Requests for diagnostic consultation occur only in countries where satisfactory services are available. Consultation services are generally inadequate and not fully recognized as indicated by the low rate of referrals. A well-organized consultation service staffed by specially trained staff is preferable to one based on the rotation of staff.

Lipowski, Z.J. 1974. Consultation-liaison psychiatry: An overview. *American Journal of Psychiatry* 131:623–630.

Lipowski reviews the history and status of consultation-liaison psychiatry. He defines its scope as the clinical, teaching, and research activities of the psychiatrist in nonpsychiatric areas of the general hospital. He notes that its activities are spreading beyond the hospital walls into all types of health-care facilities.

Lipowski distinguishes between consultation and liaison activities. Consultation refers to the provision of expert diagnostic opinion and advice on patient management at the request of another professional, whereas liaison connotes a linking up of groups for the purpose of effective collaboration.

Consultation-liaison psychiatry represents the application of the psychosomatic approach to clinical work. Lipowski feels the liaison psychiatrist is one of the few health professionals with training broad enough to be able to integrate the diverse data relevant to comprehensive evaluation and management of patients. The consultation team should be an administrative unit composed of psychiatrists, liaison nurses, social workers, and psychologists. His opinion is that the administrative head should be a psychiatrist who has equal standing with other physicians. The team members should be assigned to specific parts of the hospital to allow them to become acquainted with the staff and develop a special interest in and a knowledge of that area of medicine. The functions of the consultation staff are clinical work, teaching, and clinical research.

Lipowski sees the integration of comprehensive health care as the area in which the psychiatrist's future lies. He recommends solid training in medicine and expert knowledge about people and the essential interaction of mind and body. As other professionals provide more of the therapeutic work, the liaison psychiatrist will provide complementary services.

Martin, M.J. 1975. The role of psychiatric consultation in psychosomatic medicine. *Psychosomatics* 16:7-11.

Martin presents a general schema for performing a psychiatric consultation and then describes the variety of patients often seen in psychiatric consultation. These patients are often admitted to a medical service for diagnosis of symptoms which are found to be solely or primarily psychosomatic in origin. However, the consultant must always be alert for hidden organic problems and aware that all medical difficulties have emotional components. Martin presents a chart of medical syndromes which can present first with psychiatric symptoms.

The consultant must be alert to the dynamics of the referral. The physician may be requesting service because of pressure from other health-team members. It may occur because the physician is no longer able to cope with the problems of the patient. It may also reflect personal needs of the physician.

The consultation should be conducted in a relaxed manner and in a quiet place. The consultant should plan to review the patient's record, talk with the referring physician, and then interview the patient. A short note should be written. The consultant should include a review of longitudinal history as well as consider the life situation of the patient when the symptoms began presenting. The consultant should provide a diagnosis both because the recommendations will be clearer and because of the value most physicians place on diagnosis. Recommendations must be based on data. Therapeutic recommendations should be specific and practical.

Krakowski, A.J. 1975. Consultation-liaison psychiatry: A psychosomatic service in a general hospital. *International Journal of Psychiatry in Medicine* 6:283-292.

Krakowski reviews the role and functions of the consultation-liaison psychiatrist in a general hospital. The consultation psychiatrist interprets the psychosocial aspects of illness and correlates them with the biological-medical aspects. He or she functions in diagnostic, therapeutic, instructional, and research activities. Reasons for resistance to a psychiatric consultation include the attitude of society toward mental illness and the stigma attached to it. Frequently the referral to the psychiatrist is seen by the physician as an admission of failure. He or she may also doubt the value of the consultation and this attitude may also be seen in the patient. The consultant must be careful to provide prompt and competent service in a manner acceptable and useful to the health-team members.

Houpt, J.L.; Weinstein, H.M.; and Russell, M.L. 1976-1977. The application of competency-based education to consultation-liaison psychiatry: I. Data gathering and case formulation. *International Journal of Psychiatry in Medicine* 7:295-307.

Houpt, J.L.; Weinstein, H.M.; and Russell, M.L. 1976–1977. The application of competency-based education to consultation-liaison psychiatry: II. Intervention knowledge and skills. *International Journal of Psychiatry in Medicine* 7:309–320.

Russell, M.L.; Weinstein, H.M.; and Houpt, J.L. 1976–1977. The application of competency-based education to consultation-liaison psychiatry: III. Implications. *International Journal of Psychiatry in Medicine* 7: 321–328.

These three articles outline a competency-based model of training for consultation-liaison psychiatry. Clear, objective goals of what knowledge is expected of the psychiatry resident have been formulated and presented. This allows the resident greater flexibility in terms of how and where he or she is able to gain training. It also allows for better supervision and evaluation as both the resident and his or her supervisors have a clear understanding of what material, experience, and knowledge the resident is to have mastered.

Schniewind, H.E. 1976–1977. A psychiatrist's experience in a primary health care setting. *International Journal of Psychiatry in Medicine* 7: 229–240.

Schniewind reports on his personal experience of working primarily within a primary health-care setting. He emphasizes the importance of administrative support for the psychiatrist and of the psychiatrist being readily available and visible to health-care-team members. The psychiatrist must work toward building an appropriate relationship with the physicians and nurses in order for them to value his or her services and make appropriate referrals. Realistic expectation building is also a part of this process. The psychiatrist must also work to build a satisfactory relationship with other mental-health workers. Schniewind feels this is a satisfactory experience because patients are felt to be more accepting of the psychological aspects of their illness when the psychiatrist is a part of the primary medical-care setting.

Wise, T.N. 1977. What to expect from a psychiatric consultant. *Primary Care* 4:661–668.

Wise presents three major reasons to consult with a psychiatrist:

1. to clarify a confusing diagnosis;
2. for assistance in explanation and management of difficult psychological symptoms;
3. to clarify specific reaction to physical disease.

He presents case examples of each of these types of referrals. Further, he advises the physician on how to make a referral. Wise advises that the physician should expect personal contact from the psychiatrist regarding the patient and communication that is understandable. Management suggestions should be practical and sensible.

The Role of the Psychologist as a Health Professional

Wright, L. 1967. The pediatric psychologist: A role model. *American Psychologist* 22:323–325.

Wright discusses the emerging role of the psychologist within a medical setting. He notes that there are significant differences between treating patients in a psychiatric setting and in one where the patients do not have significant problems of mental illness. Wright recommends that the pediatric psychologist be well trained in both child development and clinical child psychology. The majority of referrals are for developmental/cognitive appraisals, questions of child rearing, especially behavioral problems, and information regarding normal growth and development. Wright recommends that beyond a competency in these areas, the pediatric psychologist should also have a disposition toward economy and the applied science. He hopes that knowledge will be extended in these areas through practice, but feels that research per se will follow a clearer delineation of the role. Wright sees three trends that need to be established in the future: (1) delineation of the role of the pediatric psychologist, (2) more specific training for psychologists in this area, and (3) an extension of knowledge in pediatric psychology. He especially recommends the establishment of internship training in pediatric psychology.

Schofield, W. 1969. The role of psychology in the delivery of health services. *American Psychologist* 24(6):565–584.

Schofield reviews and discusses the role of psychologists as health practitioners in the areas of maintaining health as well as preventing and treating illness. Within his formulation, Schofield views health as a generic term, subsuming mental health. Due to its study, prevention and treatment of nonhealth (for example, mental illness), psychology is viewed as both a health and a life science. Psychologists contribute to health through direct and indirect contact with individuals, through teaching, training, and consultation. Schofield sees expanding opportunities for psychologists in the study of physical illness and the psychological concomitants of both the disease and the conditions of patients. He recommends a need for a different kind of psychologist, trained in the scientist-clinician tradition, but with specialized knowledge of physical illness. Schofield feels that psychologists need to turn from their almost-solitary interest in psychiatric problems to these other areas in order to become fully functioning health practitioners.

Barlow, D.H. 1974. Psychologists in the emergency room. *Professional Psychology* 5(3):251–256.

Barlow reports on the experiences of psychology interns at the University of Mississippi Medical Center who were placed in rotation with psychiatric residents on call to the emergency room twenty-four hours a day, seven days a week. The interns were responsible for patients from admission to discharge. When called, the intern reported to the emergency room, checked the patient's chart and was briefed by the medical intern on duty. The psychology intern then interviewed the patient, formulated the problem presented, and made a disposition, which included writing nonmedical orders, working with families and various agencies, and initiating the recommended intervention. Initial difficulties included anxiety on the part of interns, which was replaced with increasing confidence within five to six months. Interns felt that the positive aspects of the program included the opportunity to see a wide variety of patients in acute distress, the necessity for making rapid assessments and formulations, and the opportunity to use various intervention strategies under stressful circumstances. Another result of the experience is the heightened respect for psychologists by non-psychiatric medical personnel.

Saunders, T.R. 1975. Toward a distinctive role for the psychologist in neurodiagnostic decision making. *Professional Psychology* 6:161–166.

Saunders reviews the literature regarding the usefulness and accuracy of neuropsychological techniques. He notes that psychological procedures are frequently more standardized, produce more meaningful quantifiable data, and provide more understanding of brain-behavior relationships than traditional neurological techniques. Saunders points out that neurologists most frequently ask psychologists to distinguish between organic and functional illness. However, as Lipowski has previously noted, there are five possible ways in which physical and psychological factors can interact. These include: (1) psychological presentation of a physical disorder, (2) psychological complication of an organic illness, (3) psychological reaction to a physical illness, (4) somatic presentation of a psychological disorder, and (5) true psychosomatic conditions. Thus, the distinction between functional and organic illness is viewed as a simplistic one, probably not truly possible to make on an absolute basis. Saunders goes on to review the accuracy with which organic conditions can be inferred from neuropsychological data and to note the less-intrusive nature of psychological versus neurological assessment procedures.

Schofield, W. 1975. The psychologist as a health care professional. *Intellect* 255:258.

Schofield looks ahead to the likelihood that the 94th Congress will vote for some type of comprehensive health-care insurance for all citizens. He pre-

dicts that this will allow a unique opportunity to establish a truly innovative health-care-delivery system, especially if it includes services for the
mental or emotional component of the individual's health. Schofield
reviews the efforts of psychologists to present themselves as legitimate
health-care professionals and notes that psychologists have traditionally
been trained to recognize the interactive effect of physical and psychological difficulties. In contrast, the medical community has yet to have successfully trained physicians who recognize that all illness is psychosomatic and
somatopsychic although recent efforts have been made to integrate the
behavioral sciences into the medical curriculum. Schofield reviews the
growing acceptance of psychologists by state legislatures and insurance
companies. He notes that APA has established a Task Force on Health
Research and sees psychology's expansion into research in the health-
illness domain as a way to facilitate the acceptance of more holistic practice
and philosophy.

Schofield, W. 1976. The psychologist as a health professional. *Professional
Psychology* 7:5–8.

Schofield discusses the role of the psychologist within a health maintenance organization. He states that psychologists have traditionally been
associated only with clinical psychology, psychiatry, and mental illness. In
order for psychologists to play a functional role as health professionals
they must reexamine their interests and roles in clinical and research areas.
Schofield notes that a comprehensive collection of care components does
not guarantee comprehensive care. All diseases are psychologically stressful to some degree and psychologists must begin to examine how best to
provide services and educate others to respond to the patient in a comprehensive manner. Several research examples are given.

Wiggins, Jack G. 1976. The psychologist as a health professional in the
health maintenance organization. *Professional Psychology* 7:9–13.

Wiggins discusses the growth of the health maintenance organization
movement nationally and states that the biggest danger to psychologists is
that health maintenance organizations (HMOs) will be run within the
structure of the traditional medical model. He calls for psychologists to
demonstrate their usefulness as health professionals by forming local
panels of psychologists interested in health care and its psychological concomitants and to provide for strong legislative advocacy. Wiggins
expresses concern that unlicensed persons may be hired to perform professional functions within HMOs and argues for clinical psychologists to set
professional standards. Clinical psychologists are defined as health professionals within the HMO legislation, but need to work with medical personnel and state lawmakers to define their role within health-care systems.
Additionally, Wiggins advocates broadened definitions of clinical psychology and mental health to include interest in all conditions that have psychological aspects which could have an adverse effect upon the health of
the individual.

APA Task Force on Health Research. 1976. Contributions of psychology to health research: Patterns, problems, and potentials. *American Psychologist* 31(4):263–274.

The Task Force reviews the role of psychologists within the health-care-delivery system. It begins with the assumption that one's health is paramount to the achievement of other goals and values. In reviewing the status of health care, it notes that the health-care industry is the single largest service industry in the United States, but that it cannot be viewed as an integrated system. Research shows that many people do not have adequate access to basic health-care services and that health, or the lack of it, is related to socioeconomic factors. The Task Force acknowledges that the presence of psychological factors in illness is generally accepted on a philosophical level, but is frequently not dealt with in the actual practice of medicine. Also, as health-care-delivery systems are developing emphasis is being given to the prevention of illness and to health maintenance. Psychologists have been slow to become involved in health-care issues, but because of their training and research background, they can play an essential role in investigating such issues as what motivates health-related behavior, what are the psychological dimensions of persons who follow through with treatment recommendations, and what are the most productive methods of rehabilitation. They call for psychologists to take a more active interest in health-care areas and the need for the APA to provide a "suitable home" for them within the organization.

Drotar, D. 1977. Clinical psychological practice in a pediatric hospital. *Professional Psychology* 8(1):72–80.

Drotar reports on the pediatric psychology program at the Case Western Reserve University School of Medicine. Over a three-year period 528 hospitalized patients were referred to pediatric psychologists out of 20,320 hospital admissions. More than 40 percent of these were five years old or younger and nearly one half concerned questions of intellectual development. Other referrals concerned questions of psychological adaptation to chronic physical disease or handicap, evaluation of behavior problems, and management of psychological crises. Drotar notes that the time pressures of an acute hospital setting require rapid assessment and screening by the pediatric psychologist. Initial referrals were made primarily by physicians in training, with the medical school faculty's acceptance following eventually. Pediatric psychological services have been directed initially toward problems with a high level of physician interest. Services have included assessment, consultation with the medical team, and psychotherapeutic intervention.

Lothstein, L.M. 1977. Role of the clinical psychiatrist and psychologist in primary care medicine. *Primary Care* 4:343–354.

Lothstein discusses the appropriate use of psychiatric and psychological consultation by the primary-care physician and outlines different types of

consultation models. He reviews the educational backgrounds of each profession and the types of services typically within their purview. Lothstein
concludes by giving suggestions regarding when psychiatrists and/or psychologists should be involved in primary-care medicine and gives suggestions for making a successful referral.

Budman, S.H., and Del Gaudio, A.C. 1979. A survey of psychologists at
health maintenance organizations and community mental health centers. *Professional Psychology* 10:244–248.

Budman and Del Gaudio compare the activities of psychologists within
HMOs and traditional community-mental-health centers. They have found
that psychologists in HMOs are involved in the provision of direct clinical
services to a greater degree than psychologists in community-mental-health
settings. Inservice training and supervisory activities are less emphasized
within HMOs. Relatively little research is done in either setting. Com-
munity-mental-health-center psychologists are more likely to be involved
in administrative activities. HMO psychologists provide significantly more
individual psychotherapeutic services while community-mental-health-
center psychologists see more patients in group therapy. Almost one half
of the HMOs responding to the survey had no psychologists on staff.

**The Training and Practice of Psychology in Medical
Settings**

Routh, D.K. 1970. Psychological training in medical school departments of
pediatrics: A survey. *Professional Psychology* 1:469–472.

Routh surveyed 100 medical schools to determine what types of training
were available for psychology students. He found that the majority of
medical schools have at least one psychologist affiliated with their pediatric
service and that fifty-two schools are participating in some type of pediatric psychology training. The four basic areas of training are developmental, clinical, developmental clinical, and psychological pediatrics.
Seventeen schools reported that psychologists in their schools are involved
in teaching the medical curriculum.

Fischer, H.L., and Engeln, R.G. 1972. How goes the marriage? *Professional Psychology* 3(1):73–79.

Fischer and Engeln review the development of collaborative efforts
between psychologists and pediatricians, and describe their experiences in a
large pediatric outpatient practice using a psychology trainee to provide
consultation to physicians. The psychologists were available to patients

during a two-hour time period each week and they met with the physicians in the practice for one hour every other week. This conference provided for feedback to the physicians and time for discussions on a general level. Typically, referrals to the psychologists occurred also at this meeting. Over the course of one year the psychologists saw twenty-two patients, the majority of whom were male. Two major issues that arose were the method and amount of payment for the psychologist, and training for the physician in the role and professional capabilities of psychologist. The trainees felt that the experience allowed them to broaden their experience and to be able to form a professional identity.

Hafner, A.J. 1973. Innovations in clinical psychology internship training. *Professional Psychology* 4(1):111–118.

Hafner reviews a survey of 541 internship training centers regarding the types of training given to psychology interns. The major areas of emphasis are diagnostics, psychotherapy, and consultation to other professionals. Some centers provide training experiences in supervision and administration; research activities are limited. Some of the innovative training experiences are working as a psychiatric technician, living on the ward with patients for five days a week, and working as a child-care worker.

Wexler, M. 1976. The behavioral sciences in medical education: A view from psychology. *American Psychologist* 31(4):275–283.

Wexler reviews the history of the body-mind dichotomy within medical services and education. He notes that the study of human behavior within medicine was initially introduced through the discipline of psychiatry and that it has not been accepted without a struggle. Wexler feels that this struggle continues because the behavioral sciences have not provided physicians with specific skills which can be applied to specific problems. Curriculum development has occurred without a clear study and recognition of final goals. Wexler recommends that behavioral scientists determine what information is basic and necessary for physicians to know. Then medical curricula can be designed to meet the needs of these areas without overloading the curriculum.

Blanchard, C.G., and Barlow, D.H. 1976. Psychologists and psychiatrists in a department of psychiatry. *Professional Psychology* 7(3):331–338.

Blanchard and Barlow review the results of the 1972 APA Committee on Psychology in Medical Schools. Those findings indicated that psychologists were primarily involved in teaching and research, with many also providing clinical service. One of the disadvantages cited by the group surveyed was the difficulty in obtaining an effective and respected position within a department established for another profession. The APA Committee recommended that psychology either be given the status of a separate department or that psychology become an autonomous unit within a department of behavioral sciences. Blanchard and Barlow report on the program at the University of Mississippi Medical Center in which the object of the program was to test the limits of the abilities of a psychologist within a psychiatric setting. This was accomplished primarily through the establishment of an internship program. Patients admitted to the inpatient service were assigned randomly to psychiatric residents and psychology interns, with interns assuming full responsibility for patient assessment and the designing of the treatment program. Interns took turns with psychiatric residents on the emergency rotation schedule. Requests for consultation to medical units were also assigned to both groups. In evaluating the program, psychiatric faculty pointed to the differences in role responsibilities and functions, emphasizing the psychiatrist's medical education. Psychologists, however, saw less role differentiation. Psychology interns felt themselves to be better trained for their internship. Residents felt that psychology interns were not adequately clinically oriented and that they had not developed a full sense of patient responsibility. Both trainee groups expressed concern regarding the development of professional identification and role models. Conflict between the two groups was usually resolved as they became better acquainted.

Matarazzo, J.D.; Lubin, B.; and Nathan, R.G. 1978. Psychologists' membership on the medical staff of university teaching hospitals. *American Psychologist* 33(1):23-29.

Psychologists from 115 schools of medicine were surveyed to determine their faculty status following the 1974 JACH accreditation reviews. From 1952 until 1972, psychologists who worked within medical-school settings indicated that they were fully functioning members of the medical staffs and that many were full voting members. However, beginning in 1974 JACH began to note the fact that psychologists had been written into the bylaws of medical schools as potential full staff as a deficiency. In July 1976, APA filed formal suit with the Federal Trade Commission questioning those actions. The current survey indicates that between February 1976 and January 1977 significantly fewer psychologists were accorded full membership status within medical schools. Of the forty-two psychologists earlier reporting full status, only six retained that status. The number of psychologists who indicated that they held special membership status increased from three to thirty-one. The authors encourage the membership of psychologists on medical-school faculties in the interest of the profession and of the public.

Index

Abbott, M.A., 262
Abnormal psychology, 65
Abortion, habitual spontaneous and
    therapeutic, 205, 208, 325, 380
Abram, H.S., 287
Abroms, G.M., 82
Absenteeism, problem of, 231
Abstinence, 243, 250-251, 262
Abuse: alcohol, 242-244, 299; child, 149;
    drug, 97-98, 340; insurance coverage, 9;
    polydrug, 247; substance, 140, 157;
    verbal, 99
Academy of Behavioral Medicine Research,
    161
"Acceptance," feeling of, 129, 132
Accreditation of the Education and Training
    Board, Committee on, 5-6
Acculturation, impact of, 213-215, 360
Acetaminophen, 36
Achievement, striving for, 44
Acupuncture, practice of, 314, 370
Acute myllogenous leukemia (AML), 409,
    413
Adair, J., 353, 360
Adams, R.N., 360
Administration and administrative concerns,
    234-235; on aging, 220; emergency-room,
    100; hospital, 418
Adolescents, 134, 136, 195; handicapped,
    135; psychiatry for, 6; sexuality of, 135,
    256, 293-294, 320-321
Adult: disability, 7; psychiatry, 6; sexuality,
    322
Affection, demonstrations of, 149
Aftercare, need for, 106
Agencies: social-service, 107, 297, 306;
    traditional, 297
Aggression, passive, 157
Aging and age: administration of, 220;
    attitudes on, 213; the elderly, 212, 217,
    222, 298-299, 367; gay men and lesbians,
    307-308; groups, 6; homes for, 218-219;
    of immigrants, 369; of intercourse, 318;
    and masturbation, 318; myths on, 213; of
    parents, 217; of patients, 197; premature,
    193; problems of, 9, 43, 82, 94, 262, 302,
    326; and sexuality, 256, 294-295,
    321-322; study of, 211
Agism: attitudes and eradicating, 211-225
Agle, D.P., 144, 146, 156
Agras, Stewart, 139, 160
Aides, need for, 325
Alcohol, 64, 72, 157, 233; abuse of, 242-244,
    299; and drugs, 248-249; interviewing on,
    241-251; problems with 241-251
Alcoholics Anonymous (AA), 242, 250, 309
Alcoholism and alcoholics, chronic, 57, 97,
    214, 340
Alfert, E., 49
Allport, G.W., 299
Ambulatory patients, 62; care of, 86, 103
Amebiasis, 297, 305
American Board of Family Practice, 28
American Cancer Society, 383
American College of Physicians, 242
American Historical Association, 366
American Hospital Association, 242
American Medical Association (AMA), 242,
    244, 383
American Psychiatric Association, 242
American Psychological Association, 5-6, 8
Ames, Louise Bate, 106
Amish people, 349
Amniocentesis, 207
Amputations, trauma of, 287
Anal sex, 259
Analgesic medication and usage, 36, 45, 57,
    61, 89-90, 144, 157
Ancestral spirits, 351
Anderson, C., 257, 259
Andrew, J.M., 45
Anger: issue of, 14, 62-63, 97-98, 117, 129,
    133-134, 268, 305, 331, 333; repressed,
    340
Angiogram, need for, 397-398
Angleitner, A., 215
Anglo culture, 365
Annon, J.S., 258-259, 261, 264
Anonymity, protection of, 108
Anorexia nervosa, 139
Anthropology and anthropologists, 323
Antidepressant medication, 182
Antihypertensive therapy, 36, 262
Anxiety: arousing of, 277; attacks of, 309; of
    castration, 268; defenses against, 235;
    factor of, 49, 63, 70, 85, 94, 116, 119,
    156, 187, 198, 214, 246, 266, 396; mastery
    of, 124; neurotic, 60; parental, 125;
    performance, 258-259; reduction
    techniques, 170-171, 176; sexual, 263
Applied social sciences, 1
Arizona, 339
Arnold-Chiari Malformation, 394-396
Arthritis: condition of, 144-148, 287; in
    joints, 157; rheumatoid, 177
Asian-American: background of, 365-367

Asians, 323; female modesty, 372-373; immigration of, 366-367, 370; infant mortality, 373; pregnancy and childbirth, 373
Assault, physical and sexual, 298, 308
Assertiveness, development of, 143, 156, 159
Assessment, 8, 95-96, 141; methods of, 59-60; psychological, 5, 100; techniques, 22
Asthma, attacks of, 142
Attitudes, 237; on aging, 211-225; cultural, 224; family, 199; homosexual, 303-305; Indian, on illness, 349; moral, 313; of nurses, 40; professional, 60, 216, 303-305; racial, 325, 334; sexual, 318; sibling, 318; social, 334; societal, 313
Authoritarianism, paternal, 342
Authority: factor of, 328-329, 352; "lover," 316-317; parental, 342
Autogenic training, 156, 171
Automatic stress, 230-233
Autonomic nervous system instability, 197
Autonomy, 225; loss of, 14; self-, 344; sense of, 218; surrender of, 135; threat to, 21
Avoiders, philosophy of, 45
Awareness, level of, 57

Bacteriology and bacteriologists, 1
Bahnson, C.B. and M.B., 116
Bahr, D.M., 353
Bandura, A., 120, 251
Barbach, L.G., 261, 265, 274-276
Barlow, G.H., and Barlow, D., 17-18, 22, 139, 160
Barnes, A.B., and Barnes, M.R., 142-143, 205
Barsky, A.J., 74
Bashshur, R., 361
Bean, L.J., 361
Beatty, J., 142
Bedside manner, importance, of, 1-2, 379
Beecher, Henry K., 170
Behavior: adaptive, 47; child, 103, 143-145; coronary-prone, 44; cultural, 40; deviant, 131; dysfunctional, 106; focus on, 140-141; human, 40, 43-44, 105; interactional bases of, 118-119; interpersonal, 45; maladaptive, 42, 47-48, 55; neurotic, 64; oppositional, 118; pathological, 60; rational, 109-111; social, 40, 131; therapy, 124, 139, 160; training, 109-111
Behavior Therapy and Health Care (Katz and Zlutnick), 160
Behavioral: data, 33; management, 59, 178-182; medicine, 30, 56; perspective, 169-182; psychology, 56, 139; science, 2, 28-29, 41, 49, 105, 113, 115, 124

Behavioral Medicine Research, Academy of, 161
Bellack, A.S., 141
Benadryl, 395
Benson, H., 143, 156, 187, 192, 194
Bereavement. See Loss, concept and issue of
Berger, M.M., 68
Bergler, Edmund, 313
Bernal, G.A., 147
Bernstein, D.A., 49, 204
Bibring, G.L., 72
Bieber, I., 268, 298, 300-301
Bigelow, G., 160
Biggs, M., 287
Binder, C., 301
Biochemistry and biochemists, 26, 47, 169
Biofeedback procedures, 49, 59, 82, 142, 146-147, 171, 181, 330
Biological sciences, 1
Biology and biologists, 21, 25, 30, 55, 60, 332
Biomeasurable symptoms, 140
Biopsy, need for, 386
Biopsychosocial orientation, 3, 40, 52, 57
Biosocial activities, 2
Bird, B.L., 141-142
Birk, L., 139
Birrer, Cynthia, 377, 391-406
Birth control, techniques of, 192, 205, 306, 325
Birthing and births, problem of, 206-207. See also Childbirth
Bisexuality, problem of, 302, 319
Bjornsson, S., 124
Black, R.G., 147
Black ethnic group: discrimination against, 299, 334; family compactness, 327-329; health care of, 323-337; social survival of, 327
Blanchard, E.B., 146
Blank, J., 261
Blood: clotting disorders, 144-145; pressure, 65, 231, 249; transfusions, 117
Boke of Chyldren, The, 103
Bone cancer, 7; transplant procedures, 422
Bonica, J.J., 169, 177
Bonn, University of, 215
Boone, D.C., 145, 157
Borkovec, T.D., 49
Bornstein, P., 159
Bower, S.A., and Bower, G.H., 143, 156
Bowers, J., 369
Boyer, J., 142
Brain syndrome, chronic, 42-43
Breast: cancers, 190, 379-381; development, 195, 271; feeding, 203, 380
Breath testers, use of, 248
Breslow, L., 142
Brockway, Jo Ann, 57, 169-182

Bross, M.G., 356, 361
Brown, M.M., 45, 142
Buddhism, philosophy of, 370
Budgets, 341; cuts in, 236; management of, 223
Bureaucracy: hospital, 85, 121; medical, 379, 382, 385–386, 388; staff setting, 358, 417
Burnap, D.W., 263, 284
Burnout, incidence of, 229–233, 236, 239
Butler, Robert N., 213, 215, 218–219, 262

Caesarian sections, 206
Cahalan, D., 244
Calhoun, G., 285
California, 107, 339, 366; University of, 272
Canada, 355
Cancer: bone, 7; breast, 190, 379–381; cervical, 306; detection of, 142, 383; impact of, 18–20, 113–115, 124, 177; in Japanese-Americans, 367–368; terminal, 409–424; treatment for, 293–294. *See also* Acute myllogenous leukemia (AML)
Caplan, G., 71, 94
Cardiac: arrythmias, 142; disease, 287; insufficiency, 65
Cardiovascular: disease, 142, 229, 262, 368; system, 231, 288, 368
Carkhuff, R.R., 48
Carlson, K., 207
Carrillo, Carmen, 339–345
Cartwright, C., 48
Cassata, Donald M., 55, 67–76
Cassell, S., 120
Castelnuovo-Tedesco, P., 76
Castration anxiety, 268
Cataldo, M.F., 139–143, 159
Cedars-Sinai Medical Center, 185
Center for Disease Control, 305
Centers: clinic, 29; community, 116, 197; counseling, 229, 307; crisis, 298, 308
Central nervous system (CNS), 125, 247
Cerebral palsy (CP), 292–293
Cervical cancer, 306
Chan, C., 368–369, 372
Chang, J.K., 372
Chemical-dependency services, 6, 179, 297, 309
Chemotherapeutic agents, 117
Chemotherapy, use of, 293, 385, 387, 412–414, 416, 421–422
Childbirth, 199–200, 380; and Asian pregnancy, 373; natural, 201
Childhood: experiences of, 256, 269–270; and masturbation, 293, 320–321
Childrearing practices, 341–344; and sexuality, 320–321
Children and child's needs; abuse, 149; behavior, 103, 143–145; delivery of, 18;

health services, 7, 139; hospitals for, 106, 113, 116–117; inpatient psychiatric units for, 11; long-term disabilities, 133–134; malignant diseases, 116–118; maternal relationship, 130; parental interpersonal dynamics, 268; personality inventory, 109; physically handicapped, 7, 133; psychology for, 62, 105; psychosocial care, 113; rehabilitation of, 134; self-control skills, 159; sociocultural forces on, 104; welfare of, 63
Chicano ethnic group, 342
Chilgren, R., 262
China and Chinese-Americans, 366–369
CHLA hematology-oncology patient, 120–121
Chrisman, N., 369
Christmas disease, 144
Christian influence and the church, 327, 350–352
Chronic: alcoholics, 57, 97, 214, 340; brain syndrome, 42–43; disability, 129–137; diseases and illnesses, 9, 51, 56, 70, 141–145, 285–287, 354, 406; fatigue, 229–230; pain, 7, 146–157, 169, 174–175, 178–182; stress, 230–231, 239
Cigarette smoking, effects of, 64–65, 141, 246
Cisin, I., 244
Citizens' Commission on Graduate Education, 27
Civil Rights, Commission on, 367; and gays, 298, 308
Classical: conditioning, 44; psychoanalysis, 267
Clerical supervisory personnel, 5
Cleveland, Ohio, 222
Clinics and clinicians: behavioral science, 2; centers, 29; counseling, 123, 236; experience, 13–20; family practice, 11–13; free, 236; guidance, 108; health-care, 13–20, 233; need for, 6, 56, 143, 335, 348; neuropsychological, 6–7; observations by, 50; and pain, 170, 172; psychiatrical, 6–8; psychological, 5–6, 9, 13–20, 22, 41, 59–65, 233; sex, 272–273
Clitoris: size, 260; stimulation, 261, 269
Codeine, use of, 36
Cognitive behavior-modification (CBM) processes, 100, 284
Cohen, Barry T., 283–295
Cohen, William S., 216, 255
Cole, T.M., 262
Coleman, E., 300
Colorado, 339
Comatose conditions, 50, 424
Communal living, 218
Communication: barriers, 371–372; doctor

and patient, 79–80; of feelings, 134; gaps
in terminology, 417; sexual, 269–270;
techniques in, 28, 37, 48, 258, 264, 333;
training, 264; value of, 130; verbal and
nonverbal, 271
Community: centers, 116–197; health-care
delivery, 5; hospitals, 11; medicine, 2, 28;
mental health, 64, 116; planning and
planners, 223; psychology, 64
Community Health Service, Bureau of, 139
Compatability, sexual, 194
Competence and competitiveness, 44, 72–73
Complaints: emotional, 387; medical, 100;
patient's, 86; physical, 14, 87, 98, 178;
psychological, 14; psychosomatic, 13;
sexual, 264; somatic, 309
Conditional stimuli (CS), 118
Confidentiality, issue of, 306–307
Confrontation, problems of, 48
Confucianism, philosophy of, 370
Confusion and congruence, 13, 48
Congenital diseases, 208
Conroe, R.M., 28, 76
Conspiracy of silence, 285, 291
Consultation and consultants, medical and
psychological, 5, 7–12, 22, 107–108, 114,
186, 317
Contraceptions, use of, 192, 380–381
Convalescence, period of, 9
Conversion hysteria, 59
Cooper, I.M., 122, 405
Coping: capacity for, 93–94, 119, 130; and
death, 409; degrees of, 90–91, 159;
emotional, 246; and illnesses, 365;
mechanisms, 56, 96, 231; resources,
68–70; styles, 44–45, 359; sexual feelings
toward patients, 315–317
Core information and content, 27, 298–302
Coronary heart disease, 44, 141
Cosmic rules, 347, 351–353
Costs, medical, 325
Cotherapy and cotherapists, 32, 274, 287
Cottrell, H.L., 261
Counseling: centers, 229, 307; marital, 207;
patient, 12, 266; professional, 204, 231;
sessions, 64, 123, 270, 315, 317; sex, 35,
257–278, 313; student, 6; supportive
approach to, 81, 123
Counselors, 29, 106, 314; free clinic, 236;
homosexual, 319; trained, 31
Couple sexual behavior therapy, 270–274
Crane, P.S., 366
Crasilneck, H.B., 122
Creer, T.L., 142
Crewe, N.M., 285
Crisis: intervention centers and techniques,
11, 62–63, 94–97, 100, 298, 308;

maturational, 97; situations and theories,
49, 85
Cross-cultural factors, 323; sex-role
differences, 344; tribal comparisons, 347
Cruikshank, W.M., 106
Cuban American ethnic group, 339
Cullen, S.C., 122
Cultural: attitudes, 224; backgrounds, 91;
barriers, 373; behavior, 40; differences,
323; expectations, 199; factors, 119–120;
groups, 341; habits, 326; influences, 95;
variations, 339, 354
Culture, 366; American, 212, 216; Asian,
371–373; Euroamerican, 347–348,
358–359; Hispanic, 341, 344; Indian, 360;
peasant, 369
Cummings, N.A., 107
Curettage, need for, 193
Curriculum models, 50–52; graduate, 28
Curtin, Sharon R., 219
Curtiss, K.A., 159
Cystic fibrosis, 7

Dabrowski, K., 107
Danaher, K., 406
Dash, J., 122
Data: behavioral, 33; collection, 153, 157;
demographic, 345; psychometric, 125
Davis, M.S., 157, 160
Davison, L., 49
Dean, R., 298
Death: approaching awareness of, 129, 221,
422–424; coping with, 409; issue of dying,
7, 71, 90, 132, 136
Debilitation, 223, 225; emotional, 391
DeCecco, J., 301
Decision-making functions, 74, 192, 202,
328; social, 334
Decompression, periods of, 234
D'Costa, A., 104
Defense mechanisms and defenders, 45, 63
Delivery: health-care, 5, 143–144, 159–160;
labor, 32, 199–203, 207
Delusions, somatic, 59
Dembroski, T.M., 44
Demography, variables of, 299, 345
Denial, factor of, 96
Depression: chronic, 70; factor of, 94,
116–118, 129, 132, 143, 147, 196–197,
246, 309, 314; incapacitating, 47; mood,
156–157; and pain, 182; postmastectomy,
388; respiratory, 34; situational, 134
Deprivation, sensory, 124
Dermatology, conditions of, 142
Desensitization techniques, 122, 156
Despair, factor of, 117, 396
Deterioration, physical, 220

Determinants, biological, 60
Deuschle, K., 353, 360
DeVellis, B.M., 46
Developing continuums (or Clusters) of Care, 222–223
Developmental psychology, 2, 42–43, 62, 104
Deviant behavior, social, 131
Diabetes, 290, 348; Amish, 349; and erectile dysfunction, 261–262
Diabetes mellitus, 287, 368
Diagnostic information and techniques, 12–13, 28, 76, 80–81, 85, 93, 140, 192, 198, 215; of cancer, 142, 383; psychological, 32
Diet and dietary habits, 65, 233, 246
Dietrich, Shelby L., 139, 144
Differential psychology, 9
Dignity: human, 290; personal, 136
Dilation and curettage procedure, 193
Dillehunt, Harold Q., 256, 313–322
Disability: adult, 7; children's, 133–134; chronic, 129–137; learning, 64, 105; long-term, 130, 133–134; orthopedic 146; overcoming, 135; physical, 263, 285, 287; prevention of, 141; problems of, 9, 159, 217, 221, 231, 406
Discrimination: black ethnic group, 299, 334; in education and housing, 329; factor of, 213, 256, 308, 334, 340; job, 125, 329
Disengagement and disorganization, 94–95, 214
Distress: emotional, 68–70, 75–76; 174–175, 221, 318; endoscopic, 49; physical, 79; somatic expression of, 36; status, 68–70; tension-related, 81; treatment-induced, 117–118
Divorce, trauma of, 71
Doctoral programs, 10–11
Doctors, 325, 330, 335; female relationship of, 197–198; patient interaction with, 12–13, 79–80, 192, 256, 316, 379
Donovan, J., 187, 192, 194, 200, 203, 205
Double vision, 392–393, 397
Dreikurs, R., 72
Drugs: abuse of, 97–98, 242, 340; and alcohol, 248–249; antihypertensive, 262; dependency, 64; effectiveness evaluation, 118, 142, 160; industry, 169; interactions, 248, 395; pain killing, 423; prescription, 247; on sexuality, 262; and therapy, 398; and tranquilization, 214; use of, 9, 47, 72, 198, 221, 233, 255, 262
Dualism, 119, 286; trend away from, 1–3
Durability, academic, 31

Eaton, J., 367
Ebersold, M.J., 147

Ecology, human, 60
Economy and economic concerns, 326–327, 368; social, 298, 325, 332
Education and educators, 28, 106, 313–314, 340; accreditation, 5–6; discrimination in, 329; doctoral programs, 10–11; family practice, 28–31; nursing, 39–52; prophylactic, 9; public-health, 64; sex, 255, 278, 318
Egalitarianism, factor of, 358
Egan, G., 80
Egbert, L.D., 170
Egoism and ego development, 134, 63
Einstein, Albert, 26
Eisdorfer, Carl, 215
Eiser, C., 125
Eisler, R.M., 156–157
Ejaculation, 257, 262; premature, 264–266, 268, 318, 381; rapid, 277; retrograde, 294
Elderly persons. See Aging and age
Electrical stimulation, 147
Electrodermal treatments, 146
Electroencephalographic treatments (EEG), 146, 393, 395–397
Electromyographic tests (EMG), 140, 146–147
Ellis, Albert, 109
Embarrassment, trauma of, 187
Emergency: medical services, 85; medicine, 87; room treatment, 12, 15, 17–18, 32, 56, 85–87, 96, 99–100, 298, 308, 317, 333
Emotion and emotional situations: anguish, 294; behavior, 344; complaints, 387; conflicts, 269; coping, 246; debilitation effects of, 391; difficult disorders, 68–70, 75–76, 146, 174–175, 318; etiology, 79, 83; hazards, 94–95; health and family needs, 15–17, 314, 383, 414–416; maturity, 204; normal, 198, 422; pain, 419, 421; problems of, 28, 88, 146, 170, 180, 217; rehabilitation, 399; secondary, 146; stress, 156; supports, 197, 327
Empathy, 48, 80, 185
Emphysema, 287
ENCORE, YMCA sponsored, 389
Endler, N.S., 44, 118
Endoscopy, 45, 49
Enelow, A.J., 68
Engel, B.T., 142
Environment: factor of, 40, 55, 67, 139, 142; Gnotobiotic (germ free), 124; home, 218–219, 422–424; hospital, 149; influence of, 153–156; interest in, 44; physical, 1, 141; problems of, 291; social, 141, 147, 153, 160, 323; and stress, 118–119, 299; work, 229, 239
Epictetus, 110

Epidemics, problem of, 297
Epidemiology and epidemiologists, 9, 140, 159, 297
Epigenesis, concept of, 42
Epileptic seizures, 142
Epstein, L.H. and M.H., 142–143, 147
Equilibrium, state of, 94–96, 131–133
Erectile dysfunction, 257, 261–267, 277
Erection, 272; uncontrollable, 315–316
Erotic stimulation, 271
Ersner-Hershfield, Seth, 57, 241–251
Eskimo, 351
Ethanol, tolerance to, 246
Ethics, factor of, 300–301
Ethnicity and ethnic minority groups, 94, 119–120, 303, 329, 335–336, 339, 365, 373
Ethnocentric stereotypes, 341
Ethnohistory and historians, 349
Etiology: emotional, 79–83; psychogenic, 79–82
Euroamerican: culture, 347–348, 358–359; medicine, 351, 353, 356–357; theories, 352–353, 354
Euthanasia, factor of, 325
Evaluation procedures, 7, 13
Evans, A.E., 125
Evil spirits, factor of, 369
Examination(s): bimanual, 191; gynecological, 21–24, 188–192; medical, 15, 394; mental-status, 67; pelvic, 186, 189–192, 195, 197, 202, 260; physical, 74, 188–192; proctological, 315; self, 260
Excitement, sexual, 268
Exercise: sensual exploration, 274; homework, 270–272, 276–277; sessions, 180–181
Expectations: cultural, 199; societal, 294
Experience: of anguish, 16–17; collaborative teaching, 36; emphasis on, 5; field placement, 9–10; homosexual, 316; internship, 11–22; of pain, 16–17; sexual, 270, 273; training, 6
Experimental psychology, 59, 169
Exploration: sensual, 274; surgical, 117
Expressiveness, factor of, 72
Extrapyramidal dysfunction, 34

Fabrega, H., 147
Failure, trauma of, 62
Fallibility, human, 110
Family, 60, 64, 140–141; adjustment problems, 9; attitudes, 199; black, 327–329; emotional needs, 414–416; extension of, 341, 344–345; income, 328; medical conferences, 21; organizational structure, 2, 28, 371; physician of patient, 2, 12, 27–28, 32, 79, 140–141; planning,

192; premorbid functioning, 119–120; relationships, 70, 233; stability, 125; surrogate, 345; traditional, 327; therapists, 63, 82
Family Practice and Community Health, Department of, 12
Family practice and psychological medicine, 25–37, 284; clinics, 11–23; graduate curricula, 28; interns and residents, 31–33; and rotation, 7–8; and teachers, 30, 32
Fantasies and fantasizing, 122, 259, 316, 318; patient, 380; sexual, 190, 314
Fatherhood, authoritarian, 342
Fatigue, 203, 291, 391, 393; chronic, 229–230, 233; neurotic, 396
Fazaari, Patrick, J., 56, 129–137
Fears and phobias, 139, 198, 201, 309; of hospitalization, 372–373; sexual, 267; of strangers, 88, 93
Fecal incontinence, 142
Federal Council on Aging and the Aged, The, 216, 220, 222
Feedback: factor of, 68–69, 157, 271, 274, 303; visual, 181
Feelings, communication of, 134
Fees, 82
Female: breasts, 271; depression in, 314; and doctor relationship, 197–198; genitals, 189–190, 260–261; Lamaze-trained, 44; modesty in Asia, 372–373; peer group, 388; physically disable, 263; problems, 185; sexuality, 274–275; unmarried, 199, 204, 208
Fenichel, O., 47
Fenwick, R., 305
Field placements, factor of, 9–10
Filipino, 366–367
Fine, H.L., 287
Fink, R., 142
First intercourse, age of, 318
Fisher, Bernard, 385
Fisher, J.C., 79
Flexibility, need for, 215
Flint, M., 196
Fogelson, R.D., 360
Folk medicine, 120
Follette, W., 107
Fordyce, Wilbert E., 143, 147, 149, 153, 169, 172, 178–179, 181
Fowler, G.R., 45
Frank, E., 257, 259
Frank, J.D., 82
Fraumeni, J.F., 368
Free clinics, need for, 236
Freud, Sigmund, 42, 268, 284, 313–314, 320
Friar, L.R., 142

Friedman, J.M., 262
Friends and friendship, 37, 140-141
Frustration: factor of, 2, 62, 88, 98-99, 131, 133, 233, 305; toleration of, 65
Fuchs, M., 361
Fuller, G.D., 49, 146
Funding and financial resources, 6, 367, 371

Gaarder, K.R., 146
Gambrell, E., 263
Gambrill, E.D., 156
Gardner, G.G., 122
Gay Health Guide, The (Rowan and Gillette), 305
Gay men, 256, 297-310; and civil rights, 298, 308; community services, 308; core information on, 298-302; medical information about, 305-307; Minnesota Committee on, 308; older age group, 307-308; as parents, 307; working with, 319-320
Gebhard, P., 259, 299
General Accounting Office (GSO), 222
General practitioners, 25-26, 219.
Genetics, determinants of, 60
Genitals, 190, 195, 271; female, 189-190, 260-261; size and shape of, 260; stimulation of, 291; system of, 288
Gentry, W.D., 147, 160
Geriatrics and gerontology: medicine for, 219; research in, 42; social, 211
Germ-free environment, 124
Geropsychiatry and geropsychiatrists, 213
Gestalt therapy, 82
Ghetto, existance of, 366
Gillette, P., 305
Gillum, R.F., 74
Ginott, Haim, 320-321
Glynn, E.L., 159
Gnotobiotic environment, 124
Goal(s): of intervention, 47; nursing, 45; performance, 272; psychological, 40
Golden, J.S., 262-263, 274-275, 283-285, 287, 291, 295
Goldfarb, A., 262
Goldstein, M.J., and Goldstein, M.K., 45, 142
Gomperts, Edward, 139
Gonorrhea, cases of, 297, 304-306, 348-349
Gonsiorek, John C., 256, 297-310
Goodenough Draw-a-Man test, 109
Goodman, J., 159
Gorden, T., 367
Grachow, F., 368
Graduate schools, 6, 8; family-practice curricula, 28; training programs in, 10, 28
Grants, hospital, 345

Gray, M.J., 197
Green, R., 189
Greenhill, J.P., 187
Grief: acute, 91, 97; burden of, 129-130, 419; expressions of, 61, 63, 89, 136; issue of, 13-14, 214
Group: dynamics, 48; hypnotic-training, 122; therapy, 82, 124, 274, 276
Guamanian ethnic group, 366
Guidance clinics, 108
Guilt: feelings of, 13, 60, 63, 90, 93, 97, 117, 169, 199, 259, 267-268, 351; of patients, 315-316; unnecessary, 263
Gynecology and gynecologists, 57, 185-208, 284, 379; and physical examinations, 21-24, 188-192

Haar, E., 185
Haenszel, W., 368
Hafner, A. Jack, 5-12, 22, 106
Halevy, Jehudah, 1
Half-way houses, 340
Hall, C.S. and J.A., 43, 122
Halpern, L.M., 147, 181
Hamburg, D.A., 142
Hammersmith, M., 301
Handicap, physical, 7, 47, 133, 135
Harris, J., 147
Hatterer, L., 301
Hauck, P.A., 109-110
Hawaii, 366
Hayes, Donald, 404
Headaches, problem of, 231
Healing and healers: approach to, 357-359, 415; indigenous, 356; and organic disorders, 2; and patient relationship, 1; practicing powers of, 354, 369
Health, Education, and Welfare, Department of (HEW), 328, 365-367
Health care: behavior research, 8; clinics, 6, 13-20, 233; community, 5; delivery, 5, 143-144, 159-160; emotional, 314; insurance; maintenance organizations, 9; management, 139; plans, 37; professionals, 56-57; psychology, 1, 5-6, 8, 13-20, 32, 59-60; and sexuality, 314-316
Health Care Psychology, Division of, 8, 11
Health Education Monographs, 46
Health Professionals Educational Assistance Act, 103, 105
Health Resources Development Act of 1975, 365
Heart disease, 255; attacks, 13, 232; chronic, 145
Heinman, J., 276
Heinrich, R., 274-275

Helplessness: mastery of, 124; sense of, 143, 330

Hematology, 113–114

Hemophilia and hemophiliacs, 56, 139–161; behavioral-medicine approach to, 143, 146

Henderson, J.B., 142

Henker, B., 159

Hepatitis, 297, 305

Herbal remedies, native, 350, 354–355, 370

Hersen, M., 141, 160

Hess, R.J., 395

Hessler, R.M., 368–369

Hetler, J.H., 106

Hierarchy, structure of, 122, 418

Higgins, G.E., 287

High blood pressure, 65, 231, 249

Hilgard, E.R., 122

Hilgartner, M.W., 144–145

Hill, R.B., 327–328

Hilliard, Ronald D., 55, 79–83

Hillman, R.W., 244

Hinshaw, A.L., 186

Hispanic ethnic group, 323; culture, 341, 344; heritage, 339–340; lifestyles, 345; population, 339–341, 345

Hodgkin's disease, 113, 121

Holistic approach to illness, 1–2, 31, 33, 40, 420

Holland, J., 118, 124

Holmes, F.F., Holmes, H.A., and Holmes, T.H., 71, 113, 230

Holmes Stress Scale, 36

Home: cures, 120; environment, 218–219, 422–424; visits, 108

Homeostasis, loss of, 131

Homes for the aged, 218–219

Homework exercises, 270–272, 276–277

Homicides, potential for, 95, 348

Homosexuality: behavior, 256, 298, 309; counselors, 319; experiences, 316–318; latent, 344; societal attitudes, 299, 303–305

Hooker, E., 298

Hopelessness, feelings of, 263, 266

Hopkins, J., 298

Horner's syndrome, 403

Hospital(s), 56, 143, 218, 221, 235, 333, 335, 350; administration, 418; bureaucracy, 85, 92, 121; children's, 106, 113, 116–117; community, 11; environment, 149; of Native Americans, 359–360; private, 12; services, 139; state, 41; university affiliated, 270

Hospitalization, 219, 295, 340; fear of, 372–373

Hostility, 88

House Select Committee on Aging, 216

Housing, 340; discrimination in, 329; substandard, 366

Huang, C., 368

Huard, P., 369

Human: adaptive processes, 47; behavior problems, 8, 40, 43–44; dignity, 290; ecology, 60; fallibility, 110; service fields, 229–232, 234, 236; sexuality, 272, 283–285, 293, 313, 316; suffering, 14

Humanism and humanitarianism, 31, 51, 304, 411

Hurvitz, Carole, 185

Hyman, Carol, 139

Hyperemesis Gravidarum, 205

Hypercholesterolemia, 141

Hyperglycemia, 349

Hypertension, 36, 46, 262, 348; control of, 141–142

Hyperventilation, 231

Hypnosis: group training, 122; use of, 59, 82, 124, 156, 171

Hysterectomy, 193–194, 334, 380

Hysteria, conversion, 59

Identity: operant pain, 177–178; personal, 196; racial, 326–327, 335; sexual, 199, 208

Illness: adjustment to, 56; chronic, 9, 159, 287; coping with, 365; fear of, 85; impact of, 67; Indian attitude toward, 349; organic, 55; psychological nature of, 1; terminal, 40

Imagination. See Fantasies and fantasizing

Immigration and immigrants, 366–368, 370

Immunology and immediacy, 48, 61

Impotence, trauma of, 318

Inadequacy: feelings of, 16, 233, 273, 299; sexual, 270, 287

Incapacitation. See Handicap, physical

Ince, L.P., 146

Incest, problem of, 268, 351

Income: family, 328; subsistance level, 366

Incontinence, fecal, 142

Independence, sense of, 72, 134

Indian Affairs, Bureau of, 348–350, 360

Indian Health Service (IHS), 348, 359–361

Indians. See Native Americans

Individualization, 6, 216; power of, 354, 356

Indonesia, 366

Industrial: injuries, 230; organizational psychology, 61; societies, 212, 358

Infant: feeding, 203; maternal bond, 203, 206–208; mortality, 368, 373; sexuality, 320

Infertility, problem of, 208

Inflexibility, myth of, 214

Information: limited, 258, 260–264;

psychosocial, 67
Inpatient care, 107, 179, 291; psychiatrical,
    6-8, 11; services, 293
Insomnia, factor of, 246
Institute of Medicine, 161
Institutions: research, 345; social, 9, 225,
    upgrading, 220-221
Insurance programs, medical, 9, 104, 335
Integrity, narcissistic, 88, 93
Intelligence: factor of, 42-44; performance
    tests for, 43, 125
Interaction: behavior bases, 55, 118-119;
    environmental, 44; interpersonal, 40, 63;
    social, 3
Intercourse and coitus, 200, 261; age at first,
    318; attempts at, 271-272; painful,
    264-265
Interdisciplinary: endeavors, 140; research,
    65; studies, 9; team approach, 7, 12, 56
Interns, internships, and internists, 25;
    hospital, 219; psychology, 31-33; training
    programs, 5-8, 10-22
Interpersonal: behavior, 45; child-parent
    dynamics, 268; interactions, 40, 63;
    problems, 85; risks, 60
Intervention: behavioral medicine, 141-142;
    goals of, 47; procedures, 7-8, 48-49, 92,
    117, 141; psychological, 5, 16, 32-33, 89,
    94, 113-125; strategies, 59, 108-111,
    141-142; therapeutic, 22, 96
Interviews and interviewing, 67-76, 193, 317,
    333; on alcohol, 241-251; behavioral
    analysis, 178; gynecological, 186-187;
    psychological, 115; skills required for, 12,
    177; techniques of, 64, 241, 249
Intestinal diseases, 305
Intimacy, degrees of, 316
Intolerance, homosexuality, 299, 303-305
Intragroup conflicts, 230
Iophendylate, use of, 401-402
Ireton, Harold R., 11-12, 22, 28, 31, 55,
    67-76
Is Sex Necessary? (Thurber and White), 255
Isolation: protective, 125; social, 124, 291,
    335

Jacob, R.G., 142
Jacobs, L., 122
Jacobson, E., 156
Jamison, K., 262-263
Janis, I., 120
Japanese ethnic group, 366-367; cancer in,
    368
Javet, Pierre, 397
Jealousy, factor of, 196
Jellinek, E.M., 242, 244
Jewish ethnic group, prejudice against, 299

Jilek, W.G., 352
Jobs: discrimination, 125, 329; promotion in,
    230; stress in, 236-239, 246
Jogging, popularity of, 65
Johnson, J.E., 49
Johnson, Malcolm, 215
Johnson, Samuel, 377
Johnson, V., 255, 257, 261, 264, 266-267,
    270-272, 283-284, 286, 294, 313, 321
Jones, D.E., 361
Jorgensen, R.L., 357
Jospe, Michael, 2, 11-22, 255, 283-295
Journal of American Medical Association,
    383
Journal of Behavioral Medicine, 161
Judeo-Christian tradition, 320
Judges and courts, 108, 233
Judgments, moral and social, 97
Julty, S., 261

Kagen-Goodheart, L., 113
Kahana, R., 72
Kalish, R.A., 367
Kamin, Jules H., 185
Kamiva, J., 146
Kaplan, H.S., 261-262, 264-266, 274-275,
    283
Karon, M., 120
Kase, S.V., 160
Kasper, C.K., 144
Kass, D.J., 277
Katz, E.R., 113, 118, 124, 160
Kaufman, R.M., 22
Kellerhals, J.M., 196
Kellerman, Jonathan, 56, 113-125
Kemnitzer, Luis S., 347-361
Kerner Commission Report, 333
Kidney diseases, 142
King, S.H., 1-2, 368
Kinsey, A., 249, 301-302
Kiowa Apache Indians, 356, 361
Kissin, B., 244
Kitano, H., 366
Knapp, M.L., 68
Knaus, W.J., 109
Koch, C.R., 113
Kohle, K., 124
Kohlenberg, R.J., 42, 142
Korea and the Koreans, 366, 368
Korman, M., 8
Korsch, B.M., 80
Krasner, L., 172
Kroger, W.S., 156
Kubler-Ross, Elizabeth, 129

LaBarre, M., 204
LaBaw, W., 122

Labor, 199, 207; delivery process, 32, 199, 201–203, 207; as painful experience, 201
Laboratory procedures, 9, 142, 372, 379; research, 47; studies, 10, 49; technicians, 31; tests, 15, 50, 79, 187, 269
Lakota Indians, 354–355, 360
Lalonde, M., 142
Lamaze trained women, 44
Laminar-airflow studies, 124–125
Language barriers, 339–341, 366–368, 371
Lansdown, R., 125
Lansky, S.B., 113, 118
Latent homosexuality, 344
Latino group, 326
Lawler, Edward, 234
Laws on human sexuality, 313
Lazarus, R.S., 49, 139
Leadership, types of, 48
Learning: collaborative, 31–32; disabilities, 64, 105; holistic, 31; self-directed, 30; theories, 7, 47
LeBarr, W., 370
Lefebre, Ludwig, 316
Leiblum, S.R., 274
Leisure time, use of, 299
Lesbians: age factor, 307–308; and civil rights, 298, 308; core information, 256, 297–310; medical facts on, 305–307; and spinal-cord injuries, 307; working with, 319–320
Leshner, M., 287
Leukemia, 7, 120; dying of, 409–424; lymphoblastic, 113. See also Acute myllogenous leukemia (AML)
Leventhal, H., 49
Levin, Les, 26
Lewinsohn, P.M., 47, 143, 157
Lewis, S., 114, 218–219, 262
Li, F.P., 367
Liaison functions, 2
Liberman, R.P., 139
Libet, J., 47
Libido, loss of, 309
Licensure and relicensure, professional, 285–286, 340
Life situations, 67–68, 70–72
Lifespan expectancy, 113, 211; sexuality throughout, 293–295
Lifestyle, 47, 232–234, 265–266, 319, 414; alterations in, 40, 57, 368; Hispanic, 345; sexual, 301–303, 305–307
Lindzey, G., 43
Lippman, Cathie-Ann, 57, 185–208
Lippman, Helen, 185n
Lipowski, L.J., 2, 22, 26, 68
Lithotomy position, 190–191
Liver diseases, 142

Living with Chronic Neurologic Disease (Cooper), 405
Lobbying and lobbiests, professional, 325
Lobitz, W.C., 258, 265–266
London, P., 122
Loneliness, factor of, 315, 320, 419
Long, A.E., 187, 189
Long-term disability, 130, 133–134
LoPiccolo, L., 258, 265, 275–276, 283
Los Angeles Children's Hospital, 113
Los Angeles County Occupational Health Service, 229
Loss, concept and issue of, 14, 129–133, 222
Lothstein, L.M., 22
"Lover authority," 316–317
Lovitt, T.C., 159
Lowman, J.T., 113
Loya, F., 262
Lucas, M.J., 272
Luckey Laboratories, 248
Lurie, H.J., 263
Lymphoblastic leukemia, 113

McCue, K., 121
McDonald, J.S., and McDonald, H.H., 194, 395
McGuire, L., 274–275
MacDougall, J.M., 44
Machismo among Raza groups, 344
McKenzie, J., 369
MacPhillamy, D.J., 47
McWhinney, I.R., 30, 68
McWhirter, D.P., 262
Magnusson, D., 44, 118
Magrab, P.R., 143
Mahon, Robert, 325–337
Mahoney, M.J., 157
Maisto, S.A., 248
Maladaptive behavior, 42, 47–48, 55
Maladjustment: marital, 266; personal, 68, 72–74
Male: chauvinism, 382; sexuality, 261, 274–277
Malignant diseases, 113, 116–118. See also Cancer
Malnutrition, problem of, 214, 350
Mammography, 382
Management, 234; behavioral, 59, 178–182; budget, 223; health, 139; of pain, 169–182
Manuals: on alcoholism, 244; on sex, 293
Margolis, S., 141
Marital: conflicts, 73, 249, 266, 351; counseling, 207; disolution, 132; relationships, 201
Marks, I.M., 139
Marston, M.V., 160
Martin, C.E., 259

Masek, B.J., 139, 142-142
Mason, T.J., 368
Mass-murder suicides, 63
Massage, use of, 370, 392
Mastectomy, psychemotional problem of, 379, 386-389
Master of Science degree, 11
Masters, W.H., 255, 257, 261, 264, 267, 270-272, 283-284, 286, 294, 313, 321
Masturbation, age at, 318; childhood, 293, 320-321; conflicts over, 259, 265, 272, 315, 322
Maternal and Child Health Service, 139n
Maternal instincts, role of, 130, 203-208, 321
Matriarchial status, black families, 327-328
Mattsson, A., 156
Maturity: emotional, 15-17, 204; sexual, 204
Maultsby, Maxie C., 109
Meadows, A.T., 125
Measurement, reliance on, 141
Medicaid and medicine programs, 220-221
Medical: bureaucracy, 379, 382, 385-386, 388; centers, 105-106; complaints, 100; crisis situations, 90, 93; emergency services, 85; evaluation processes, 7, 35, 175-176; examination, 15, 394; hemophilia aspects, 143-146; information on gays and lesbians, 305-307; nursing services, 13, 51, 86, 113, 115; records, 12; rehabilitation, 7; schools, 100-105, 334, 345; scientists, 30; second opinions, 198; sexual concerns, 283, 286; sociology, 2, 28-29; specialization, 25; underserved populations, 340
Medication: analgesic, 160; narcotic, 181; pain, 176; prescriptions for, 172; resistance to, 9; traditional, 369; tranquilizing, 230; use of, 45, 91-92, 178-179, 248, 262, 328
Medicine, 1, 11, 130; behavioral, 30, 56, 139-161; biological, 30; community, 2, 28; emergency, 87; Euroamerican, 351, 353, 356-357; family-practice, 7-8, 11-22; folk, 120; geriatric, 219; herbal, 370; history of, 2; nonpsychiatric, 2; power of, 354; psychological, 2, 25-37, 284; scientific, 32
Meditation, benefits from, 370, 414
Meichenbaum, D.H., 110, 156, 159
Melamed, B.G., 120
Melzack, Ronald, 169
Menlove, F.L., 120
Menopause, response to, 195-196, 262, 321, 380
Menstruation, 192, 196
Mental: illness, 11; retardation, 64, 105; status examination, 67

Mental health: community, 6, 64, 116; problems, 5, 8-9, 317; professionals, 2; rural communities, 6; student services, 6; training, 103
Menzies, Isabel, 235
Merrit, A.D., 145
Merskey, H., 147, 182
Methotrexate, 118
Mexicans and Mexican-Americans, 120, 333, 339, 341
Meyer, A.J., and Meyer, J.K., 142, 272
Militancy, factor of, 299
Miller, N.R., 172, 275
Millis, John, 27
Milne, J.F., 287, 295
Minnesota, University of, 6, 8; Division of Health Care Psychology, 11; Health Science Center training programs, 5-10; hospital, 7
Minnesota Child Development Inventory, 109
Minnesota Committee for Gay Rights in Minneapolis, 308
Minnesota Multiphasic Personality Inventory (MMPI), 36, 109, 178
Minipsychiatrists, 29
Minority: groups, 303, 339, 373; patients, 336; population, 297; professionals, 335-336; racial, 365-367
Miscarriages, trauma, 263
Mobility, social, 328
Modesty in Asian women, 372-373
Moment and Other Essays, The (Woolf), 377
Montgomery, P.S., 146
Moods, factor of, 156-157
Mooney, J., and Mooney, T.O., 262, 361
Moore, D.C., 124
Moral: attitudes, 313, 325, 351-354; code, 347, 352, 356
Morale, factor of, 62, 230
Morales, R.F., 366
Morgan, A.H., 122
Moriwaki, S., 367
Morphine, use of, 417, 423
Morrissey, J.F., 49
Mortality, infant, 373
Mosak, H., 72
Motherhood. *See* Maternal instincts, role of
Motivation, 40, 170, 266, 304; lack of, 97, 107, 233; unconscious, 269
Mourning, fundamental process of, 129, 131-136, 206
Moxa treatment, 370
Multiple sclerosis, 403-406
Murphy, John Benjamin, 109
Muscle: relaxation, 156; tension, 49, 231, 233, 237

Musculoskeletal structures, 160
Myelogram, 394, 401, 403
Myocardial infarction, 71, 286
Myths: on aging, 213; on inflexibility and disengagement, 214; of unproductivity, 213

Nadelson, D., 199–201, 208
Narcissism, factor of, 88, 93
Narcotic substances, 157, 181; postoperative, 170
National Academy of Sciences (NAS), 161
National Center for Health Statistics, 104
National Council on Alcoholism, 244
National Institute on Aging, 213, 220
National Institute on Alcohol Abuse and Alcoholism (NIAAA), 242
National Institute of Mental Health (NIMH), 6
National Multiple Sclerosis Society, 405
Native Americans (Indians): attitudes toward illness, 349; Bureau for, 348, 350, 360; culture, 360; disease patterns of, 348–349; health services, 347–348, 359–361; herbal use, 350; historical background, 347–351; medicine and physicians, 323, 333, 350–354
Navajo tribe, 351, 353, 361
Nee, V.G., 366
Negrete, V.F., 80
Nemiah, J.C., 132
Neo-Freudians and neoanalytic views, 42, 284
Nervous system and nervousness, 197, 246, 288, 393
Neurology and neurologists, 6–7, 105, 391–406
Neuromuscular disease, 142
Neuropsychology and neurophysiologists, 6–7, 47, 169
Neurosis, obsessive and compulsive, 139–140
Neurasthenia, 396
Neurosurgery, 6–7, 105
Neuroticism and neurotics, behavior and fatigue, 60, 64, 72, 269, 299, 304, 389, 396
New York State, 339
Nieberding, Joseph E., 2, 11–22
Nielson, I., 199, 201
Niswander, K.R., 205
Nonbiofeedback behavioral procedures, 146–147
Noncoital sexual activities, 264, 271
Nonpain behavior, 180
Nonpsychiatric areas of medicine, 2
Nontraditional sexual behavior, 256
Norris, C., 263
Notman, M., 196

Nursing and nurses, 130, 200, 233, 325; attitudes and goals, 39–40, 45; district, 219; education and schools, 39–52, 100; patient interactions, 46; pediatric, 51; personnel, 18, 34, 114, 153; professional, 2–3; psychiatric, 41, 51, 101; psychological, 39–52; public-health, 41, 106; students, 31; surgical, 51; time involved, 61
Nursing homes, 33–34, 62, 219; admission to, 220
Nutrition, factor of, 244

Obesity, factor of, 34, 65, 141, 157, 193, 249, 290
Obler, M., 274
Obsessive-compulsive actions, 139
Obstetrics and obstetricians, 25, 57, 185–207, 379
Occupations and occupational stress, 229–231, 319; therapy, 63, 130, 358
O'Connor, J.F., 268
Olbrechts, F.M., 361
Older Americans Act, 216–217
Olin, B., 262
O'Malley, F., 114
Omnipotence, feelings of, 93–94
Oncology, 7, 56, 105, 113–125
Operant pain, behavioral management of, 172–173, 177–182
Operating procedures, 187
Opinions, medical, 186, 198
Oppositional behavior, 118
Oppression, societal, 299–300
Optimism, factor of, 72–73, 83
Oral sex contact, 259, 305
Organic diseases, 2, 28–29, 55, 177, 287
Organizational: family structure, 2, 28, 371; industrial psychology, 61
Orgasm and orgasmic dysfunction, 200, 257, 272, 275; attainment of, 276–277, 294; lack of, 264–265; multiple, 259, 261–262
Oriental ethnic groups, 366–367
Orthopedic: disabilities, 25, 146; surgery, 292
Ostomy Association, 263
Ostracism, trauma of, 308
Our Right to Love (Vida), 306
Outpatient: clinics, 6–8, 21–22; departments, 103; medical services, 15, 86, 107, 171, 291; psychiatry and psychotherapy, 6–8, 11, 179
Overeating. See Obesity, factor of
Overstreet, E., 197

Pain, 49, 91, 117; alleviation of, 169; avoidance of, 176; behavioral, 175,

178–182; clinical, 170, 172; chronic, 7, 146–157, 169, 174–175, 178–182; control, 57, 124; and depression, 182; and drugs, 182; emotional, 419, 421; experience of, 16–17; identification of, 177–178; and intercourse, 264–265; learning approach to, 171–173; management of, 169–182; medications, 176; narcotics for, 178; operant, 172–182; pattern of, 177–179; psychogenic, 175; severe, 89; and tension, 147
Palmer, P., 156
Palos, S., 369
Pap smears, 197
Papadopoulou, Z.L., 143
Parallelism, factor of, 131
Paranoia, 59, 214
Paraplegia and paraplegics, 56, 262, 291, 294, 320
Paraprofessionals, 297, 340, 371
Parents and parenthood: aged, 217; anxiety, 125; authoritarianism, 342; gay, 307; involvement, 410; overdependence, 344; prohibitions, 268
Parlee, M.B., 196
Pasnau, Robert O., 205–206, 262–263
Paternalism, factor of, 134
Passivity and passive aggression, 156–157, 299, 372
Pathology, 25; behavior, 60; organic, 177; reports, 20; speech, 7; speculative, 177
Pathophysiology of disease, 9
Patient(s): activities, 119; aged, 197; comfort, 62; complaints, 86; counseling, 12, 266; and death, 129; doctor relationship, 12–13, 27–28, 79–80, 192, 256, 316, 379; economic status, 326; emotional needs, 383; evaluation, 7; family and friends, 140–141; fantasies, 380; guilt feelings, 315–316; holistic care, 1, 33; impression of, 46; minority, 336; paranoid, 59; psychogenic etiology with, 79–81; sexuality of 286, 315–317; in shock, 50
Patronizing attitudes, 134
Patt, S.L., 205
Patterson, G.R., and Patterson, R.T., 159, 205
Pattison, E.M., 241, 243, 251, 352
Peace, emotional, 422
Peasants, culture of, 369
Pediatric Psychology, Society of, 106
Pediatrics, Department of, 7
Pediatrics and pediatricians, 11, 25, 130; and chronic pain, 149; health-care, 103–111; and intensive-care unit, 143; and psychologists, 106–111; neurology, 7;

oncology, 56, 113–125
Peebles, J.J., 114
Peer: group support, 48, 380–381, 388; relationships, 204
Pelvic: examination, 186, 189–192, 195, 197, 202, 260, 271–272
Penis and penile gonorrhea, 265, 305
Perfectionism, 110
Performance: anxiety over, 258–259; goals, 272; intellectual, 125, 269, 271
Perlman, A., 262
Permission, granting of, 258–260
Personal: dignity, 136; identity, 196; maladjustments, 68, 72–74; resources, 72–74
Personality, 9, 68–69, 72, 232; changes, 268–269; differences, 298; dynamics, 129; inventory, 109; of practitioners, 325; psychology of, 42–47; style, 46–47, 135–136; tests, 108; trait characteristics, 132, 156
Personnel: medical, 115; nursing, 18, 34, 114, 153
Perspectives and perception, behavioral medicine, 46, 169–182
Perversion, 259
Pessimism, factor of, 72
Phaire, Thomas, 103
Pharmacological agents, 147
Pharyngeal gonorrhea, 304–305
Phobias. See Fears and phobias
Physical: assaults, 298, 308; complaints, 14, 87, 98, 178; deterioration, 220; development, 195, 211; disabilities, 263, 285, 287; distress, 79; environment, 1, 141; examinations, 21–24, 74, 79, 98, 188–192, 269; fitness, 200; handicaps, 7, 133, 135; illnesses, 5, 287–293; injuries, 147, 170; restraints, 97; sciences, 50–51; stress, 147; therapy, 130, 149, 153, 160, 180, 383; trauma, 330
Physical Medicine and Rehabilitation, Department of, 7
Physicians, 1, 3, 329; family, 2, 12, 27–28, 30, 32, 79; Indian, 350; Mexican-American, 341; patient relationship, 12–13, 79–80, 192, 256, 316, 379; primary care, 12, 21–22, 27, 103, 284–285
Physiology, 140, 274
Piaget, Jean, 42
Pierce, D., 274
Pilipino community, 366–368
Placebo, use of, 170
Placement opportunity, 6
Plans, planners, and planning, 223; family, 192; prepaid health, 37
Plasek, Marily, 185

Play therapy. *See* Recreation
Pneumonia, 348, 350, 353
Politics and political activities, 28, 333, 356
Polydrug abuse, 247
Pomeroy, W.B., 259
Population: Hispanic, 339–341, 345; minority, 297; patient, 7; underserved medically, 340; psychiatric, 5, 25, 29
Postmastectomy depression (PMD), 388
Postoperative difficulties, 170, 194
Postpartum psychosis, 206–208
Potency, problems of, 262
Poverty, factor of, 340, 365
Power: healing, 354; idea of, 354–357; individual, 354, 356; political, 333; repository of, 355; spiritual, 354, 356–357
Practice and practitioners, medical, 1, 13, 25–26, 219, 325, 369
Precepts (Hippocrates), 1
Pregnancy, 196, 263, 380; in Asia, 373; complicated, 205–207; normal, 199; teenage, 204–205
Preisler, H.D., 124
Prejudice(s): against blacks, 299; against the elderly, 213–214; on Jews, 299. *See also* Discrimination
Premature: aging, 193; ejaculation, 264–268, 318, 381
Premorbid family functioning, 119–120
Prescription drugs and medication, 172, 247
Pressure, periods of, 237–238, 272
Preston, Terry Anne, 185
Prevention, techniques of, 64–65, 140–142, 145–146
Price, Susan C., 255, 257–278, 286
Primary: physicians, 12, 21–22, 27, 103, 284–285; teachers, 29–31
Privacy and confidentiality, issues of, 306–307
Private hospitals, 12
Proctological examination, 315
Professional: consultation, 319; counseling, 204, 231; health-care, 2–3, 56–57, 175–181, 314–316; licensing, 285–286, 340; lobbyist, 325; mental-health care, 1–2, 116; minority-group members, 335–336; nursing, 2–3; organizations, 334; skill training, 9, 100, 313; stereotyping, 21
Professionalism: attitudes, 60, 216, 303–305; sense of, 189, 336, 410
Prophylactics, 5, 9
Prostatitis, 305
Protective isolation, 125
Provider-client relationship, 302–305
Pseudocyesis, history of, 208
Psychiatric: nursing, 41, 51, 101;

populations, 5, 25, 29; wards, 41
Psychiatry and psychiatrists, 82, 284, 314, 388; adolescent and adult, 6; clinical treatment, 6–8, 11, 64
Psychic tension, 107
Psychoanalysis, classical, 267
Psychodynamics, knowledge of, 97
Psychoemotional problems, 318, 386–389
Psychogenic etiology, 79–82, 175–176, 180, 269
Psychological Institute at the University of Bonn, 215
Psychological Systems Review (PRS), 67–68, 74, 76
Psychology and psychologists: abnormal, 65; assessment, 5, 100; behavioral, 56, 139; child, 62, 105; clinical, 5, 9, 22, 41, 59–61, 64–65; complaints, 14; community, 64; diagnostic techniques, 32; developmental, 2, 42–43, 62, 104; differential, 9; educational factor, 39–52; experimental, 59, 169; goal of, 40; health-care, 1–2, 5–8, 13–20, 25–37, 59–60, 113, 284; industrial, 61; interns and residents, 2, 21, 31–33; intervention, 5, 16, 32–33, 89, 94, 113–125; interviewing techniques, 115; issues, 1, 29, 314, 388; junior, 29; nursing, 39–52; pediatric, 106–111; personality factor, 42–47; research task forces, 8; social, 42–46, 61, 63, 65; supervisory, 5; testing, 12; vocational, 9, 62–63
Psychology Today (Renwick and Lawler), 234
Psychometry and Psychometrists, use of, 32, 36, 64, 109, 125
Psychopathology, 9, 47–48, 56, 59–60, 62, 135, 212, 298
Psychosexual development, 268
Psychosis, 139–140; postpartum, 206–208
Psychosocial: care, 113, 116; changes, 196; and children, 113, 116–117; context, 55, 64; information, 67, 297; problems, 79, 86, 406; programs, 116–117; stresses, 368
Psychosomatic: complaints, 13, 396; illnesses, 214, 368
Psychotherapeutic techniques, 250–251, 316
Psychotherapy and psychotherapists, 11, 29, 64, 115, 124, 169, 174–175, 266, 269, 315–316, 327
Puberty, period of, 208
Public-health: education, 64; nursing, 41, 106
Public Health, Department of, 197
Public Health Service (PHS), 348, 350; hospital, 353
Puerto Rican ethnic group, 339
Pulse rate, 49

Quadriplegia and quadriplegics, 56, 130–131, 135, 262, 291, 294
Quality, sensory, 170
Quasi-social workers, 29
Quast, Wentworth, 56, 103–111
Questionnaires, use of, 103
Quevillon, R., 159
Quinn, J.R., 369

Racer, Harley J., 2, 11–12, 22, 25–37, 76
Racial identity, 32, 303, 319, 326–327, 335
Racism, 213; attitudes, 325, 334; minority groups, 365–367; and practitioners, 333–335; vulnerability, 329–333
Radiation, use of, 125, 293, 385, 387
Radiology, studies on, 86
Radiotherapy, 117
Rahe, R.H., 71, 230
Rape, heterosexual, 308–309
Raphael, B., 193
Rapid ejaculation, 277
Rapport, establishment of, 186–190
Rational Behavior Training (RBT), 109–111
Rationalization, habit of, 63
Rau, D., 246
Raymaud's disease, 142
Raza group, sex role of, 341–343
Reach to Recovery program, 383–384, 386
Reality testing, 60
Recreation: activities, 70–71; skills, 181; therapy, 123, 221
Rectal gonorrhea, 304–305
Referral and treatment problems, 250–251
Regression, factor of, 96
Rehabilitation: of children, 134; emotional, 399; long-term, 153; medical programs, 6–7, 105, 140; old-age, 211; optimal, 113; sexual, 262; vocational, 262
Rehabilitation Services Administration, 169
Reich, Wilhelm, 284
Reichard, G., 360
Reinforcers, level of, 182
Rekers, G.A., 139
Relaxation: muscle, 156; patterns of, 239; progressive, 49; techniques, 156, 237; training, 181, 274
Religion and religious life, 28, 70–71, 303, 309, 319, 326, 351, 356, 366; backgrounds, 299; beliefs, 199; clergy, 101; cults, 63; organized, 382; preferences, 82
Remission, factor of, 417, 419
Renal: colic, 35–36; diseases, 368; failure, 290, 295
Renne, C.M., 142
Renshaw, D., 262, 287
"Repeater" file, 99–100

Reports and records: medical, 12; pathology, 20
Repression, 308; anger, 340; of sexual urges, 313
Reproductive Research Foundation, 271
Research and researchers, 110, 301; activities, 2, 9; behavioral-medicine, 161; contributions, 22; epidemiological, 159; genius, 31; in gerontology, 42; institutions, 345; interdisciplinary, 65; investigations, 49; laboratory, 47; reproductive, 271; studies and theories, 3, 82
Research and Training Center Mart, 169
Residents and residency programs, 2, 21, 31–33
Resistance to medication, 9
Respiratory depression, 34
Respondent pain behavior, 172
Resources: coping, 68–70; economic, 368; financial, 367, 371; personal, 72–74
Responsibility and respect, 37, 72–73, 195, 235
Responsiveness, sexual, 294
Restraints, physical, 97
Retardation, mental, 64, 105
Retirement, 81; communities, 218
Retrograde ejaculation, 294
Reyes, E., 246
Reynolds, Barry S., 255, 257–278, 286
Rheumatoid arthritis, 177
Richardson, H., 298
Richey, C.A., 156
Ricker-Smith, Katherine, 221
Rimoin, D.L., 348
Ringold, E., 262
Risks, taking of, 60, 145, 160, 198
Risley, T.R., 141
Roberge, L., 352
Robins, E., 299
Robinson, C.H., 259
Roeske, N., 194
Rogers, C.R., 48, 80
Roman, P.M., 244
Room, R., 244
Rosalki, S.B., 246
Rosen, G., 265, 274
Ross, Marcia, and Ross, Alvin P., 377, 409–424
Rotation, family-practice medicine, 7–8, 11–22
Rotter, J.B., 46
Rowan, R., 305
Rubinstein, D., 257, 259
Rural areas and communities, 6, 108
Russo, Dennis C., 56–57, 139–161
Rutter, M., 159

Sadoughi, W., 287
Saghir, M., 299
Samoa and Samoans, 366
Scalzi, C.C., 262
Schaie, K.W., 42
Schechter, M.D., 352
Scheingold, L.D., 287
Schizophrenia, 63, 72, 178
Schmidt, C.W., 272
Schneidman, B., 274–275
Schochet, B.R., 68
Schoener, G., 309
Schofield, William, 5, 8, 11, 22, 32, 105
Schools, medical and nursing, 100, 103, 105, 107, 334, 345
Schwartz, G.E., 139–140, 142
Schweikert, Robert J., 241
Science and scientists: applied biological, 1; behavioral, 2, 28–29, 41, 49, 105, 113, 115, 124; and education, 11; medical, 30–32; nursing, 39; physical, 50–51; social, 39
Scotland, 219
Scott, R.W., 142
Screening, psychological, 67–76
Second medical opinions, 186, 198
Secondary emotional dysfunction, 146
Security, sense of, 130
Sedatives, use of, 34
Seduction, vulnerability to, 342
Segregation, evils of, 334
Seigler, I.C., 42–43
Self-: accusation, 329; autonomy, 344; awareness, 134; blame, 236; care, 202; confidence, 336, 420; control, 134, 159; depreciation, 196; derision, 299; destruction, 403; determination, 134, 186, 356, 358, 360; disclosure, 48; doubt, 235; evaluation, 200; examination, 260, 334; expression, 342; gratification, 320; healing, 360; hypnosis, 122–123, 414; identity, 327; image, 73, 356; liquidating programs, 182; maintenance habits, 87; management training, 159; pleasuring, 321; protection, 332; stimulation, 259, 264; sufficiency, 216, 238; treatment, 405; worth, 72–73, 217
Self-esteem: defects in, 47; exercise in, 34; factor of, 73, 196, 207, 283, 305; positive, 295; staff personnel, 85
Self-help: encouragement of, 122; groups for, 406; for sexual dysfunctions, 276–278; skills needed, 292; strategy interventions, 59, 108–111, 141–142; therapy, 255
Seligman, M.E.P., 47, 143
Selltiz, C., 367

Seminars, value of, 291
Senarclens, M.D., 195
Senility, 197; myth of, 214
"Sensate-focus" activities, 271
Sensitizers and sensitivity, 45, 185; clinical, 179; level awareness of, 57
Sensory qualities, 131, 170
Sensual: activities, 277; exploration exercises, 274; pleasure, 258
Serenity, myth of, 214
Settlage, D.S., 190–191
Sex and sexism, 82, 213; clinics, 272–273; communications about, 269–270; counseling, 35, 257–278, 313; cross-cultural differences, 344; education, 255, 278, 318; manuals, 293; oral-genital, 259, 304; Raza group roles, 341–343; steroid replacement, 322; therapy, 255, 257–278, 286–287
Sexual interests and sexuality: activities, 70, 187, 195, 198, 200, 22; of adolescents, 256, 294–295, 321–322; anatomy, 260, 274; anxieties, 263; attitudes, 318; behavior of couples, 272–273; and childbearing, 321; childhood, 320–321; compatability, 194; complaints, 264; disorders, 139; and drugs, 262; dysfunction, 13, 35, 64, 260, 262, 264, 267, 276–278; excitement, 268; experiences, 270–273; fantasies, 190, 314; fears, 267; feelings, 197; female, 274–275; functioning, 125, 135; health care, 314–316; human, 272, 283–285, 293, 313, 316; identity, 199, 208; inadequacy, 161, 270, 274–277, 287; infantile, 320; laws on, 313; lifespan factor, 293–295; lifestyle variables, 301–303, 305–307; maturity, 204; medical aspects of, 283, 286; overt, 314; of patients, and physical illness, 287–293; problems, 246, 258, 285–286; relationships, 193, 198; repression of urges, 313; response cycles, 260; revolution, 259; surgery effects on, 285; taboos, 285
Selye, Hans, 234
Shamans, effectiveness of, 350–353, 355–357
Shame, factor of, 93
Shea, M.J., 106
Shigellosis, trauma of, 297, 305
Shively, M., 301
Shock, patients in, 50
Shure, M.B., 110
Sibling rivalry, 318
Siegel, S.E., 120
Siegelman, M., 298
Silence, conspiracy of, 285, 291
Situational depression, 134

Skills: self-help, 292; social, 47, 156–159, 181, 274; vocational, 181
Skinner, B.F., 172
Smallpox, 349–350
Smith, Barbara L., 57, 229–239
Smith, E., 272
Smith, Roberta Ann, 3, 39–52
Smoking. *See* Cigarette smoking, effects of
Sobell, Mark B., and Sobell, Linda, C., 57, 149, 241–251
Socarides, C., 2928, 301
Social: adversity, 213; agencies, 107; attitudes, 334; backgrounds, 319; balance, 28, 55, 347, 354; behavior, 40, 131, 143; change, 211; class, 299–300; contacts, 216–217, 301; cultural habits, 326; decisions, 334; economic concerns, 298, 325, 332; environment, 141, 147, 153, 160, 323; gerontology, 211; groups, 60; history, 67; institutions, 9, 225; interactions, 3, 40, 61–62, 147; isolation, 124, 291, 321, 335; learning theories, 46; life, 26, 125–126; mobility, 328; network, 380, 385; problems, 224; psychology, 42, 45–46; reaction, 65; reinforcement, 47; relationships, 204, 358; sciences, 1–2, 41, 39, 51, 125; services, 86, 219, 225, 297, 306, 366–367; skills, 47, 156–159, 181, 274; status, 94; structure, 308; support systems, 68, 301, 308; survival, 327; skills, 274; welfare, 297; withdrawal, 309; workers, 22, 29, 31, 35, 63, 82, 101, 104, 108, 114, 119, 219, 233, 307, 314, 329, 382, 388
Social Services, Department of, 197
Socialization and sociability, 34, 72–73
Society and societal attitudes: behavior, 212, 313; expectation, 294; homosexuality intolerance, 299, 303–305; industrial, 212, 258; oppression, 299–300; priestly, 355; subcultures of, 317; Western, 314
Sociocultural characteristics, 104, 341, 369
Socioeconomic factors, 31, 86, 217, 326, 339, 387
Sociology, 61, 140, 255; medical, 2, 28–29
Sociopolitical motivations, 242, 342
Solnit, A.J., 133
Somatic: complaints, 309; delusions, 59; distress expressions, 20, 36; symptoms, 178
Sorcery and sorcerers, traits of, 356
South Dakota, 360
Southeastern Asian countries, 366
Speculative pathology, 177
Spear, F.G., 182
Specialization and specialists, medical, 6, 25, 28

Speech pathologists, 7
Speisman, J.C., 49
Spencer-Peet, J., 246
Sphygmomanometer, use of, 50
Spinal-cord injury, 171–172, 255, 291–295; chronically disabling, 129–137; and gays and lesbians, 307
Spinetta, J.J., 120
Spiritual forces and power, 352, 354, 356–357
Spitz, R., 287
Spivack, G., 110, 287
Stability, family, 125
Staff: morale of, 62, 85; obstetric, 202; social-work, 307
Stanford University School of Medicine, 160
Stark, M.H., 133
State hospitals, 41
Status: emotional distress, 68–70; social, 94; socioeconomic, 86, 326
Stauss, F.E., 277
Steinman, Richard, 211–225
Stephens, G.G., 25, 30
Stereotyping, professional, 21
Sterilization, 334; voluntary, 194
Stern, L.O., 268
Sternbach, R.A., 170
Steroid replacement, sex, 322
Stimulation: clitoral, 261–262, 269; conditioned, 118; electrical, 147; erotic, 265, 271; genital, 291; noxious, 170; self-, 259, 264; timing of, 272–273; transcutaneous, 179
Stoicism, factor of, 114, 371, 373
Strangers, fear of, 88, 93
Strategies: self-control, 159; self-help intervention, 59, 108–111, 141–142
Stravino, V.D., 147
Strengths of Black Families (Hill), 328
Stress: adaptation to, 48; automatic, 230–233; avoidance of, 175; chronic, 230–231, 239; emotional, 156; environmental, 118–119, 299; Holmes scale for, 36; illness-related, 229; job, 233–239, 246; management, 171, 233–234; occupational, 229–231; physical, 147; psychosocial, 368; reaction to, 65, 116–118, 231; reduction of, 404; results of, 17–18, 85, 87, 131, 156, 181, 198; sources of, 81; vulnerability to, 56, 57; work effects of, 229–239, 246
Stress Without Distress (Seyle), 234
Stroke, effects of, 287
Stuart, R.B., 157
Students: counseling bureau, 6; medical, 104; mental-health-service, 6; nursing, 31
Studies: on aging, 211; CWPS, 105; interdisciplinary, 9; laboratory, 10, 49;

laminar airflow, 124–125; research, 82; radiological, 86; on students, 104

Stunkard, A.J., 157

Subcultures, 317, 323

Subsistence-level incomes, 366

Substandard housing, 366

Suchman, E.A., 365

Suffering, exposure to, 14, 169

Suicide: ideation, 206; incidence of, 95, 98, 340, 348; mass-murder, 63; risk of, 70

Superstitions, 369

Supervision and supervisors, 5, 235

Support systems and supportive care, 13, 68, 72, 197, 225, 301, 308, 327

Surgery and surgical operations, 11, 25, 32, 179, 193, 294, 372; elective, 198; exploratory, 117; for injuries, 290; major, 18–19, 206; nursing for, 51; oncologists, 383; orthopedic, 292; and patient care, 15; specialities and procedures, 130, 147; sexual problems after, 262–263, 285

Surrogate families, 345

Survival of black people, social, 327

Surwit, R.S., 142

Suspiciousness, 179, 215

Swanson, D.W., 147

Sweden, 219

Swisher, S.N., 68

Sympathy, feelings of, 61

Symptomatology, changes in, 160

Syphilis, cases of, 349

Taboos, 259, 294; sexual, 285

Taoism, philosophy of, 370

Task forces, health-behavior research, 8

Teachers and teaching activities, 2, 29–32, 36

Team interdisciplinary factor, 7, 12, 56

Technicians, 325; laboratory, 31; X-ray, 379

Technological practices, 323, 356–357

Teenagers, 195; pregnancy of, 204–205

Telephone conversations and terminology, 276–277, 417

Tension: factor of, 85, 95, 181; muscle, 49, 231, 233, 237; pain-cycle, 147; psychic, 107; relife of, 201; and somatic distress, 81

Terminal illnesses, 40, 409–424. See also Cancer

Tests and testing: givers of, 109; instruments for, 6; intelligence, 43, 125; laboratory, 15, 50, 79, 187, 269; personality, 108; psychological, 12; rigorous, 60

Texas, 339

Thannatology, growth of, 113

Therapeutic: abortion, 205; assistance, 7; intervention procedures, 22, 96; techniques, 5, 120–124

Therapy and therapists, 6, 13, 157, 233; antihypertensive, 36; behavior, 124, 139, 160; couple, 270–274; drug, 398; family, 63, 82; Gestalt, 82; group, 48, 82, 124, 274, 276; occupational, 63, 130, 358; physical, 130, 149, 153, 160, 180, 383; recreational, 123, 221; referral for, 17; response to, 9; self-help, 255; sex, 255, 257–278, 286–287; short-term, 12; supportive, 225

Thermal biofeedback, 147

Third World people, 335

Thomas, J.D., 159

Thurber, James, 255

Time and timing: leisure, 299; nursing, 61; of stimulation, 272–273; urgency of, 44

Tobacco, use of, 64–65, 141

Toister, R.P., 103

Tokenism, philosophy of, 134

Trachoma, 348, 350

Tradition and traditional activities: agencies, 297; family, 327; Judeo-Christian, 320; medication, 369

Trager, Brahna, 221

Training: assertiveness, 143; autogenic, 156, 171; communication skills, 264; of counselors, 31; experience needed, 6; graduate, 10, 28, 64; group hypnotic, 122; internship, 5–8, 10; Lamaze woman, 44; mental-health, 103; professional, 9, 313; programs, 1, 5–10; relaxation, 181, 274; sexual, 286; skills, 9, 274, 313; teaching, 1–3

Tranquilizers: drug, 214; medication, 230; use of, 34, 239, 247

Transfusions, blood, 117

Transplant procedures, bone-marrow, 105, 422

Transportation problems, 367, 371, 373

Transcutaneous stimulation, 179

Trauma, physical, 88, 330

Treatment, 85; cancer, 293–294; distress, 117–118; modalities, 13; outpatient, 179; psychiatric, 64; self-, 405; stress, 57

Tribal cultures, 347

Trice, H.M., 244

True, Reiko Homma, 365–373

Trust: element of, 37; mutual, 130

Tseng, W.S., 368

Tuberculosis, 348–350, 368

Turk, D., 156

Tyma, S., 147

Ullman, L.P., 172

Unassertiveness, factor of, 156–157

Unconditioned stimulus (UCS), 117–118

Unconscious motivations, 269

Uncontrollable erections, 315–316
Underhill, R., 360
Unemployment, 340, 366
United Kingdom, 216
University-affiliated hospitals, 270
Unmarried status, factor of, 199, 204, 208
Unproductivity, myth of, 213
Urban areas, 13
Urges, sexual, 3, 13
Urology and urinary tract infections, 284, 304, 349

Vacations, need for, 230
Vaginal gonorrhea, 306
Vail Conference, 8, 10
VanKeep, P.A., 196
Varni, James W., 56–57, 139–161
Venereal Disease Control Division, 305
Verbal responses, 50, 99, 271
Vernick, J., 120
Victimization, traits due to, 299
Vida, G., 306
Vietnam and the Vietnamese, 366
Vincristine, 118
Visiting Nurse Association, 197
Visitor approvals and home visits, 62, 108
Visual feedbacks, 181
Vocational: planning, 6; psychology, 9, 62–63; skills, 181
Voluntary sterilization, 194
Von Willebrand's Disease, 144
Vulnerability, sense of, 329–333

Wagner, N.L., 287
Walker, D.E., 360
Wallace, H., 361
Waller, J.A., 244
Wallston, Kenneth A., 3, 39–52, 285–286
Washington, State of, 366
Waters, V., 110
Weaver, J.L., 367–368
Weight, reduction of, 34–35
Weil, R.J., 367
Weinberg, M., 301
Weiss, S.M., and Weiss, T., 139–140, 142, 161
Weissenberg, M., 149, 169–170
Welfare: of children, 63; social, 297; workers, 108, 233

Wellish, D., 262–263
Wentz, A.C., 196
Werkman, S.L., 79
Weschler, D., 43
West Germany, 215
Western society, 314
White, E.B., 255
Whiteman's diseases and Native Americans, 356–360
Williams, C.L., 142, 301
Williamson, J.D., 406
Wilm's tumor, 113
Winkler, Win Ann, 377, 379–389
Wirt, Robert D., 59–65
Wisconsin, 108
Wiseman, S.M., 246
Withdrawal, trauma of, 96, 309
Wolpe, J., 139, 156
Womanhood: movement for, 342; responsibilities of, 195. See also Female
Wong, K., 367, 369
Wood, C.S., 349
Woods, N.F., 287, 288–290, 349, 361
Woolf, Virginia, 377
Work and workers, 29, 229–231, 239, 319–321, 377. See also Social
Workshops, 110, 221, 291
World Health Organization (WHO), 242
Worley, L.M., 103
Wright, L., 104
Wrightsman, L.S., 45
Wustman, Elaine, 85–101

X-rays, 372, 397, 401; technicians, 31, 379

Yale Conference on Behavioral Medicine, 139–140, 161
Yancik, R., 104
Yin-Yang forces, 370
Yoga activities, 370
Young Women's Christian Association (YWCA), and ENCORE, 389
Yule, W., 159

Zander, A., 48
Zeiss, R., and Zeiss, A., 265–266, 277
Zifferblah, S.M., 160
Zilbergeld, B., 261, 266, 274–275, 277
Zlutnick, S., 142, 160

About the Contributors

Cynthia Birrer, M.A., B. Ed., was until recently a member of the academic staff at the Department of Education, University of the Witwatersrand, Johannesburg. She has studied and lectured there and in the United States, Australia, and Europe. She is the author of *Medical Cop-out, Multiple Sclerosis,* and numerous journal articles, specializing in psychological aspects of medical care.

Jo Ann Brockway, Ph.D., is on the staff of the Department of Rehabilitation, School of Medicine, University of Washington, Seattle. Dr. Brockway received the Ph.D. from the University of Iowa and completed her internship in health-care psychology in the Division of Health Care Psychology, University of Minnesota, Minneapolis. Her professional interests include pain and analgesia, and the sexual problems of spinal-cord-injured patients.

Carmen Carrillo, Ph.D., is a licensed clinical psychologist. Currently, she is executive director of Mission Mental Health Center in San Francisco and chairperson of the State of California's Citizens Advisory Council for Mental Health. Dr. Carrillo is a member of the Board of Directors of the Mexican American Legal Defense and Educational Fund, Nueva Luz Resources, Inc., and BASSTA (Bay Area Spanish-Speaking Therapists Association). Long active as an advocate and clinician in the Raza community, she has written numerous articles on issues relevant to the Spanish-speaking population in the United States.

Donald Cassata, M.A., Ph.D., is coordinator of behavioral medicine for the family-practice residency-training program in the Department of Family Medicine, University of North Carolina, Chapel Hill. Dr. Cassata received the M.A. from the University of Denver and the Ph.D. from the University of Minnesota. For the past six years, his responsibilities have included teaching physician-patient relationship, medical interviewing and counseling skills, and psychological medicine to medical students and family physicians. His research interests include medical-interview assessment, effects of videotape feedback, nursing-care systems, and psychosocial evaluation.

Harold O. Dillehunt, Ph.D., is a clinical psychologist in private practice in San Francisco and San Mateo. He received his education at the University of California, Berkeley, and the California School of Professional Psychology. Dr. Dillehunt has served as consultant to Nueva Learning Center in Hillsborough, California, since 1968 as well as consulting with numerous public schools in the area of affective education. He has also served as board member and consultant to the California Association of the Gifted. Recently, he has published *Self Science Education—The Subject Is Me,* an affective-education curriculum.

Seth Ersner-Hershfield, Ph.D., is a staff psychologist at the Center for Mental Health, Newton Memorial Hospital, Newton, New Jersey. He was formerly a psychologist at the Dede Wallace Center Alcohol Programs, Nashville, and adjunct assistant professor of psychology, Vanderbilt University. Dr. Ersner-Hershfield received the Ph.D. in 1978 from Rutgers University. His research and clinical interests are in behavior-therapy approaches to alcohol abuse and insomnia.

Patrick J. Fazzari, M.D., is director of rehabilitation medicine at Mount Sinai Hospital, Hartford, one of the teaching hospitals of the University of Connecticut Health Center, where he is also a member of the faculty.

John C. Gonsiorek, Ph.D., is currently clinic supervisor of Walk-In Counseling Center, a crisis and short-term counseling center in Minneapolis. He was previously a clinical psychologist in the Department of Physical Medicine and Rehabilitation at the University of Minnesota Medical School. He received the Ph.D. in clinical psychology from the University of Minnesota in 1978. Dr. Gonsiorek's research and clinical interests include behavioral medicine, sexual orientation, schizophrenia, and community mental health.

A. Jack Hafner, Ph.D., received the doctorate in clinical psychology from Indiana University. He is currently professor and acting director of the Program in Health Care Psychology in the School of Public Health, University of Minnesota, Minneapolis. Dr. Hafner is the newsletter editor for the Association of Psychology Internship Centers, a Fellow of the American Psychological Association, and a Diplomate in Clinical Psychology of the American Board of Professional Psychology.

Ronald D. Hilliard, Ph.D., received the doctorate in clinical psychology from the University of Iowa. From 1972 to 1978 he was a clinical psychologist at the Des Moines Child Guidance Center. In 1979 he became coordinator of behavioral-sciences training at the Broadlawns Family Practice Residency Program in Des Moines.

Harold Ireton, Ph.D., is a clinical psychologist, consultant, and teacher of behavioral medicine and pediatric psychology for residents in family medicine, medical students, and other physicians in the Department of Family Practice and Community Health, University of Minnesota Health Sciences Center, Minneapolis. He has coauthored articles on psychological methods in medical practice. His other interests include parent education and developmental assessment of young children. He is coauthor of the Minnesota Preschool Child Development Inventory, the Minnesota Preschool Inventory, and the Minnesota Infant Development Inventory.

Jonathan S. Kellerman, Ph.D., is associate clinical professor of pediatrics (psychology), University of Southern California School of Medicine, and director, Psychosocial Program, Division of Hematology-Oncology, Childrens Hospital of Los Angeles. He received the Ph.D. in clinical psychology in 1974 from the University of Southern California. Dr. Kellerman's major interests are pediatric psychology, the treatment of anxiety and sleep disorders in children, pediatric hypnosis, psychological aspects of severe and chronic disease, and development of objective measurement of distress behavior in children. He has written numerous articles and presentations on various aspects of pediatric psychology and is the editor of *Psychological Aspects of Childhood Cancer*. Dr. Kellerman is a member of the Psychological Committee, Children's Cancer Study Group.

Luis S. Kemnitzer, Ph.D., is associate professor of anthropology, San Francisco University. He received the Ph.D. from the University of Pennsylvania. Dr. Kemnitzer's research interests include Native American urbanization, Lakota religious healing, health needs of urban Native Americans, aging and identity, and traditional and modern medicine in Palau (Micronesia). He is a consultant in methodology of medical-care research to Native American organizations. His publications are in Q-sort methodology and value conflict, Lakota healing ritual, Native American perception of medical encounters, health and healing among Plains Indians, and research methods in aging and Native American migration.

Cathie-Ann Lippman, M.D., is a child psychiatrist in Los Angeles. She is a consultant to the pediatric liaison service at Cedars-Sinai Hospital, maintains a private practice, and has a clinical appointment at the Neuropsychiatric Institute of the University of California at Los Angeles. She helped establish "A Model Liaison Program for the Obstetrics Staff: Workshop on the Tragic Birth" (with Ken Carlson), for training obstetrics staff, which was published in *The Family in Mourning*.

Robert Mahon, Ph.D., is a clinical psychologist working in community-mental-health services in San Francisco. His primary experience and interest is in crisis intervention, minority issues in psychology, program evaluation, and consultation and teaching. He received his undergraduate education at Yale University and received the Ph.D. in clinical psychology from the University of California, Berkeley. Since 1968, he has taught at the elementary, high-school, and college levels. He was the first intern at Westside Community Mental Health's National Institute of Mental Health funded psychology-intern training program. He currently is employed as a staff psychologist at San Francisco General Hospital.

Linda J. (Tik) Menefee, M.S., did graduate work at the University of Washington and is currently enrolled in a doctoral program at The Pacific Graduate School of Psychology. She is employed as a psychological consultant at the Regional Center of the East Bay in Oakland, California, specializing in work with developmentally disabled individuals and their families. Her interests include health psychology, neuropsychology, and forensics.

Susan Price, Ph.D., is codirector of the Human Sexuality Program, Neuropsychiatric Institute, University of California at Los Angeles, and the Professional Training Program in Human Sexuality, UCLA Extension, and is in private practice with the Institute for Sex and Marital Therapy, Los Angeles. She has specialized in training and supervising sex therapists to meet the needs of patients who have not been reached by traditional sex-therapy programs. Dr. Price has lectured and published articles on group treatment for rapid ejaculation and female orgasmic dysfunctions, and techniques for providing cost-efficient sex education and therapy.

Wentworth Quast, Ph.D., is a professor in the Program in Health Care Psychology, School of Public Health, University of Minnesota. He received the Ph.D. from the University of Minnesota with emphasis on both clinical psychology and child development. Dr. Quast's major interests are in primary prevention, working with families, schools, and community agencies; and his research interests are in the life history of psychopathology of adolescents and in the application of cognitive behavior modification with young children.

Harley J. Racer, M.D., is a family practitioner and teacher at Hennepin County Medical Center, Minneapolis. He was formerly an associate professor in the Department of Family Practice and Community Mental Health, University of Minnesota Health Sciences Center, Minneapolis. Dr. Racer has taught in the graduate and undergraduate programs of the University of Minnesota Medical School since 1967. He has served as a consultant in faculty development for the Society of Teachers of Family Medicine.

Barry S. Reynolds, Ph.D., is a staff psychologist with the Human Sexuality Program of the Neuropsychiatric Institute at the University of California at Los Angeles, and is in private practice with the Institute for Sex and Marital Therapy, Los Angeles. He utilized individual, couple, and group methods for treating common sexual dysfunctions. Dr. Reynolds has recently specialized in the development and scientific evaluation of new procedures for the treatment of sexual dysfunctions experienced by men without partners. He has lectured and published articles on sexual dysfunction, male sexuality, biofeedback, and cognitive behavior therapy.

Alvin P. Ross, Ph.D., is a college administrator. He received the doctorate in educational administration. A former dean at International College, Los Angeles and at Northrop University, Inglewood, California, he is now president of Ryokan College, a humanistic-alternative college in Los Angeles.

Marcia Ross is a management consultant. She is self-educated in intuitive human behavior through experiential learning gained at seminars and workshops exploring and emphasizing the potentialities and values of human existence.

Dennis C. Russo, Ph.D., is chief of behavioral psychology, Children's Hospital Medical Center, Boston, and assistant professor of psychiatry, Harvard Medical School. He was formerly assistant professor of pediatrics and medical psychology at Johns Hopkins University School of Medicine and associate director, Department of Behavioral Psychology, John F. Kennedy Institute, Baltimore. He received the Ph.D. from the University of California, Santa Barbara, in 1975 and has been on the faculty of the Johns Hopkins University School of Medicine since then. Dr. Russo's research and clinical interests are in behavioral medicine and health-care interventions and the treatment of chronic medical disorders. He has written numerous articles in behavioral psychology and is associate editor of *Education and Treatment of Children.*

William Schofield, Ph.D., is a professor in the Departments of Psychiatry and Psychology and in the School of Public Health, University of Minnesota, Minneapolis. He received the M.A. and Ph.D. from the University of Minnesota. His seminal article on the role of psychologists in the delivery of health-care services established him as one of the leading proponents of professional psychology as an important force in health care.

Barbara Smith, Ph.D., is community psychologist at La Puente Mental Health Center, Los Angeles County Department of Mental Health. She was formerly head psychologist for Los Angeles County's employee programs, directed the Occupational Alcoholism Grant, and has instituted stress-management programs for executives, district attorneys, judges, sheriffs, fire fighters, nurses, therapists, welfare workers, and librarians. Dr. Smith received the Ph. D. in clinical psychology from Indiana University and took a postdoctoral fellowship at the Neuropsychiatric Institute at the University of California at Los Angeles. She spent five years in community mental health agency consultations and crisis services.

Roberta A. Smith, R.N., Ph.D., is a member of the faculty of the School of Nursing at Vanderbilt University, Nashville. A clinical psychologist, she has recently been associated with the Dede Wallace Community Mental Health Centers, also in Nashville. Dr. Smith's research interests include ways of altering the effects of stressful experiences and issues related to the mental health of the elderly.

Linda C. Sobell, Ph.D., is head of Behavioural Intervention Research, Clinical Institute, Addiction Research Foundation, Toronto. She was formerly director of alcohol programs at the Dede Wallace Center and adjunct associate professor of psychology at Vanderbilt University, Nashville. Dr. Sobell received the Ph.D. from the University of California at Irvine. She has written numerous articles and chapters on behavioral treatment of alcohol problems and treatment-outcome evaluation. She is on the editorial board of several journals and has coauthored three books, *Emerging Concepts of Alcohol Dependence* (with E.M. Pattison and M.B. Sobell), *Behavioral Treatment of Alcohol Problems* (with M.B. Sobell), and *Evaluating Alcohol and Drug Abuse Treatment Effectiveness: Recent Advances* (with M.B. Sobell and E. Ward).

Mark B. Sobell, Ph.D. is head of Sociobehavioural Treatment Research, Clinical Institute, Addiction Research Foundation, Toronto. He was formerly associate professor and director of graduate studies on alcohol dependence in the Department of Psychology at Vanderbilt University, Nashville. Dr. Sobell received the Ph.D. from the University of California at Riverside. He has written numerous articles and chapters on behavioral treatment of alcohol problems and other alcohol studies. He is on the editorial boards of several journals and has coauthored three books, *Emerging Concepts of Alcohol Dependence* (with E.M. Pattison and L.C. Sobell), *Behavioral Treatment of Alcohol Problems* (with L.C. Sobell), and *Evaluating Alcohol and Drug Abuse Treatment Effectiveness: Recent Advances* (with L.C. Sobell and E. Ward).

Richard Steinman, Ph.D., is professor of social welfare and specialist in social gerontology at the University of Southern Maine. He has done casework, community organization, or consultation on behalf of older people in Indiana, Massachusetts, Maine, and Scotland, and has lectured widely on psychosocial aspects of aging. At the University of Edinburgh Medical School, he served as Research Fellow on a study of lay response to myocardial infarction. In 1977 he chaired Maine's first Symposium on Geropsychology, Geropsychiatry and Geriatric Medicine.

Reiko Homma True, Ph.D., is a mental-health consultant for the National Institute of Mental Health, Region IX, San Francisco. She received her training in social work at the University of California, Berkeley, and in clinical psychology at the California School of Professional Psychology, San Francisco.

James Varni, Ph.D., is codirector, Behavioral Pediatrics Program, Orthopaedic Hospital, Los Angeles. He is assistant clinical professor, Department of Pediatrics, University of Southern California School of Medicine. Dr. Varni is also associated with the Division of Hematology-Oncology at Children's Hospital of Los Angeles. He received the doctorate in psychology from the University of California at Los Angeles and was a postdoctoral Fellow in the Department of Pediatrics, Johns Hopkins University School of Medicine, and the Division of Behavioral Psychology, John F. Kennedy Institute, Baltimore. Before joining the faculty at the University of Southern California, he was instructor in medical psychology, Department of Psychiatry and Behavioral Sciences, Johns Hopkins University School of Medicine, and director of the Behavior Therapy Clinic, Behavioral Medicine Center, Johns Hopkins Hospital. His clinical and research interests include behavioral medicine, biofeedback, and the application of behavioral principles to chronic medical disorders. He has published a number of articles on behavioral psychology.

Kenneth A. Wallston, Ph.D., is associate professor of psychology in nursing at Vanderbilt University, Nashville. He is also codirector of Vanderbilt's Psychology Department's Weight Management Program. His research interests are in the measurement of individuals' health beliefs, values, and attitudes and their relationship to health behaviors. He is also interested in the interaction between health-care consumers and providers.

Win Ann Winkler is a journalist, author, and lecturer. She has written *Post-Mastectomy* and several articles relating to mastectomy. She specializes in the needs of postmastectomy women, including their return to full physical and psychological functioning, choice of special clothes, exercise, and other special postmastectomy needs. She is on the Advisory Committee of the ENCORE program of the national YWCA and on the Rehabilitation Committee of the Upper New York State Breast Cancer Commission.

Robert Wirt, Ph.D., is professor and director of graduate education in clinical psychology at the New School for Social Research, New York. He was formerly the director of the Program in Health Care Psychology in the School of Public Health, University of Minnesota, Minneapolis. After receiving the doctorate in clinical psychology from Stanford University, he remained on the faculty there, directing the Psychology Clinic for a year, before moving to Minneapolis. At the University of Minnesota he established the nation's first graduate program in clinical child psychology, of which he was director until he became director of the program in Health Care Psychology. He was chairperson of the Minnesota State Mental Health Advisory Council. He has published extensively in children's mental health and clinical psychology and is senior author of *Personality Inventory for Children*.

Elaine Wustman, R.N., M.N., is a psychiatric clinical nurse specialist. She is presently providing outpatient treatment in the Evaluation and Treatment Unit, Neuropsychiatric Institute at the University of California at Los Angeles. She was formerly the coordinator of psychiatric services in the University of California at Los Angeles Medical Center's emergency room. She received the bachelor's degree in nursing from the University of Illinois Medical Center and the master's degree in community-mental-health nursing from the University of California at Los Angeles. Her professional experience includes positions as a staff nurse in medical-surgical nursing, a staff nurse and supervisor in inpatient psychiatry, and a community-mental-health nurse in a community-mental-health center in Los Angeles.

About the Editors

Michael Jospe, Ph.D., is coordinator of pediatric consultation and liaison psychiatry at Kaiser-Permanente Medical Center, Los Angeles, and assistant clinical professor of medical psychology, Department of Psychiatry and Biobehavioral Sciences, School of Medicine, University of California at Los Angeles. He also teaches medical psychology, behavioral medicine, and clinical psychology at the California School of Professional Psychology and at Pepperdine University. Dr. Jospe was formerly chief psychologist at Newington Children's Hospital, Hartford, and clinical associate in psychology at the University of Hartford. He received his undergraduate education at the University of the Witwatersrand, Johannesburg, and the University of Leeds, England. He received the Ph.D. from the University of Minnesota, Minneapolis, in 1974, and was one of the first people to complete the internship program in health-care psychology at the University of Minnesota Medical School. Dr. Jospe's interests include clinical work, teaching, writing, and research. He is the author of *The Placebo Effect in Healing* (Lexington Books, 1978) and a number of articles and papers on medical psychology, handicapped children, and the placebo effect. His main clinical interests currently focus on psychological aspects of oncology; he is writing a textbook on the psychology of cancer and conducting research on the psychological adjustment of mastectomy patients and their children.

Joseph Nieberding, Ph.D., is in private practice in psychology in Oakland and San Francisco. He specializes in multidisciplinary approaches to the treatment of illness and illness behavior, psychotherapy with developmentally disabled persons, and consultation to small group homes for individuals with multiple disabilities. Dr. Nieberding's research interests include psychological correlates of sexually communicable diseases and psychophysiological disorders in the elderly. A graduate of Oklahoma State University, he completed an internship in clinical psychology in the Division of Health Care Psychology of the University of Minnesota Medical School, where he received training that focused on innovative interfaces between psychology and medicine. He is a consultant/lecturer in psychiatry at the Naval Regional Medical Center, Oakland, and an adjunct faculty member at the Pacific Graduate School of Psychology.

Barry D. Cohen, Ph.D., is a clinical psychologist in the Department of Psychiatry, Southern California Permanente Medical Group, Harbor City, California. He is also in private practice in Los Angeles and is a research associate in the Human Sexuality Program, Department of Psychiatry and Biobehavioral Sciences, School of Medicine, University of California at Los

Angeles. He completed an internship in the Division of Medical Psychology at the University of California at Los Angeles Medical School. He received the Ph.D. from George Peabody College of Vanderbilt University. Dr. Cohen's clinical and research interests include consultation/liaison program development and evaluation, innovative treatment approches in sexual dysfunction therapy, and hypnotherapy. He has published several articles in health psychology and is particularly interested in the inclusion of human sexuality as a professional concern of the health-care practitioner.